AF780835

Marine Bioactive Peptides—Structure, Function, and Application

Marine Bioactive Peptides—Structure, Function, and Application

Editors

Chang-Feng Chi
Bin Wang

MDPI • Basel • Beijing • Wuhan • Barcelona • Belgrade • Manchester • Tokyo • Cluj • Tianjin

Editors
Chang-Feng Chi
Zhejiang Ocean University
Zhoushan, China

Bin Wang
Zhejiang Ocean University
Zhoushan, China

Editorial Office
MDPI
St. Alban-Anlage 66
4052 Basel, Switzerland

This is a reprint of articles from the Special Issue published online in the open access journal *Marine Drugs* (ISSN 1660-3397) (available at: https://www.mdpi.com/journal/marinedrugs/special_issues/marine_peptides_structure_function_application).

For citation purposes, cite each article independently as indicated on the article page online and as indicated below:

LastName, A.A.; LastName, B.B.; LastName, C.C. Article Title. *Journal Name* **Year**, *Volume Number*, Page Range.

ISBN 978-3-0365-8260-3 (Hbk)
ISBN 978-3-0365-8261-0 (PDF)

Contents

About the Editors

Chang-Feng Chi

Chang-Feng Chi. PhD studied Forestry Science at the College of Forestry, Shandong Agricultural University (Taian, China) from 1997 to 2001, and obtained her bachelor's degree in Agronomy. From 2001 to 2004, she studied Plant Pathology at the College of Plant Protection, Shandong Agricultural University (Taian, China), and earned her master's degree in Agronomy. From 2004 to 2007, she continued her studies and research on Marine Biology and earned her PhD degree from the Ocean University of China (Qingdao, China) under the guidance of Prof. Qing-Yin Wang. From 2007 to 2009, she worked as a Biology Postdoctoral Fellow at Zhejiang University. She joined the Marine Science and Technology College, Zhejiang Ocean University (Zhoushan, China) as a lecturer in July 2009 and has been a professor since July 2015. Her current research focuses on the isolation, cloning, identification, functional evaluation and action mechanisms of marine neuropeptides.

Bin Wang

Bin Wang. PhD studied Forestry at the College of Forestry, Shandong Agricultural University (Taian, China) from 1997 to 2001, and earned his Bachelor's of Agronomy. From 2001 to 2004, he studied Biochemistry and Molecular Biology at the College of Life Science, Fujian Agriculture and Forestry University (Fuzhou, China). From 2004 to 2007, he continued his studies and research on Pharmaceutical Chemistry and earned his PhD degree from Ocean University of China (Qingdao, China) under the guidance of Prof. Hua-Shi Guan. He joined the School of Food and Pharmacy, Zhejiang Ocean University (Zhoushan, China), as a lecturer in June 2007 and has been a professor since January 2015. His current research focuses on the preparation, identification, activity evaluation and action mechanisms of marine active peptides.

Preface to "Marine Bioactive Peptides—Structure, Function, and Application"

Marine organisms live in harsh marine habitats, causing them to possess significantly different and more diverse proteins than those of terrestrial organisms. The unique amino acid sequences hidden in marine proteins can be released via proteolytic hydrolysis and present a variety of biological activities, which provide multiple benefits to human health. Recently, diverse bioactive peptides have been prepared from marine organisms and their processed byproducts. Beyond their important nutritional benefits, bioactive peptides have shown remarkable bioactivities and pharmacological functions, including antioxidant, anti-inflammatory, cytotoxic, neurotoxic, antiphotoaging, anticoagulant, antidiabetic, antifreeze, endotoxin-binding, lipid-lowering and immune-modulating. These functions make marine peptides an attractive molecular basis for the design of innovative hepatoprotective drugs, anti-aging drugs, immune-enhancing products, hypolipidemic drugs, antiphotoaging skin care products, etc. Therefore, marine-derived bioactive peptides are drawing great attention from consumers and researchers due to their possibilities for being applied in functional foods and medicines.

This Special Issue "Marine Bioactive Peptides—Structure, Function and Application" aims to collect papers on up-to-date information regarding the preparation, structural identification, activity, functional evaluation and application of marine bioactive peptides.

Chang-Feng Chi and Bin Wang
Editors

marine drugs

Editorial

Marine Bioactive Peptides—Structure, Function and Application

Chang-Feng Chi [1,*] and Bin Wang [2,*]

1 National and Provincial Joint Engineering Research Centre for Marine Germplasm Resources Exploration and Utilization, School of Marine Science and Technology, Zhejiang Ocean University, Zhoushan 316022, China
2 Zhejiang Provincial Engineering Technology Research Center of Marine Biomedical Products, School of Food and Pharmacy, Zhejiang Ocean University, Zhoushan 316022, China
* Correspondence: chichangfeng@hotmail.com (C.-F.C.); wangbin@zjou.edu.cn (B.W.)

Marine organisms live in harsh marine habitats, causing them to have significantly different and more diverse proteins than those of terrestrial organisms. The unique amino acid sequences hidden in marine proteins can be released via proteolytic hydrolysis and present a variety of biological activities, which provide multiple benefits to human health [1–3]. Recently, diverse bioactive peptides have been prepared from marine organisms and their processing byproducts [4–6]. Beyond their important nutritional benefits, bioactive peptides showed remarkable bioactivities and pharmacological functions, including antioxidant, anti-inflammatory, cytotoxic, neurotoxic, anti-photoaging, anticoagulant, antidiabetic, antifreeze, endotoxin-binding, lipid-lowering and immune-modulating [1,7,8]. These functions make marine peptides an attractive molecular basis for the design of innovative hepatoprotective drugs, anti-aging drugs, immune-enhancing products, hypolipidemic drugs, anti-photoaging skin care products, etc. [8–10]. Therefore, marine-derived bioactive peptides draw great attention to consumers and researchers due to their full possibilities applied in functional foods and medicines.

This Special Issue "Marine Bioactive Peptides—Structure, Function and Application" (https://www.mdpi.com/journal/marinedrugs/special_issues/marine_peptides_structure_function_application, accessed on 3 March 2022) published 10 peer-reviewed research papers on different topics related to marine bioactive peptides, including isolation and structure identification, pharmacological functions and mechanisms and applications in medicines and foods. Herein, we introduce a brief overview of the main achievements contributed by the authors.

Excessive reactive oxygen species (ROS) destroy cell membranes and biomacromolecules in humans, which further trigger a series of chronic diseases. However, the applications of synthetic antioxidants are limited because of their underlying damage [11]. Therefore, looking for potential natural antioxidants from fish-processing byproducts to replace synthetic products has become a research hotspot. At present, polypeptides of *Urechis unicinctus* are mainly extracted from the body's wall muscle, and the internal organs are directly thrown away as waste, which not only causes environmental pollution but also leads to a waste of resources. Therefore, Li et al. [12] extracted three polypeptides (including VTSALVGPR, IGLGDEGLRR and TKIRNEISDLNER) from the viscera of *U. unicinctus* to improve the utilization value of *U. unicinctus*. Moreover, VTSALVGPR, IGLGDEGLRR and TKIRNEISDLNER can concentration-dependently protect RAW264.7 cells against H_2O_2-induced oxidative damage. This research suggested that VTSALVGPR, IGLGDEGLRR and TKIRNEISDLNER might serve as potential antioxidants applied in health-derived food or beverages. In addition, this study further developed a new use for the byproduct of *U. unicinctus*, which improved the comprehensive utilization of marine biological resources.

Non-alcoholic fatty liver disease (NAFLD) refers to a clinicopathological syndrome characterized by inflammation of the liver lobule and hepatic parenchymal steatosis [13].

Citation: Chi, C.-F.; Wang, B. Marine Bioactive Peptides—Structure, Function and Application. *Mar. Drugs* **2023**, *21*, 275. https://doi.org/10.3390/md21050275

Received: 18 April 2023
Accepted: 27 April 2023
Published: 28 April 2023

Lipid accumulation (or lipotoxicity), oxidative stress and inflammation exert critical impacts in the development of NAFLD [14]. Ye et al. [15] reported that monkfish peptides could ameliorate high-fat diet (HFD)-induced NAFLD in mice, and the mechanism demonstrated that monkfish (*Lophius litulon*) peptides can first improve the lipid metabolism in NAFLD mice via an upregulation of p-AMPK protein to reduce lipid synthesis and accelerate fatty acid β-oxidation. Secondly, monkfish peptides showed strong antioxidant activity to decrease oxidative damage by regulating the Nrf2 pathway to increase HO-1 and NQO1 levels in mouse livers. Finally, monkfish peptides can reduce the levels of inflammatory factors (TNF-α, IL-1β, IL-6 and IFN-γ). Therefore, monkfish peptides can be used as health functions or supplements to prevent and treat NAFLD.

Sturgeon is the common name for 27 kinds of cartilaginous fish of the family Acipenseridae, and its farmed production in China was about 4.4 million tons, accounting for approximately 80% of the world's production [16,17]. Cartilages accounting for 10% of sturgeon's weight became byproducts during the receiving process of sturgeon eggs. In recent years, bioactive ingredients in sturgeon cartilage were studied constantly for replacing shark cartilage used in health and functional products. Therefore, Sheng et al. [18] isolated and identified thirteen antioxidant peptides from the collagen hydrolysate of Siberian sturgeon (*Acipenser baerii*) cartilage, and GEYGFE, PSVSLT and IELFPGLP showed high antioxidant activity and protective capacity on H_2O_2-damaged plasmid DNA. More importantly, GEYGFE, PSVSLT and IELFPGLP displayed notable cytoprotection on vascular endothelial cells against H_2O_2 injury by regulating the intracellular antioxidant system to decrease the contents of ROS and malondialdehyde (MDA). Therefore, this research provides technical support for the higher-valued utilization of sturgeon cartilages. More importantly, GEYGFE, PSVSLT and IELFPGLP might act as antioxidant additives for developing health products to treat chronic diseases caused by oxidative stress, including cardiovascular, atherosclerosis, hypertension, etc.

O/W emulsion is a classic form of oil commonly used in foods, but it is easily oxidized. Some antioxidative proteins and hydrolysates can be used as emulsifiers and antioxidants in different types of oils to increase the nutritional value of emulsions. Therefore, Liu et al. [19] prepared the neutral protease chlorella protein hydrolysate (NCPH) and the alkaline protease chlorella protein hydrolysate (ACPH) and systematically studied their antioxidant activities and physicochemical properties in krill oil-in-water emulsions. NCPHs and ACPHs could significantly increase SOD activity to reduce H_2O_2-induced oxidative stress on MDA-MB-231 cells in a dose-dependent manner. Moreover, the NCPHs or ACPHs could inhibit linoleic acid oxidation, suppress the growth of the peroxide value (POV) and thiobarbituric acid reactive substances (TRABS) and remain physically stable in krill O/W emulsion for at least one month. The study suggests that protein hydrolysate from chlorella pyrenoidosa has the potential to be applied in krill oil-in-water emulsions, as both emulsifiers and antioxidants.

Wound healing involves three stages: inflammation, cell proliferation and tissue reconstruction [20]. The three phases of this lengthy procedure can involve a number of symptoms, including infection, discomfort and the development of thicker scars. To make matters worse, slow wound healing not only affects the patient's aesthetics but also seriously affects the patient's quality of life. Therefore, screening original drugs with functions of speeding up skin wound closure and inhibiting scar formation are essential for patients with tissue defects. In this regard, Zhang et al. [21] prepared the best fraction PMPs-4 (PMPPs) from the ultrafiltration fraction (<3 K Da) of shellfish *Pinctada martensii* mantle (PMPs) via gel chromatography. Cellular assays proved that PMPPs could promote the proliferation of HSF and HaCaT cells, and in vivo animal experiments indicated that PMPPs could achieve scarless healing by regulating the TGF-β/Smad pathway to inhibit the inflammatory response, accelerate the epithelialization process and regulate the collagen I/III ratio. Finally, the most promising peptide sequence FAFQAEIAQLMS in PMPPs can promote wound healing through easy docking with protein receptors of

EGFR1/FGFR1/MPP-1. This research enriches the pro-healing mechanism of marine peptides and provides candidate drugs for treating wound healing.

Various internal and external factors, such as viral infections, cancer, obesity, smoking, excessive alcohol consumption, and very little exercise, show negative effects on the normal functioning of the immune system. Immunotherapy can improve or suppress the body's immunological responses for returning the immune system to its physiologic status. In previous research, a novel immune-enhancing pentadecapeptide (RVAPEEHPVEGRYLV) was isolated from protein hydrolysates of the bivalve *Cyclina sinensis*, and it showed significant immunomodulatory effects on RAW264.7 cells and an ameliorating effect on cyclophosphamide-induced nephrotoxicity [22,23]. In the study, Zhao et al. [24] found that RVAPEEHPVEGRYLV could enhance immunity in CTX-induced immunosuppressed mice, and the mechanism indicated that RVAPEEHPVEGRYLV could activate the MAPK/NF-κB and PI3K/Akt pathways to elevate the phosphorylation levels of p38, ERK, JNK, PI3K and Akt, upregulate IKKα, IKKβ, p50 NF-κB and p65 NF-κB protein levels and downregulate IκBα protein levels. The study supports RVAPEEHPVEGRYL serving as a novel immunomodulator candidate or immune adjuvant.

Hypertension seriously affects the morbidity and mortality of cardiovascular and renal diseases. Angiotensin (Ang) I-converting enzyme (ACE) is the key protease in participating in the regulation of blood pressure through the renin–angiotensin system, and inhibiting ACE activity is an ideal method in hypertension treatment [25]. The consumption of red algae is actually expanding because they are a good source of essential nutrients, minerals and vitamins, and they also contain bioactive compounds with attractive biological activities. In this study, Mune et al. [26] used thermolysin to hydrolyze water-soluble proteins of red alga *Gracilariopsis chorda* to prepare a hydrolysate with high ACE inhibitory activity. Furthermore, two novel peptides (IDHY and LVVER) were isolated from the prepared hydrolysate, and molecular docking analysis revealed that IDHY was a promising ACE inhibitor. From these results, it could be expected that a water-soluble protein hydrolysate of *G. chorda* could serve as an ingredient in the prevention of hypertension and a good source of bioactive peptides, especially ACE inhibitory peptides.

Brown algae *Laminaria digitata* contains a variety of functional components with significant pharmacological activity, such as alginate, fucoxanthin, fucoidan, phlorotannins and vitamins. The mechanism of the antihypertensive effect of bioactive peptides is thought to inhibit enzyme activity within the renin–angiotensin–aldosterone system (RAAS), including ACE-1 and renin. In silico analysis is a useful technique to speculate on the potential bioactivity of peptides before the chemical synthesis of peptides. Previously, Purcell et al. [27] generated a protein hydrolysate of *L. digitata* with an IC_{50} value of 590 μg/mL on ACE-1. In this paper [28], 130 peptides were identified from the 3 kDa permeate of this hydrolysate using mass spectrometry. Among them, two new ACE-1 inhibitory peptides of IGNNPAKGGLF and YIGNNPAKGGLF with Peptide Ranker scores of 0.81 and 0.80 were chemically synthesized and inhibited ACE-1 by 80 ± 8% and 91 ± 16%, respectively. The observed ACE-1 IC_{50} values for IGNNPAKGGLF and YIGNNPAKGGLF were determined as 174.4 μg/mL and 133.1 μg/mL. What is interesting is that IGNNPAKGGLF and YIGNNPAKGGLF have the potential to inhibit dipeptidyl peptidase IV (DPP-IV) by mimicking sequences produced after digestion. The study highlights that *L. digitata* is an excellent material for preparing peptides with ACE and DPP-IV inhibitory activity.

Prolonged skin exposure to Ultraviolet B (UVB) radiation can result in detrimental intracellular physiological effects and produce superfluous ROS, which can injure intracellular bioactive molecules and further cause oxidative stress and cell apoptosis [29]. Then, inhibiting the photoaging induced by UVB can delay skin aging and provide a reasonable basis for studying cosmetic products to treat diseases caused by UV radiation. Recently, bioactive peptides from marine organisms have exhibited great possibilities for the adjuvant treatment and prevention of skin photoaging due to their outstanding antioxidant function. In previous research, PKK, YEGGD and GPGLM from skipjack tuna cardiac arterial bulbs were found to have excellent radical scavenging ability and a prominently protective function on H_2O_2-damaged DNA and HepG2 cells [30]. Therefore, this paper discussed the protective effects of PKK, YEGGD and GPGLM on the cells damaged by UVB oxidation from two aspects: antioxidant and apoptosis inhibition [31]. The results indicated that PKK, YEGGD and GPGLM could significantly increase the cellular antioxidant capacity through activating the Nrf2 signaling pathway and suppressing cell apoptosis through downregulating Bax-dependent mitochondrial apoptosis. This work lays a theoretical foundation for employing PKK, YEGGD and GPGLM to attenuate UVB-irradiated photoaging.

Oxidative stress can cause DNA mutation, enzyme inactivation and membrane phospholipid oxidation, which significantly increase the incidence of some chronic non-communicable diseases, such as neurological dysfunction, hypertension, cardiovascular, atherosclerosis, diabetes, cancer and auto-immune diseases [32–34]. Sheng et al. [35] utilized processing byproduct swim bladders of monkfish (*L. litulon*) to produce eighteen novel antioxidant peptides, and YDYD, QDYD, GRW, ARW, DDGGK and YPAGP revealed remarkable radical scavenging activity, lipid peroxidation inhibition ability, ferric-reducing antioxidant power and protective function on oxidation-damaged DNA and HepG2 cells. Furthermore, the stability of eighteen novel antioxidant peptides is systematically discussed. This research provides a good perspective and offers technical support for the higher-valued utilization of monkfish byproducts. More importantly, YDYD, QDYD, GRW, ARW, DDGGK and YPAGP might act as antioxidant additives for developing health products to cure chronic non-communicable diseases.

The papers included in this Special Issue deal with bioactive peptides from evolutionarily distant species, including *U. unicinctus*, monkfish (*L. litulon*), Siberian sturgeon (*A. baerii*), *C. Pyrenoidosa*, *P. martensii*, *C. sinensis*, *G. chorda*, *L. digitate* and skipjack tuna (*K. pelamis*). Among them, three of the papers involved the preparation of bioactive peptides from seaweed. These results suggest that seaweed is not only an important raw material for the preparation of polysaccharides but also a potential resource for the preparation of peptides. This should be a phenomenon of concern. Moreover, most of the identified peptides displayed broad-spectrum biological activities. To our surprise, the papers included in this Special Issue pay more attention to the functions and mechanisms of peptides in addition to the conventional isolation and identification of peptides. This means that more marine bioactive peptides will be used in pharmaceutical, cosmeceutical and nutraceutical industries in the future.

In conclusion, the Guest Editors thank all the authors who contributed to this Special Issue, all the reviewers for evaluating the submitted manuscripts and the Editorial board of *Marine Drugs*, especially Florine Wang, Assistant Editor of this journal, for their continuous help in turning this Special Issue into a reality.

Funding: Co-financed by grants from the National Natural Science Foundation of China (No. 82073764) and the Ten-thousand Talents Plan of Zhejiang Province (No. 2019R52026).

Conflicts of Interest: The authors declare no conflict of interest.

References

1. Sridhar, K.; Inbaraj, B.S.; Chen, B.H. Recent developments on production, purification and biological activity of marine peptides. *Food Res. Int.* **2021**, *147*, 110468. [CrossRef] [PubMed]
2. Ganguly, A.; Sharma, K.; Majumder, K. Food-derived bioactive peptides and their role in ameliorating hypertension and associated cardiovascular diseases. *Adv. Food Nutr. Res.* **2019**, *89*, 165–207. [PubMed]
3. Suo, S.K.; Zhao, Y.Q.; Wang, Y.M.; Pan, X.Y.; Chi, C.F.; Wang, B. Seventeen novel angiotensin converting enzyme (ACE) inhibitory peptides from protein hydrolysate of *Mytilus edulis*: Isolation, identification, molecular docking study, and protective function on HUVECs. *Food Funct.* **2022**, *13*, 7831–7846. [CrossRef] [PubMed]
4. Sila, A.; Bougatef, A. Antioxidant peptides from marine by-products: Isolation, identification and application in food systems. A review. *J. Funct. Foods* **2016**, *21*, 10–26. [CrossRef]
5. Zheng, S.L.; Luo, Q.B.; Suo, S.K.; Zhao, Y.Q.; Chi, C.F.; Wang, B. Preparation, identification, molecular docking study and protective function on HUVECs of novel ACE inhibitory peptides from protein hydrolysate of Skipjack tuna muscle. *Mar. Drugs* **2022**, *20*, 176. [CrossRef]

6. Venkatesan, J.; Anil, S.; Kim, S.-K.; Shim, M.S. Marine fish proteins and peptides for cosmeceuticals: A review. *Mar. Drugs* **2017**, *15*, 143. [CrossRef]
7. Sun, K.L.; Gao, M.; Wang, Y.Z.; Li, X.R.; Wang, P.; Wang, B. Antioxidant peptides from protein hydrolysate of marine red algae *Eucheuma cottonii*: Preparation, identification, and cytoprotective mechanisms on H_2O_2 oxidative damaged HUVECs. *Front. Microbiol.* **2022**, *13*, 791248. [CrossRef]
8. Ovchinnikova, T.V. Structure, function, and therapeutic potential of marine bioactive peptides. *Mar. Drugs* **2019**, *17*, 505. [CrossRef]
9. Zhang, S.Y.; Zhao, Y.Q.; Wang, Y.M.; Yang, X.R.; Chi, C.F.; Wang, B. Gelatins and antioxidant peptides from Skipjack tuna (*Katsuwonus pelamis*) skins: Purification, characterization, and cytoprotection on ultraviolet-A injured human skin fibroblasts. *Food Biosci.* **2022**, *50*, 102138. [CrossRef]
10. Suo, S.K.; Zheng, S.L.; Chi, C.F.; Luo, H.Y.; Wang, B. Novel angiotensin-converting enzyme inhibitory peptides from tuna byproducts-milts: Preparation, characterization, molecular docking study, and antioxidant function on H_2O_2-damaged human umbilical vein endothelial cells. *Front. Nutr.* **2022**, *9*, 957778. [CrossRef]
11. He, Y.; Pan, X.; Chi, C.F.; Sun, K.L.; Wang, B. Ten new pentapeptides from protein hydrolysate of miiuy croaker (*Miichthys miiuy*) muscle: Preparation, identification, and antioxidant activity evaluation. *LWT* **2019**, *105*, 1–8. [CrossRef]
12. Li, J.; Lu, J.; Asakiya, C.; Huang, K.; Zhou, X.; Liu, Q.; He, X. Extraction and identification of three new *Urechis unicinctus* visceral peptides and their antioxidant activity. *Mar. Drugs* **2022**, *20*, 293. [CrossRef] [PubMed]
13. Huang, D.Q.; ElSerag, H.B.; Loomba, R. Global epidemiology of NAFLD-related HCC: Trends, predictions, risk factors and prevention. *Nat. Rev. Gastroenterol. Hepatol.* **2021**, *18*, 223–238. [CrossRef] [PubMed]
14. Li, L.; Fu, J.Q.; Sun, J.; Liu, D.; Chen, C.J.; Wang, H.H.; Hou, Y.Y.; Xu, Y.Y.; Pi, J.B. Is Nrf2-ARE a potential target in NAFLD mitigation? *Curr. Opin. Toxicol.* **2019**, *13*, 35–44. [CrossRef]
15. Ye, J.; Tian, X.; Wang, Q.; Zheng, J.; Yang, Y.; Xu, B.; Zhang, S.; Yuan, F.; Yang, Z. Monkfish peptides mitigate high fat diet-induced hepatic steatosis in mice. *Mar. Drugs* **2022**, *20*, 312. [CrossRef]
16. Yuan, L.; Chu, Q.; Wu, X.; Yang, B.; Zhang, W.; Jin, W.; Gao, R. Anti-inflammatory and antioxidant activity of peptides from ethanol-soluble hydrolysates of sturgeon (*Acipenser schrenckii*) cartilage. *Front. Nutr.* **2021**, *8*, 689648. [CrossRef]
17. Zhang, Z.; Wang, Y.M.; Qiu, Y.T.; Chi, C.F.; Luo, H.Y.; Wang, B. Gelatin from cartilage of Siberian sturgeon (*Acipenser baerii*): Characterization and protective function on ultraviolet-A injured human skin fibroblasts. *Front. Mar. Sci.* **2022**, *9*, 925407. [CrossRef]
18. Sheng, Y.; Qiu, Y.-T.; Wang, Y.-M.; Chi, C.-F.; Wang, B. Novel antioxidant collagen peptides of Siberian sturgeon (*Acipenser baerii*) cartilages: The preparation, characterization, and cytoprotection of H_2O_2-damaged human umbilical vein endothelial cells (HUVECs). *Mar. Drugs* **2022**, *20*, 325. [CrossRef]
19. Liu, Y.; Qi, Y.; Wang, Q.; Yin, F.; Zhan, H.; Wang, H.; Liu, B.; Nakamura, Y.; Wang, J. Antioxidative effect of *Chlorella pyrenoidosa* protein hydrolysates and their application in Krill oil-in-water emulsions. *Mar. Drugs* **2022**, *20*, 345. [CrossRef]
20. Zhang, M.Z.; Zhai, X.Y.; Ma, T.F.; Huang, Y.K.; Yan, C.H.; Du, Y.P. Multifunctional cerium doped carbon dots nanoplatform and its applications for wound healing. *Chem. Eng. J.* **2021**, *423*, 130301. [CrossRef]
21. Zhang, T.; Yang, F.; Qin, X.; Yang, X.; Zhang, C.; Wan, Z.; Lin, H. Investigation of the in vivo, in vitro, and in silico wound healing potential of *Pinctada martensii* purified peptides. *Mar. Drugs* **2022**, *20*, 417. [CrossRef] [PubMed]
22. Li, W.; Ye, S.; Zhang, Z.; Tang, J.; Jin, H.; Huang, F.; Yang, Z.; Tang, Y.; Chen, Y.; Ding, G.; et al. Purification and characterization of a novel pentadecapeptide from protein hydrolysates of *Cyclina sinensis* and its immunomodulatory effects on RAW264.7 cells. *Mar. Drugs* **2019**, *17*, 30. [CrossRef]
23. Jiang, X.; Ren, Z.; Zhao, B.; Zhou, S.; Ying, X.; Tang, Y. Ameliorating effect of pentadecapeptide derived from *Cyclina sinensis* on cyclophosphamide-induced nephrotoxicity. *Mar. Drugs* **2020**, *18*, 462. [CrossRef] [PubMed]
24. Zhao, R.; Jiang, X.-X.; Zhao, Q.-L.; Ye, H.-W.; Lin, Y.; Huang, J.; Tang, Y.-P. Immunoenhancing effects of *Cyclina sinensis* pentadecapeptide through modulation of signaling pathways in mice with cyclophosphamide-induced immunosuppression. *Mar. Drugs* **2022**, *20*, 560. [CrossRef] [PubMed]
25. Chakraborty, R.; Roy, S. Angiotensin-converting enzyme inhibitors from plants: A review of their diversity, modes of action, prospects, and concerns in the management of diabetes-centric complications. *J. Integr. Med.* **2022**, *19*, 478–492. [CrossRef] [PubMed]
26. Mune, M.A.; Miyabe, Y.; Shimizu, T.; Matsui, W.; Kumagai, Y.; Kishimura, H. Characterisation of bioactive peptides from red alga *Gracilariopsis chorda*. *Mar. Drugs* **2023**, *21*, 49. [CrossRef]
27. Purcell, D.; Packer, M.A.; Hayes, M. Angiotensin-I-converting enzyme inhibitory activity of protein hydrolysates generated from the macroalga *Laminaria digitata* (Hudson) JV Lamouroux 1813. *Foods* **2022**, *11*, 1792. [CrossRef]
28. Purcell, D.; Packer, M.A.; Hayes, M. Identification of bioactive peptides from a *Laminaria digitata* protein hydrolysate using in silico and in vitro methods to identify angiotensin-1-converting enzyme (ACE-1) inhibitory peptides. *Mar. Drugs* **2023**, *21*, 90. [CrossRef]
29. Rabe, J.H.; Mamelak, A.J.; McElgunn, P.J.; Morison, W.L.; Sauder, D.N. Photoaging: Mechanisms and repair. *J. Am. Acad. Dermatol.* **2006**, *55*, 1–19. [CrossRef]

30. Cai, W.W.; Hu, X.M.; Wang, Y.M.; Chi, C.F.; Wang, B. Bioactive peptides from Skipjack tuna cardiac arterial bulbs: Preparation, identification, antioxidant activity, and stability against thermal, pH, and simulated gastrointestinal digestion treatments. *Mar. Drugs* **2022**, *20*, 626. [CrossRef]
31. Kong, J.; Hu, X.M.; Cai, W.W.; Wang, Y.M.; Chi, C.F.; Wang, B. Bioactive peptides from Skipjack tuna cardiac arterial bulbs (II): Protective function on UVB-irradiated HaCaT cells through antioxidant and anti-apoptotic mechanisms. *Mar. Drugs* **2023**, *21*, 105. [CrossRef] [PubMed]
32. García, N.; Zazueta, C.; Aguilera-Aguirre, L. Oxidative stress and inflammation in cardiovascular disease. *Oxid. Med. Cell. Longev.* **2017**, *2017*, 5853238. [CrossRef] [PubMed]
33. Zheng, S.L.; Wang, Y.Z.; Zhao, Y.Q.; Chi, C.F.; Zhu, W.Y.; Wang, B. High Fischer ratio oligopeptides from hard-shelled mussel: Preparation and hepatoprotective effect against acetaminophen-induced liver injury in mice. *Food Biosci.* **2023**, *53*, 102638.
34. Qiao, Q.Q.; Luo, Q.B.; Suo, S.K.; Zhao, Y.Q.; Chi, C.F.; Wang, B. Preparation, characterization, and cytoprotective effects on HUVECs of fourteen novel angiotensin-I-converting enzyme inhibitory peptides from protein hydrolysate of tuna processing by-products. *Front. Nutr.* **2022**, *9*, 868681. [CrossRef]
35. Sheng, Y.; Wang, W.Y.; Wu, M.F.; Wang, Y.M.; Zhu, W.Y.; Chi, C.F.; Wang, B. Eighteen novel bioactive peptides from monkfish (*Lophius litulon*) swim bladders: Production, identification, antioxidant activity, and stability. *Mar. Drugs* **2023**, *21*, 169. [CrossRef] [PubMed]

marine drugs

MDPI

Article

Eighteen Novel Bioactive Peptides from Monkfish (*Lophius litulon*) Swim Bladders: Production, Identification, Antioxidant Activity, and Stability

Yan Sheng [1], Wan-Yi Wang [2], Ming-Feng Wu [1], Yu-Mei Wang [1], Wang-Yu Zhu [3], Chang-Feng Chi [2,*] and Bin Wang [1,*]

1 Zhejiang Provincial Engineering Technology Research Center of Marine Biomedical Products, School of Food and Pharmacy, Zhejiang Ocean University, Zhoushan 316022, China
2 National and Provincial Joint Laboratory of Exploration, Utilization of Marine Aquatic Genetic Resources, National Engineering Research Center of Marine Facilities Aquaculture, School of Marine Science and Technology, Zhejiang Ocean University, Zhoushan 316022, China
3 Cell and Molecular Biology Laboratory, Zhoushan Hospital, Zhoushan 316021, China
* Correspondence: chichangfeng@hotmail.com (C.-F.C.); wangbin@zjou.edu.cn (B.W.); Tel./Fax: +86-580-255-4818 (C.-F.C.); +86-580-255-4781 (B.W.)

Abstract: In the study, papain was chosen from five proteases to hydrolyze proteins of monkfish swim bladders for effectively utilizing monkfish (*Lophius litulon*) processing byproducts, and the hydrolysis conditions of papain were optimized as hydrolysis temperature of 65 °C, pH 7.5, enzyme dose 2.5% and time 5 h using single-factor and orthogonal experiments. Eighteen peptides were purified from the swim bladder hydrolysate of monkfish by ultrafiltration and gel permeation chromatography methods and identified as YDYD, QDYD, AGPAS, GPGPHGPSGP, GPK, HRE, GRW, ARW, GPTE, DDGGK, IGPAS, AKPAT, YPAGP, DPT, FPGPT, GPGPT, GPT and DPAGP, respectively. Among eighteen peptides, GRW and ARW showed significant DPPH· scavenging activities with EC_{50} values of 1.053 ± 0.003 and 0.773 ± 0.003 mg/mL, respectively; YDYD, QDYD, GRW, ARW and YPAGP revealed significantly HO· scavenging activities with EC_{50} values of 0.150 ± 0.060, 0.177 ± 0.035, 0.201 ± 0.013, 0.183 ± 0.0016 and 0.190 ± 0.010 mg/mL, respectively; YDYD, QDYD, ARW, DDGGK and YPAGP have significantly O_2^-· scavenging capability with EC_{50} values of 0.126 ± 0.0005, 0.112 ± 0.0028, 0.127 ± 0.0002, 0.128 ± 0.0018 and 0.107 ± 0.0002 mg/mL, respectively; and YDYD, QDYD and YPAGP showed strong $ABTS^+$· scavenging ability with EC_{50} values of 3.197 ± 0.036, 2.337 ± 0.016 and 3.839 ± 0.102 mg/mL, respectively. YDYD, ARW and DDGGK displayed the remarkable ability of lipid peroxidation inhibition and Ferric-reducing antioxidant properties. Moreover, YDYD and ARW can protect Plasmid DNA and HepG2 cells against H_2O_2-induced oxidative stress. Furthermore, eighteen isolated peptides had high stability under temperatures ranging from 25–100 °C; YDYD, QDYD, GRW and ARW were more sensitive to alkali treatment, but DDGGK and YPAGP were more sensitive to acid treatment; and YDYD showed strong stability treated with simulated GI digestion. Therefore, the prepared antioxidant peptides, especially YDYD, QDYD, GRW, ARW, DDGGK and YPAGP from monkfish swim bladders could serve as functional components applied in health-promoting products because of their high-antioxidant functions.

Keywords: monkfish (*Lophius litulon*); swim bladders; peptide; antioxidant activity; stability

Citation: Sheng, Y.; Wang, W.-Y.; Wu, M.-F.; Wang, Y.-M.; Zhu, W.-Y.; Chi, C.-F.; Wang, B. Eighteen Novel Bioactive Peptides from Monkfish (*Lophius litulon*) Swim Bladders: Production, Identification, Antioxidant Activity, and Stability. *Mar. Drugs* **2023**, *21*, 169. https://doi.org/10.3390/md21030169

Academic Editor: Jae-Young Je

Received: 10 February 2023
Revised: 2 March 2023
Accepted: 6 March 2023
Published: 7 March 2023

1. Introduction

Bioactive peptides (BPs) comprise 3–30 amino acid (AA) residues with molecular weights (MWs) ranging from 500 to 1850 Da and are generated from diversified protein resources by enzymatic hydrolysis, chemical degradation and microbial fermentation methods [1–3]. In addition to their widely accepted nutritive value, BPs have also been proven to have important applications in promoting human health due to their significant physiological and pharmacological functions [4–6]. Then, BPs draw great interest from consumers and have been applied in a wide variety of products, especially functional food, daily cosmetics, medicinal/pharmaceutical products, and nutritional supplements [7–9].

Reactive oxygen species (ROS) are the metabolites of the respiration process and take on an important role in the physiological and biochemical reactions of organisms [10]. Normally, the body's oxidative and antioxidant defense systems are in balance, and ROS performed many specific roles including serving as cell-growth factors and regulators of signals between cells [11,12]. In contrast, an overwhelming amount of ROS will be produced in the body under adverse exogenous environmental stress or during disease episodes. Even worse, overexpression and residual ROS can disrupt the balance, lead to oxidative stress and cause damage to cellular macromolecules as confirmed by nitrotyrosine, lipid peroxidation, and DNA/RNA and protein oxidation [13–15]. Moreover, numerous examples of literature have reported that oxidative stress was a significant contributor to the emergence and progression of various chronic non-communicable diseases (NCD) such as neurological dysfunction, hypertension, cardiovascular, atherosclerosis, diabetes, cancer and auto-immune disease [16–21]. According to data released by the World Health Organization (WHO) in 2019, NCD is one of the top 10 threats to global health and led to 70% of deaths all over the world, and oxidative damage is regarded as a major cause of NCD [22]. Antioxidants can clear away excessive ROS and preserve the organisms from oxidative injury and its adverse reactions [23,24]. Therefore, several chemical synthetic antioxidants, such as butylated hydroxytoluene (BHT), butylated hydroxyanisole (BHA) and tertbutylhydroquinone (TBHQ), present powerful antioxidant functions, but they show some alarming toxic effects on body health, such as DNA damage, hepatotoxicity and carcinogenesis [25,26]. For example: Achar et al. reported that toxicity assessment on BHT revealed carcinogenic, teratogenic and mutagenic effects in animal models [27]; BHT could induce hyperactivity and alters dopamine-related gene expression in larval zebrafish (*Danio rerio*) [28]; TBHQ could cause considerable DNA fragmentation, necrosis and apoptosis [29]. Thus, actions have been taken to restrict the usage of synthetic antioxidants in consideration of their potential toxicity by consumers [30,31]. Meanwhile, the search for safe and efficient natural antioxidants has caused widespread concern.

Presently, some natural antioxidants, including flavone, quinonoid, sappanone, curcumin, phenol, melatonin and peptides have been rapidly screened and produced using animal, plant and microorganism resources [32–34]. Among those bioactive substances, antioxidant peptides (APs) are gained scientific interest for their potential advantages in preventing and treating NCD [8,35,36]. For example, VIAPW and IRWWW isolated from miiuy croaker (*Miichthys miiuy*) muscle could regulate the AMPK pathway to control the expression levels of some proteolytic enzymes in lipid synthesis and oxidation process and further decrease the intracellular levels of TG and TC [37]. Tripeptide WLP derived from sea squirt (*Halocynthia roretzi*) could relieve neurodegenerative disorders related to oxidative stress through attenuating cell apoptosis, decreasing ROS levels, and remarkably enhancing GSH-Px activity [38]. Oyster (*Crassostrea giga)* peptides (MW < 3500 Da) displayed prominent liver-protection ability in mice models of alcohol-caused hepatopathy via regulating the Nrf2-ARE pathway to heighten the antioxidant capability and inactivating NF-κB pathway to control the inflammatory reaction [39]. DREL from Jiuzao could activate these signaling pathways, including Nrf2/Keap1, p38/PI3K and MafK, to improve the antioxidative and anti-inflammatory ability in the AAPH-induced Sprague Dawley (SD) rat [40]. Consequently, APs have great potential in the functionality of food, nutraceutical supplements and pharmaceutical products for preventing and treating chronic and degenerative diseases.

Monkfish (*Lophius litulon*) belongs to the members of the genus *Lophiidae*, lives at the bottom of the offshore sea, and is found mainly in the Indian, Atlantic and Pacific Oceans [41]. Presently, BPs have been produced from monkfish muscle and its processing by-products and showed significant bioactivities. For example, peptides fraction (MW < 1 kDa) from monkfish muscle could improve the antioxidant capacity of the liver to alleviate non-alcoholic fatty liver disease (NAFLD) progression mainly through modulating the intestinal flora and AMPK and Nrf2 pathways [42–44]. APs prepared from monkfish muscle hydrolysate, including EWPAQ, FLHRP, LMGQW, EDIVCW, MEPVW and YWDAW, could concentration-dependently scavenge free radicals and control lipid peroxidation [18,41]. Low MW peptides from monkfish roes could enhance the immune regulatory effect in immunosuppressive mice by activating the signaling pathways of NF-κB/MAPK in spleen tissues [45]. Collagen peptides from monkfish skin could protect mice against the kidney damage induced by a high-fat diet by regulating the signaling pathways of Nrf2/NLRP3 [46]. However, there is no study on BPs from monkfish swim bladders. Therefore, the objectives of the study were to produce and characterize APs from the swim bladder hydrolysate of monkfish for efficient utilization of monkfish processing byproducts. Moreover, we comprehensively determined and evaluated the antioxidant capability and stability of eighteen prepared APs (MSP1 to MSP18).

2. Results

2.1. Preparation of Protein Hydrolysate of Monkfish Swim Bladders (MSBH)

2.1.1. Screening of Enzyme Species

To more thoroughly hydrolyze the protein of monkfish swim bladders, five kinds of proteases, including pepsin, trypsin, alcalase, papain and flavourzyme, were selected to evaluate their hydrolyzing capacity (Figure 1). At 5.0 mg/mL, the DPPH· scavenging ratio of produced hydrolysate by papain was 43.09 ± 1.69%, and the ratio was significantly higher than those of produced hydrolysates using pepsin (26.48 ± 0.87%), trypsin (31.47 ± 0.77%), alcalase (33.84 ± 1.14%) and flavourzyme (29.06 ± 1.2%), respectively ($p < 0.05$). Therefore, papain was chosen for the preparation of hydrolysates from monkfish swim bladders.

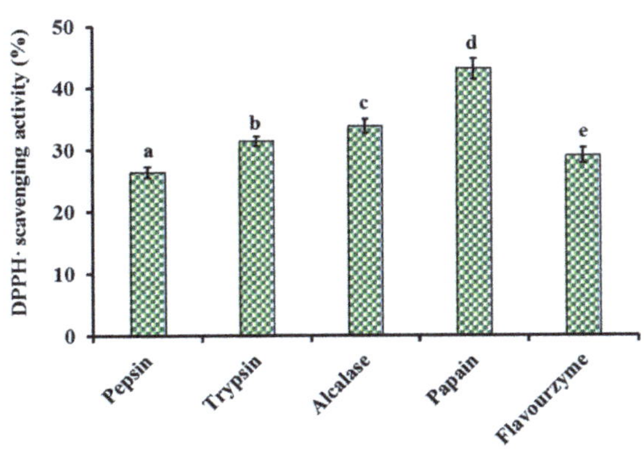

Figure 1. Influences of enzyme species on DPPH· scavenging activity of monkfish (*L. litulon*) swim bladder hydrolysates at 5.0 mg/mL. All data are presented as the mean ± SD of triplicate results. [a–e] Values with the same letters indicate no significant difference ($p > 0.05$).

2.1.2. Optimization of Hydrolysis Conditions of Papain

The hydrolysis conditions of papain including hydrolysis temperature (A), time (B), pH (C) and enzyme dose (D) on the influence of the radical scavenging activity of monkfish swim bladder hydrolysates were optimized using the single-factor experiment (Figure 2). Figure 2A depicted that hydrolysis temperature significantly affected the radical scavenging capability of swim bladder hydrolysates, and the DPPH· scavenging rate (43.47 ± 1.41%) of prepared hydrolysate at 65 °C was significantly higher than those of prepared hydrolysates at other temperature ($p < 0.05$). The DPPH· clearance rate of prepared hydrolysate showed a decreasing trend when the temperature was lower or higher than 65 °C. Figure 2B displayed that DPPH· clearance rates of swim bladder hydrolysates increased gradually with the prolongation of hydrolysis time and reached the maximum value (43.53 ± 0.96%)

at 4 h. Prolongation of hydrolysis time caused a persistent decrease in the activity of hydrolysates. Figure 2C indicated that DPPH· scavenging rate reached the maximum value (45.58 ± 0.15%) at pH 7.5. The inappropriate pH value of enzymolysis solution can affect the binding of enzyme and substrate by destroying the active center or spatial structure of papain, which further reduced its catalytic activity. Figure 2D displayed that the activity curve showed a trend of rapid rise at the enzyme dose was 1–2.0% and a slow decline when the dose was higher than 2.0%. The highest DPPH· clearance rate was 45.68 ± 0.38% when the enzyme followed by was 2.0%. According to the above experimental results, the ranges of hydrolytic conditions for papain were narrowed down to 60–70°C, 3–5 h, 7.0–8.0, 1.5–2.5% and 3–5 h for hydrolysis temperature, time, pH and enzyme dose, respectively.

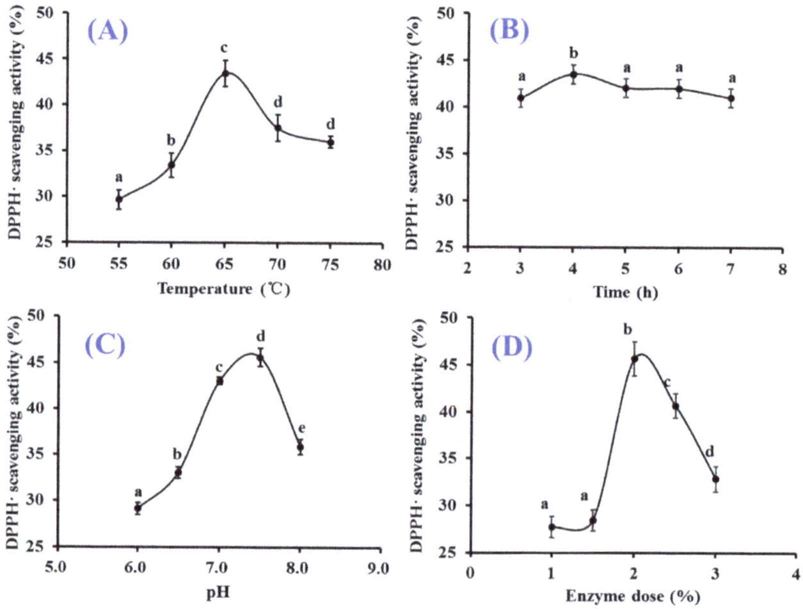

Figure 2. Effects of hydrolysis temperature (**A**), time (**B**), pH (**C**) and enzyme dose (**D**) of papain on DPPH· scavenging activity of monkfish swim bladder hydrolysates at 5.0 mg/mL. All data are presented as the mean ± SD of triplicate results. [a–e] Values with the same letters indicate no significant difference ($p > 0.05$).

The orthogonal test $L_9(3)^4$ was designed for optimizing the hydrolysis conditions of papain (Table 1). Following the *R* values, the conditions interfering with the antioxidant activity of monkfish swim bladder hydrolysates were listed in decreasing order: C (enzyme dose) > B (pH) > D (hydrolysis time) > A (hydrolysis temperature). The enzyme dose was recognized as the most important condition influencing the antioxidant activity of swim bladder hydrolysates. By verification experiments, the maximum DPPH· scavenging ratio of monkfish swim bladder hydrolysate was 47.13 ± 1.15% at 5.0 mg/mL on the optimal enzymolysis level of A2B2C3D3, that is, the optimum conditions of papain for producing monkfish swim bladder hydrolysate were hydrolysis temperature 65 °C, pH 7.5, enzyme dose 2.5% and time 5 h. In addition, the monkfish swim bladder hydrolysate produced under the optimal conditions of papain was named MSBH.

Table 1. Results of the orthogonal experiment for optimizing the hydrolysis conditions of papain.

No	Factors				DPPH· Scavenging Activity (%)
	A Temperature (°C)	B pH	C Enzyme Dose (%)	D Time (h)	
1	1 (60)	1 (7.0)	1 (1.5)	1 (3)	38.58 ± 1.39
2	1 (60)	2 (7.5)	2 (2.0)	2 (4)	43.33 ± 0.92
3	1 (60)	3 (8.0)	3 (2.5)	3 (5)	43.00 ± 0.38
4	2 (65)	1 (7.0)	2 (2.0)	3 (5)	43.47 ± 0.45
5	2 (65)	2 (7.5)	3 (2.5)	1 (3)	44.63 ± 0.65
6	2 (65)	3 (8.0)	1 (1.5)	2 (4)	41.59 ± 1.05
7	3 (70)	1 (7.0)	3 (2.5)	2 (4)	44.08 ± 0.87
8	3 (70)	2 (7.5)	1 (1.5)	3 (5)	42.67 ± 2.52
9	3 (70)	3 (8.0)	2 (2.0)	1 (3)	38.67 ± 0.52
K1	124.91	126.13	122.84	121.88	
K2	129.69	130.63	125.47	129.00	
K3	125.42	123.26	131.71	129.14	
k1	41.64	42.04	40.95	40.63	
k2	43.23	43.54	41.82	43.00	
k3	41.81	41.09	43.90	43.05	
Best level	A_2	B_2	C_3	D_3	
R	1.59	2.45	2.95	2.42	
R order		C > B > D > A			

2.2. *Preparation of APs from MSBH*

2.2.1. Ultrafiltration

The radical scavenging rates of MSBH and its four ultrafiltration fractions (MSBH-I, MW < 1 kDa; MSBH-II, 1 kDa < MW < 3.5 kDa; MSBH-III, 3.5 kDa < MW < 10 kDa; MSBH-IV, MW > 10 kDa) at 5.0 mg/mL were measured (Figure 3). The data manifested that DPPH· and HO· scavenging rates of MSBH-I were 51.57 ± 1.45% and 76.96 ± 2.40%. The rates of MSBH-I were significantly greater than those of MSBH (47.13 ± 1.18% and 58.91 ± 3.17%), MSBH-II (49.23 ± 0.42% and 68.29 ± 1.141%), MSBH-III (48.86 ± 1.00% and 60.45 ± 1.92%) and MSBH-IV (46.11 ± 0.42% and 57.54 ± 0.81%) ($p < 0.05$). Then, MSBH-I was chosen for subsequent separation.

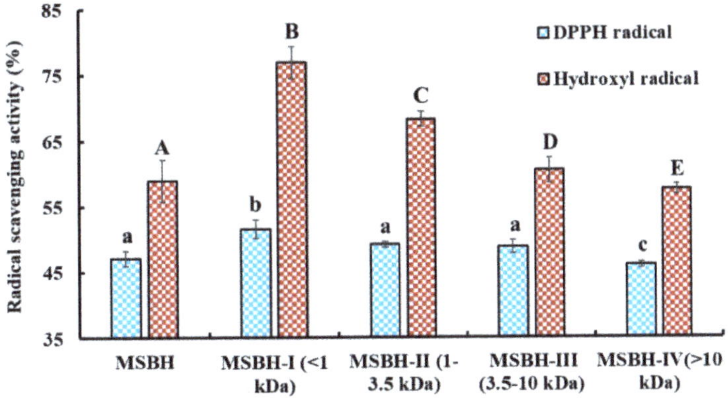

Figure 3. Radical scavenging activity of the monkfish swim bladder hydrolysate (MSBH) and its four fractions (MSBH-I to MSBH-IV). All data are presented as the mean ± SD of triplicate results. $^{a–c}$ or $^{A–E}$ Values with the same letters indicate no significant difference ($p > 0.05$).

2.2.2. Chromatography of MSBH

Using the Sephadex G-15 column, MSBH was fractionated into three subfractions (MSBH-Ia, MSBH-Ib and MSBH-Ic) according to the chromatographic diagram at 220 nm (Figure 4A). The DPPH· scavenging abilities of MSBH-Ib were 59.91 ± 0.55% at 5.0 mg/mL, which were significantly higher than those of MSBH-I (52.41 ± 1.42%), MSBH-Ia (59.91 ± 0.55%) and MSBH-Ic (47.04 ± 0.87%) ($p < 0.05$). At 1.0 mg/mL, HO· scavenging abilities of MSBH-Ib were 71.19 ± 0.85%, which were significantly higher than those of MSBH-I (18.04 ± 0.83%), MSBH-Ia (19.07 ± 1.33%) and MSBH-Ic (65.33 ± 0.79%), respectively ($p < 0.05$).

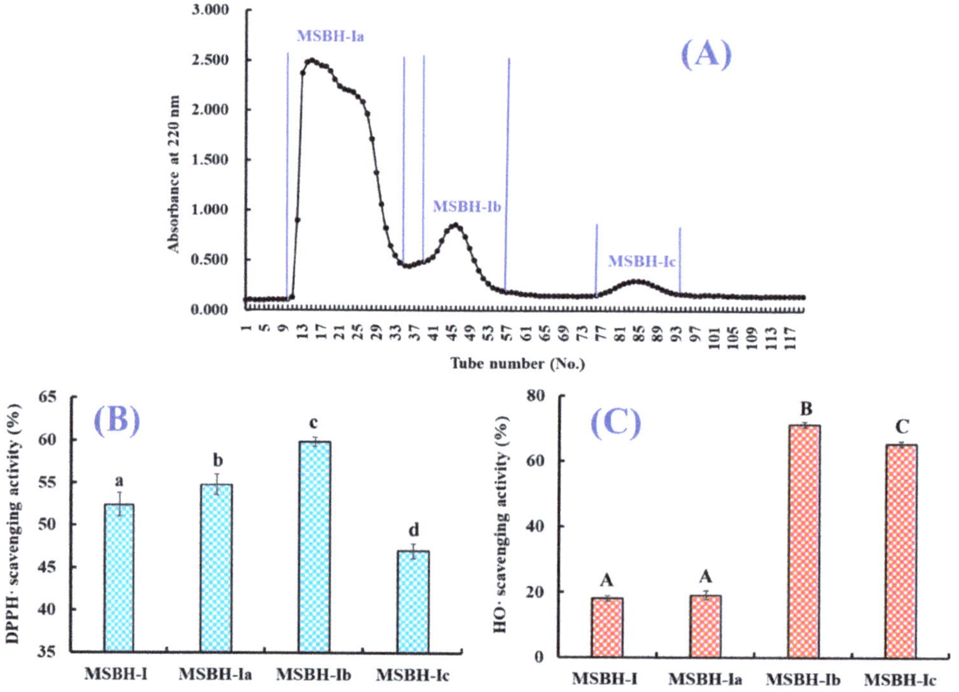

Figure 4. Chromatographic diagram of MSBH-I isolated by Sephadex G-15 and the radical scavenging activity of prepared subfractions (MSBH-Ia, MSBH-Ib and MSBH-Ic) from MSBH-I. (**A**) Chromatographic diagram of MSBH-I; (**B**) DPPH· scavenging activity; (**C**) HO· scavenging activity. All data are presented as the mean ± SD of triplicate results. $^{a–d}$ or $^{A–C}$ Values with the same letters indicate no significant difference ($p > 0.05$).

Finally, MSBH-Ib with high DPPH· and HO· scavenging abilities was isolated using RP-HPLC. By the chromatographic diagrams of MSBH-Ib at 214 and 254 nm (Figure 5), sixteen chromatographic peaks (P1–P16) with retention time (RT, min) of 6.08 (P1), 7.14 (P2), 8.22 (P3), 8.30 (P4), 8.93 (P5), 9.02 (P6), 9.87 (P7), 10.89 (P8), 10.91 (P9), 12.60 (P10), 13.92 (P11), 14.93 (P12), 15.02 (P13), 17.18 (P14), 17.99 (P15) and 20.50 min (P16) were collected lyophilized (Table 2). Then, sixteen components (P1–P16) separated by RP-HPLC were enriched for structure identification.

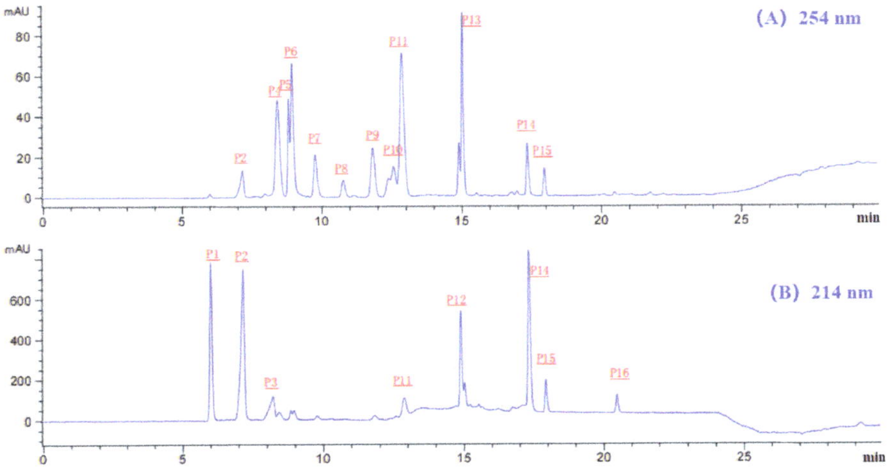

Figure 5. Chromatographic diagrams of MSBH-Ib by RP-HPLC at 254 nm (**A**) and 214 nm (**B**).

Table 2. Retention time (RT, min), amino acid (AA) sequences and molecular weights (MWs) of eighteen isolated APs (MSP1-MSP18) from MSBH.

Peaks	RT (min)	AA Sequence	Theoretical/Observed MW (Da)
P1	6.08	MSP1: Tyr-Asp-Tyr-Asp (YDYD) MSP2: Gln-Asp-Tyr-Asp (QDYD)	574.54/574.54 539.49/539.49
P2	7.14	MSP3: Ala-Gly-Pro-Ala-Ser (AGPAS)	401.41/401.41
P3	8.22	MSP4: Gly-Pro-Gly-Pro-His-Gly- Pro-Ser-Gly-Pro (GPGPHGPSGP)	858.90/858.89
P4	8.30	MSP5: Gly-Pro-Lys (GPK)	300.35/300.35
P5	8.93	MSP6: His-Arg-Glu (HRE)	440.45/440.45
P6	9.02	MSP7: Gly-Arg-Trp (GRW)	417.46/417.46
P7	9.87	MSP8: Ala-Arg-Trp (ARW)	431.49/431.49
P8	10.89	MSP9: Gly-Pro-Thr-Glu (GPTE)	402.40/402.40
P9	10.91	MSP 10: Asp-Asp-Gly-Gly-Lys (DDGGK)	490.47/490.47
P10	12.60	MSP11: Ile-Gly-Pro-Ala-Ser (IGPAS) MSP12: Ala-Lys-Pro-Ala-Thr (AKPAT)	443.49/443.49 486.56/486.56
P11	13.92	MSP13: Tyr-Pro-Ala-Gly-Pro (YPAGP)	503.55/503.54
P12	14.93	MSP14:Asp-Pro-Thr (DPT)	331.32/331.32
P13	15.02	MSP15: Phe-Pro-Gly-Pro-Thr (FPGPT)	517.57/517.57
P14	17.18	MSP16: Gly-Pro-Gly-Pro-Thr (GPGPT)	427.45/427.45
P15	17.99	MSP17: Gly-Pro-Thr (GPT)	273.29/273.29
P16	20.50	MSP18: Asp-Pro-Ala-Gly-Pro (DPAGP)	455.46/455.46

2.3. *Determination of the AA Sequences and MWs of Eighteen Isolated APs (MSP1-MSP18)*

The MWs and sequences of APs in HPLC chromatographic peaks (P1–P16) were determined by protein sequencer and ESI-MS (Table 2). Peaks of P1 and P10 contained two peptides. Therefore, eighteen APs (MSP1-MSP18) from chromatographic peaks of P1–P16 were identified as Tyr-Asp-Tyr-Asp (YDYD, MSP1), Gln-Asp-Tyr-Asp (QDYD, MSP2), Ala-Gly-Pro-Ala-Ser (AGPAS, MSP3), Gly-Pro-Gly-Pro-His-Gly-Pro-Ser-Gly-Pro (GPGPHGPSGP, MSP4), Gly-Pro-Lys (GPK, MSP5), His-Arg-Glu (HRE, MSP6), Gly-Arg-Trp (GRW, MSP7), Ala-Arg-Trp (ARW, MSP8), Gly-Pro-Thr-Glu (GPTE, MSP9), Asp-Asp-Gly-Gly-Lys (DDGGK, MSP10), Ile-Gly-Pro-Ala-Ser (IGPAS, MSP11), Ala-Lys-Pro-Ala-Thr (AKPAT, MSP12), Tyr-Pro-Ala-Gly-Pro (YPAGP, MSP13), Asp-Pro-Thr (DPT, MSP14), Phe-Pro-Gly-Pro-Thr (FPGPT, MSP15), Gly-Pro-Gly-Pro-Thr (GPGPT, MSP16), Gly-Pro-Thr (GPT, MSP17) and Asp-Pro-Ala-Gly-Pro (DPAGP, MSP18), respectively. In addition, the MWs of eighteen APs (MSP1-MSP18) were determined as 574.54, 539.49, 401.41, 858.89,

300.35, 440.45, 417.46, 431.49, 402.40, 490.47, 443.49, 486.56, 503.54, 331.32, 517.57, 427.45, 273.29 and 455.46 Da, respectively, which were quite consistent with their theoretical MWs (Table 2).

2.4. *Antioxidant Activity of MSP1 to MSP18*

2.4.1. Radical Scavenging Activity of Eighteen Isolated APs (MSP1-MSP18)

Figure 6A and Table 3 showed that the EC_{50} values of MSP7 and MSP8 on DPPH· were 1.053 ± 0.003 and 0.773 ± 0.003 mg/mL, which were significantly lower than those of the other sixteen isolated APs ($p < 0.05$).

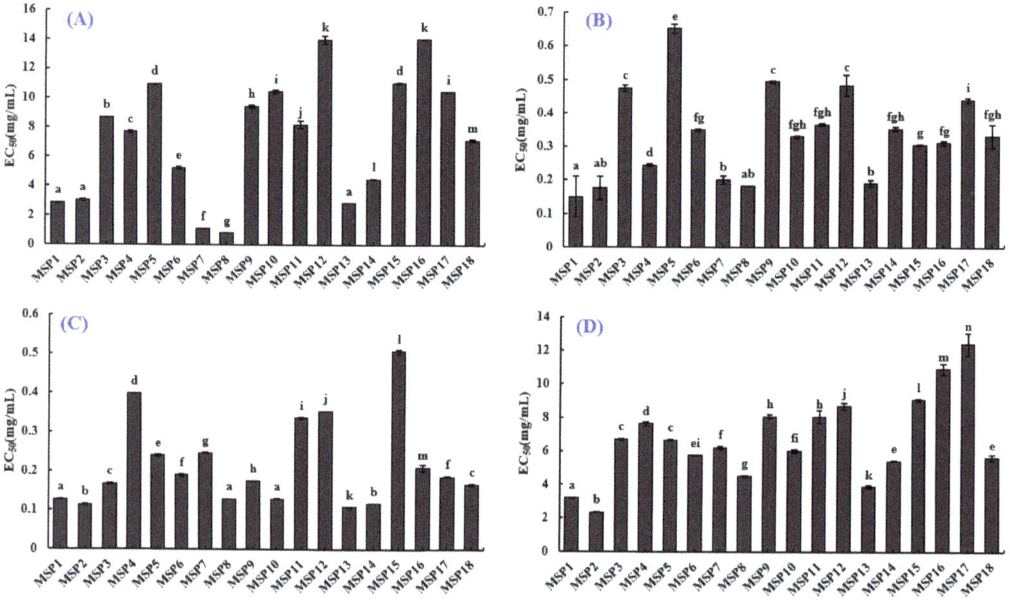

Figure 6. Radical scavenging activity of eighteen isolated APs (MSP1-MSP18). (**A**) EC_{50} values of peptides (MSP1-MSP18) on DPPH·; (**B**) EC_{50} values of peptides (MSP1-MSP18) on HO·; (**C**) EC_{50} values of peptides (MSP1-MSP18) on O_2^-·; (**D**) EC_{50} values of peptides (MSP1-MSP18) on $ABTS^+$·. All data are presented as the mean ± SD of triplicate results. [a–n] Values with the same letters indicate no significant difference ($p > 0.05$).

The data in Figure 6B and Table 3 depicted that MSP1 had the minimum EC_{50} (0.150 ± 0.060 mg/mL) on HO· among eighteen APs (MSP1 to MSP18) and followed by MSP2 (0.177 ± 0.035 mg/mL), MSP7 (0.201 ± 0.013 mg/mL), MSP8 (0.183 ± 0.0016 mg/mL) and MSP13 (0.190 ± 0.010 mg/mL).

Figure 6C and Table 3 showed MSP1, MSP2, MSP8, MSP10 and MSP13 have significant O_2^-· scavenging capability with EC_{50} values of 0.126 ± 0.0005, 0.112 ± 0.0028, 0.127 ± 0.0002, 0.128 ± 0.0018 and 0.107 ± 0.0002 mg/mL, respectively. EC_{50} values of MSP1, MSP2, MSP8, MSP10 and MSP13 on O_2^-· were significantly lower than those of the other thirteen isolated peptides.

Figure 6D and Table 3 indicated that eighteen isolated peptides (MSP1-MSP18) showed relatively weak $ABTS^+$· scavenging ability. The EC_{50} values of MSP1, MSP2 and MSP13 were 3.197 ± 0.036, 2.337 ± 0.016 and 3.839 ± 0.102 mg/mL, respectively, which were remarkably lower than those of the other fifteen isolated peptides.

Table 3. EC_{50} values of eighteen isolated APs (MSP1-MSP18) on HO·, DPPH·, O_2^-· and $ABTS^+$·.

Peptides	EC_{50} (mg/mL)			
	DPPH·	HO·	O_2^-·	$ABTS^+$·
MSP1	2.824 ± 0.019 [a]	0.150 ± 0.060 [a]	0.126 ± 0.0005 [a]	3.197 ± 0.036 [a]
MSP2	2.993 ± 0.054 [a]	0.177 ± 0.035 [a,b]	0.112 ± 0.0028 [b]	2.337 ± 0.016 [b]
MSP3	8.667 ± 0.023 [b]	0.475 ± 0.0103 [c]	0.166 ± 0.0017 [c]	6.693 ± 0.030 [c]
MSP4	7.703 ± 0.091 [c]	0.244 ± 0.0035 [d]	0.397 ± 0.0008 [d]	7.613 ± 0.133 [d]
MSP5	10.947 ± 0.031 [d]	0.652 ± 0.0132 [e]	0.239 ± 0.0026 [e]	6.641 ± 0.043 [c]
MSP6	5.231 ± 0.083 [e]	0.349 ± 0.0037 [f,g]	0.188 ± 0.0026 [f]	5.729 ± 0.025 [e,i]
MSP7	1.053 ± 0.003 [f]	0.201 ± 0.013 [b]	0.245 ± 0.0021 [g]	6.188 ± 0.084 [f]
MSP8	0.773 ± 0.003 [g]	0.183 ± 0.0016 [a,b]	0.127 ± 0.0002 [a]	4.503 ± 0.040 [g]
MSP9	9.420 ± 0.109 [h]	0.493 ± 0.0042 [c]	0.173 ± 0.0020 [h]	8.034 ± 0.124 [h]
MSP10	10.417 ± 0.110 [i]	0.329 ± 0.004 [f,g,h]	0.128 ± 0.0018 [a]	6.004 ± 0.087 [f,i]
MSP11	8.195 ± 0.271 [j]	0.366 ± 0.004 [f,g,h]	0.335 ± 0.0027 [i]	8.054 ± 0.366 [h]
MSP12	13.96 ± 0.284 [k]	0.482 ± 0.0309 [c]	0.353 ± 0.0006 [j]	8.695 ± 0.200 [j]
MSP13	2.821 ± 0.012 [a]	0.190 ± 0.010 [b]	0.107 ± 0.0002 [k]	3.839 ± 0.102 [k]
MSP14	4.450 ± 0.005 [l]	0.353 ± 0.0067 [f,g,h]	0.116 ± 0.0002 [b]	5.411 ± 0.028 [e]
MSP15	11.013 ± 0.042 [d]	0.306 ± 0.0025 [g]	0.505 ± 0.0058 [l]	9.058 ± 0.082 [l]
MSP16	13.99 ± 0.046 [k]	0.312 ± 0.0065 [f,g]	0.208 ± 0.0080 [m]	10.89 ± 0.322 [m]
MSP17	10.413 ± 0.006 [i]	0.439 ± 0.0069 [i]	0.185 ± 0.0014 [f]	12.387 ± 0.670 [n]
MSP18	7.119 ± 0.092 [m]	0.332 ± 0.035 [f,g,h]	0.166 ± 0.0020 [c]	5.621 ± 0.169 [e]

All data are presented as the mean ± SD of triplicate results. [a–n] Values with the same letters indicate no significant difference in each column ($p > 0.05$).

In addition, we comprehensively considered the radical scavenging activities of eighteen isolated APs (MSP1-MSP18), and finally selected MSP1, MSP2, MSP7, MSP8, MSP10 and MSP13 for subsequent bioactive and stability experiments.

2.4.2. Lipid Peroxidation Inhibition Ability

In organic tissues, lipid peroxidation is generally described as a process in which oxidants attack lipids containing polyunsaturated fatty acids (PUFAs), which has an important role in human health because lipid peroxidation products, including MDA and 4-HNE, play a vital cytotoxic role in promoting cell death and controlling gene expression [47]. Therefore, the assay was applied to comprehensively evaluate the activities of MSP1, MSP2, MSP7, MSP8, MSP10 and MSP13 (Figure 7A). In the linoleic acid emulsion system, the values at 500 nm of MSP1, MSP2, MSP7, MSP8, MSP10 and MSP13 were significantly smaller than that of blank control (without peptide and GSH) during 7 days. The finding demonstrated that MSP1, MSP2, MSP7, MSP8, MSP10 and MSP13 could effectively inhibit the reaction rate and efficiency of lipid peroxidation in the experimental system by reacting with H_2O_2. Moreover, the MSP8 showed a similar inhibiting capability to that of GSH, followed by MSP1, MSP10 and MSP13.

2.4.3. Ferric Reducing Antioxidant Power (FRAP)

The FRAP assay reflects the ability of compounds that serve as electron donors to decrease the oxidized intermediates in the lipid peroxidation process, and it has been used as a preferred method to evaluate the "total antioxidant content" of functional molecules [48,49]. As shown in Figure 6B, MSP8 showed a higher ability to convert Fe^{3+}/ferricyanide complex into Fe^{2+} form than the other five determined peptides, followed by MSP1, MSP10 and MSP7. However, the reducing power of MSP1, MSP2, MSP7, MSP8, MSP10 and MSP13 was lower than that of glutathione (GSH).

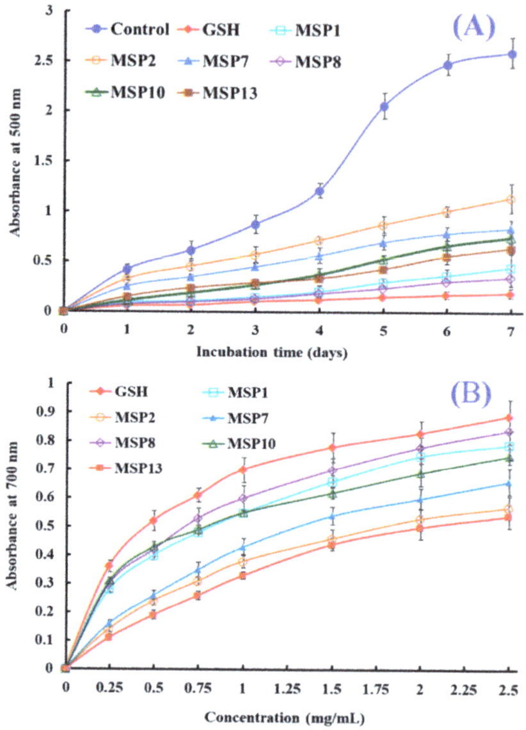

Figure 7. The lipid peroxidation inhibition ability (**A**) and ferric reducing antioxidant power (FRAP) (**B**) of MSP1, MSP2, MSP7, MSP8, MSP10 and MSP13. All data are presented as the mean ± SD of triplicate results.

2.4.4. Protective Effect on H_2O_2-Damaged Plasmid DNA

Figure 8 indicated the protective ability of MSP1, MSP2, MSP7, MSP8, MSP10 and MSP13 on pBR322DNA against H_2O_2 damage. Compared with the supercoiled (SC) form of pBR322DNA with two phosphodiester chains (Figure 8, lane 1), the phosphodiester chains of plasmid DNA were clipped by the HO· and formed a linear (LIN) or open circular (OC) structure in the model group (Figure 8, lane 8). Nevertheless, more SC structures were preserved in the pBR322DNA of MSP1, MSP2, MSP7, MSP8, MSP10 and MSP13 groups (Figure 8, lane 2–7), which indicated that MSP1, MSP2, MSP7, MSP8, MSP10 and MSP13 could protect plasmid DNA (pBR322DNA) against the damage by HO·. In addition, the protective function of MSP1 and MSP8 was similar to that of GSH and significantly stronger than those of MSP2, MSP7, MSP10 and MSP13.

2.4.5. Cytoprotective Function on H_2O_2-Damaged HepG2 Cells

Figure 9 indicated that MSP1, MSP2, MSP7, MSP8, MSP10 and MSP13 could increase the viability of H_2O_2-injuried HepG2 cells at 200 μmol/L. In addition, the viability of H_2O_2-injured HepG2 cells in MSP1 and MSP8 groups was 82.14 ± 3.28% and 81.32 ± 2.45%, which were significantly higher than that of the model group (51.08 ± 1.97%). Therefore, MSP1, MSP2, MSP7, MSP8, MSP10 and MSP13 presented cytoprotective function to H_2O_2-injuried HepG2 cells by increasing the cell viability.

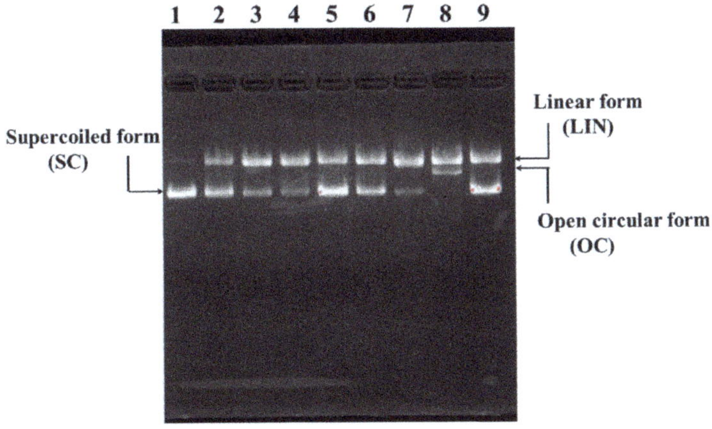

Figure 8. The protective effects of MSP1, MSP2, MSP7, MSP8, MSP10 and MSP13 on the H_2O_2-damaged plasmid DNA (pBR322DNA). Lane 1: native pBR322DNA; Lane 2–9, DNA + $FeSO_4$ + H_2O_2 + MSP1, MSP2, MSP7, MSP8, MSP10, MSP13, H_2O and GSH, respectively.

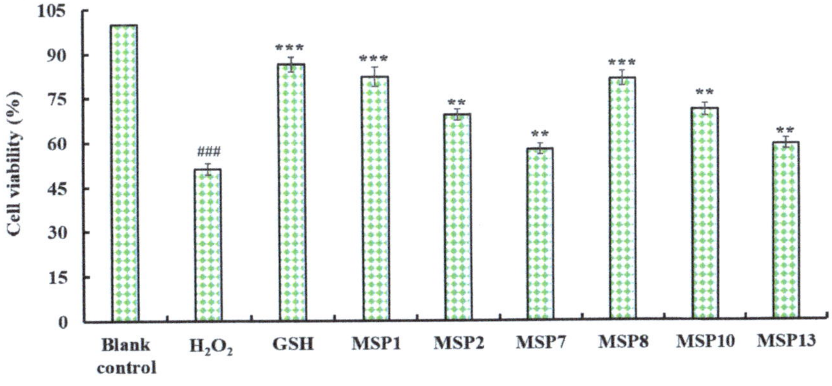

Figure 9. Cytoprotective effects of MSP1, MSP2, MSP7, MSP8, MSP10 and MSP13 on the H_2O_2-induced HepG2 cells at 200 μmol/L. GSH served as the positive control. All data are presented as the mean ± SD of triplicate results. ### $p < 0.001$ vs. blank control group; *** $p < 0.001$ and ** $p < 0.01$ vs. H_2O_2-induced model group.

2.5. Stability of MSP1, MSP2, MSP7, MSP8, MSP10 and MSP13

2.5.1. pH Stability of MSP1, MSP2, MSP7, MSP8, MSP10 and MSP13

Figure 10 and Table 4 indicated that MSP1, MSP2, MSP7, MSP8, MSP10 and MSP13 showed significant differences in tolerance to acid and alkali treatment (pH 3 to 11). MSP1, MSP2, MSP7 and MSP8 kept the highest $O_2^-\cdot$ scavenging activity at pH 7.0, but MSP10 and MSP13 kept the highest activity at pH 11.0 and 9.0, respectively. In addition, MSP1, MSP2, MSP7 and MSP8 were more sensitive to alkali treatment because their $O_2^-\cdot$ scavenging rates dropped by 35.26%, 73.07%, 69.19% and 83.05%, respectively, at pH 11.0. Conversely, MSP10 and MSP13 were more sensitive to acid treatment because their $O_2^-\cdot$ scavenging rates dropped by 26.26% and 33.05% at pH 3.0. Those data suggested that MSP1, MSP2, MSP7 and MSP8 are appropriate for the application to products in a neutral environment, but MSP10 and MSP13 are appropriate for the application to products in an alkali environment.

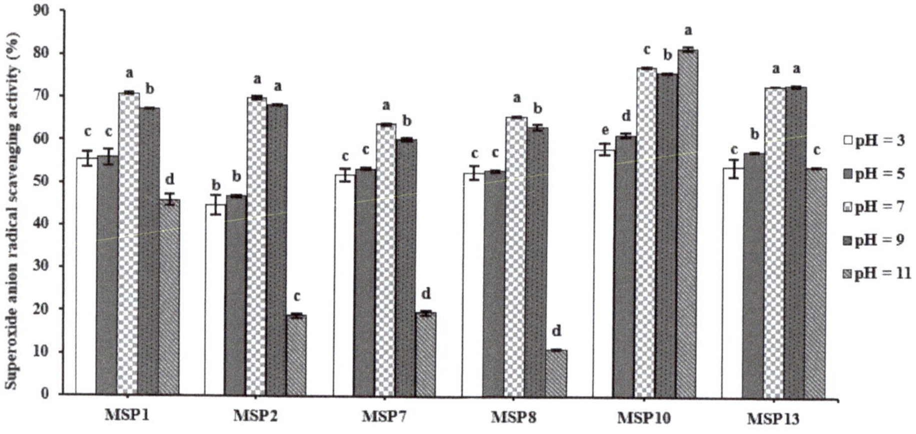

Figure 10. $O_2^-\cdot$ scavenging activity of MSP1, MSP2, MSP7, MSP8, MSP10 and MSP13 subjected to different pH treatments. All data are presented as the mean ± SD of triplicate results. [a–e] values with the same letters indicate no significant difference of the same peptide ($p > 0.05$).

Table 4. Declined percentage of $O_2^-\cdot$ scavenging activity of MSP1, MSP2, MSP7, MSP8, MSP10 and MSP13 subjected to different pH treatments.

Peptides	Declined Percentage (%)				
	pH 3	**pH 5**	**pH 7**	**pH 9**	**pH 11**
MSP1	−21.77	−21.10	0.00	−4.97	−35.26
MSP2	−36.14	−33.16	0.00	−2.29	−73.07
MSP7	−18.68	−16.43	0.00	−5.78	−69.19
MSP8	−19.97	−19.47	0.00	−3.85	−83.05
MSP10	−28.91	−24.92	−5.13	−7.06	0
MSP13	−26.03	−21.19	−0.15	0	−26.03

2.5.2. Thermal Stability of MSP1, MSP2, MSP7, MSP8, MSP10 and MSP13

The $O_2^-\cdot$ scavenging activity of MSP1, MSP2, MSP7, MSP8, MSP10 and MSP13 treated using different temperatures (25, 37, 60, 80 and 100 °C) was present in Figure 11, and the results manifested that six APs have high-temperature tolerance. Compared with MSP1, MSP7, MSP8 and MSP13, MSP2 and MSP10 were relatively affected by high temperature (100 °C), and their $O_2^-\cdot$ scavenging activity, respectively, decreased by 3.84% and 2.60%. Those data suggested that MSP1, MSP2, MSP7, MSP8, MSP10 and MSP13 are appropriate for the application to products treated by high temperatures because of their high-temperature tolerance.

2.5.3. Stability of MSP1, MSP2, MSP7, MSP8, MSP10 and MSP13 Subjected to Simulated Gastrointestinal (GI) Digestion

Figure 12 presented the effects of simulated GI digestion on the antioxidant ability of MSP1, MSP2, MSP7, MSP8, MSP10 and MSP13, and the results indicated that $O_2^-\cdot$ scavenging activities of MSP1, MSP2, MSP7, MSP8, MSP10 and MSP13 decreased gradually when they were treated with pepsin and trypsin in turn. Among six peptides, the $O_2^-\cdot$ scavenging rates of MSP2, MSP7 and MSP10 showed the most seriously affected after simulated GI digestion and decreased by 47.59%, 49.19% and 53.33%, respectively; the $O_2^-\cdot$ scavenging rates of MSP8 and MSP13 were also affected and decreased by 28.62% and 35.83%, respectively(Table 5). However, MSP1 showed good tolerance and its $O_2^-\cdot$ scavenging rate only decreased by 4.1% (Table 6). Those results suggested that MSP1 showed high stability when it was treated with simulated GI digestion.

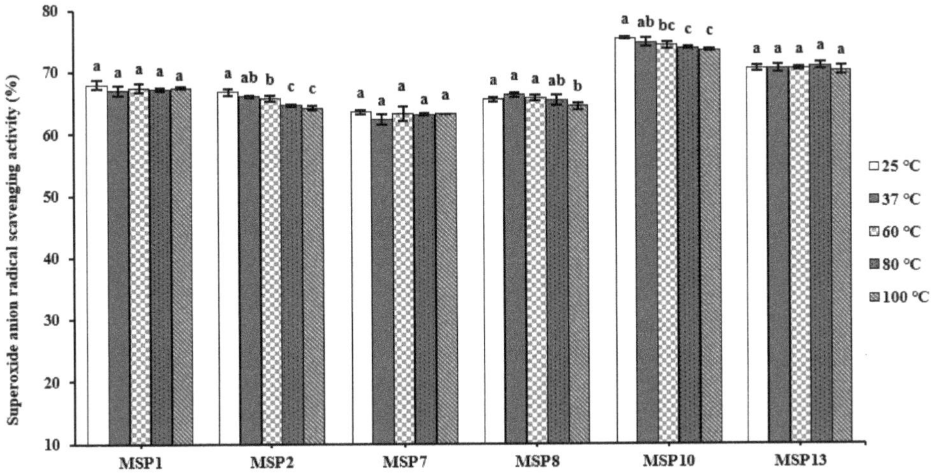

Figure 11. $O_2^-\cdot$ scavenging activity of MSP1, MSP2, MSP7, MSP8, MSP10 and MSP13 subjected to different thermal treatments. All data are presented as the mean ± SD of triplicate results. [a–c] Values with the same letters indicate no significant difference of same peptide ($p > 0.05$).

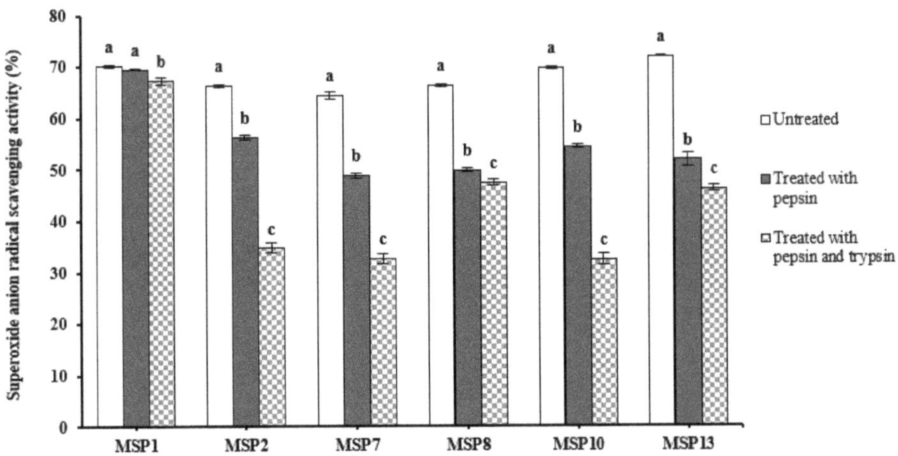

Figure 12. $O_2^-\cdot$ scavenging activity of MSP1, MSP2, MSP7, MSP8, MSP10 and MSP13 subjected to simulated GI digestion treatments. All data are presented as the mean ± SD of triplicate results. [a–c] Values with the same letters indicate no significant difference in the same sample ($p > 0.05$).

Table 5. Declined percentage of $O_2^-\cdot$ scavenging activity of MSP1, MSP2, MSP7, MSP8, MSP10 and MSP13 subjected to simulated GI digestion treatments.

	Declined Percentage (%)		
	Untreated	**Treated with Pepsin**	**Treated with Pepsin and Trypsin**
MSP1	0.00	−0.84	−4.10
MSP2	0.00	−15.13	−47.59
MSP7	0.00	−24.34	−49.19
MSP8	0.00	−24.93	−28.62
MSP10	0.00	−21.98	−53.33
MSP13	0.00	−28.02	−35.83

Table 6. Declined percentage of $O_2^-\cdot$ scavenging activity of MSP1, MSP2, MSP7, MSP8, MSP10 and MSP13 subjected to different thermal treatments.

Peptides	Declined Percentage (%)				
	25 °C	37 °C	60 °C	80 °C	100 °C
MSP1	0.00	−1.48	−0.82	−1.15	−0.82
MSP2	0.00	−1.00	−1.50	−3.17	−3.84
MSP7	0.00	−1.94	−0.52	−0.70	−0.53
MSP8	0.00	1.02	0.34	−0.17	−1.70
MSP10	0.00	−0.87	−1.58	−2.16	−2.60
MSP13	0.00	0.00	0.00	0.61	−0.46

3. Discussion

3.1. Preparation of APs from MSBH

BPs are encapsulated in the sequence of proteins and keep inactive form and can be released by a variety of hydrolysis pathways [28]. In comparison with chemical and microbiological degradation, protease degradation is known as an effective, safe and rational method for the production of protein hydrolysates because of the high controllability and reproducibility of the enzymatic process, the mild and safe conditions of enzymatic protein digestion and the absence of side reactions in the enzymatic reaction. Then, protease degradation is more widely used in the food and pharmaceutical industries [3,50,51]. Therefore, proteases including papain, alcalase, pepsin, flavourzyme, Protamex®, trypsin and their combinations are frequently used to manufacture BPs from marine organisms and their by-products [9,52,53]. In addition, many enzymes have specific cleavage sites (papain: Arg-, Lys- and Phe-; alcalase: Ala-, Leu-, Val-, Tyr-, Phe- and Try-; trypsin: Arg- and Lys-; pepsin: Phe- and Leu-), and different cleavage sites will have a certain effect on the activity of hydrolysates [54,55]. Ktari et al. found that hydrolysates from cuttlefish (*Sepia officinalis*) by-products obtained by alcalase and sardinelle crude enzyme exhibited the strongest activity among eight hydrolysates [52]. Alcalase hydrolysate of Antarctic Krill had the highest radical scavenging ability among the five hydrolysates [56]. Nangnoi strain hydrolysate generated by alcalase showed the highest activities among the three hydrolysates [57]. In the study, MSBH produced by papain shows the highest activity further proving this conclusion that specificity and conditions of proteases are the key factors for the generation of APs.

The hydrolysate profile is also influenced by enzyme concentration, digestion time, digestion temperature, ambient pH and other factors. At the optimum pH and temperature, the cleavage rate of protease is accelerated and non-specific digestion sites are less likely to occur. In addition, insufficient enzymatic digestion may occur with too short a digestion time and too low an enzyme concentration [3,12]. Jang et al. found that the optimal hydrolysis conditions for alcalase 2.4 L were pH 6.0, temperature 70 °C, enzyme concentration 5% (w/w), and hydrolysis time 3 h. The optimal hydrolysis conditions for Collupulin MG were pH 9.0, temperature 60 °C, enzyme dose 5% (w/w), and the DPPH· radical scavenging activity of the two hydrolysates under optimal conditions was 60.04 and 79.65%, respectively [58]. In the study, the optimum conditions of enzymatic hydrolysis of papain were temperature 65 °C, pH 7.5, enzyme dose 2.5%, enzymatic hydrolysis time 2 h and the DPPH· scavenging rate of enzymatic hydrolysis product was 47.13 ± 1.15%. It was further proved that the enzymatic hydrolysis condition of papain significantly influenced the generation of APs.

Protein hydrolysates consist of peptides with different chain lengths, and MW is also a key factor affecting the separation and production of BPs [28,59]. In consequence, membrane ultrafiltration and gel permeation chromatography become the most popular methods for peptide isolation from different hydrolysates, such as salmon byproduct [32], Antarctic Krill [56], miiuy croaker muscle [49], Skipjack tuna (*K. pelamis*) bone [51], seahorse (*Hippocampus abdominalis*) [60], oyster (*C. giga*) [61] and *E. cottonii* [62]. Refering to the existing literature, we designed the separation method and eighteen APs (MSP1-MSP18) were prepared from MSBH using radical scavenging activity as the screening index. Among eighteen peptides (MSP1-MSP18), MSP1, MSP2, MSP7, MSP8, MSP10 and MSP13 presented remarkable antioxidant activity.

3.2. Antioxidant Activity of MSP1, MSP2, MSP7, MSP8, MSP10 and MSP13

DPPH· is a very stable radical and is commonly used as a substrate to assess antioxidant activity. MSP7 and MSP8 have a strong hydrogen donating capacity and can reduce stable DPPH·. A review of the literature found that the EC_{50} values of MSP7 and MSP8 on DPPH· were lower than those of marine APs from scalloped hammerhead sharks (*Sphyrna lewini*) muscle (WDR: 3.63 mg/mL; SAP: 3.06 mg/mL; PYFK: 4.11 mg/mL) [63,64], seaweed (*Eucheuma cottonii*) (YSKT: 1.71 mg/mL; FYKA: 2.56 mg/mL) [31], tuna (*Katsuwonus pelamis*) cardiac arterial bulbs (GEQSN: 2.054 mg/mL; GEGQR: 2.257 mg/mL) [50] and Spanish mackerel (*Scomberomorous niphonius*) skin (GPTGE: 1.42 mg/mL; PYGAKG: 3.02 mg/mL) [62]. However, the EC_{50} values of MSP7 and MSP8 on DPPH· were higher than those of marine APs from Spanish mackerel skin (YGPM: 0.72 mg/mL) [62], monkfish muscle (EDIVCW: 0.39 mg/mL; YWDAW: 0.51 mg/mL) [18] and tuna roes (AEM: 0.250 mg/mL; YVM: 0.288 mg/mL) [65]. This finding suggests that MSP7 and MSP8 can convert DPPH· to less harmful or non-harmful products, breaking the free radical chain reaction.

HO· is a kind of strong free radical, which can not only cause lipid peroxidation in vivo but also attack polysaccharides, nucleic acids and other macromolecules, causing serious damage to cells. MSP1, MSP2, MSP7, MSP8 and MSP13 have strong HO· scavenging ability and their EC_{50} values were lower than those of marine APs from tuna roes (AEM: 0.456 mg/mL; YVM: 0.413 mg/mL) [65], monkfish muscle (EDIVCW: 0.61 mg/mL; YWDAW: 0.32 mg/mL) [18] and skin (GPY: 3.22 mg/mL; YGPM: 0.88 mg/mL) [62], Antarctic krill (*Euphausia superba*) (VEKT: 1.53 mg/mL; IDSQ: 2.57 mg/mL) [29], loach (*Misgurnus anguillicaudatus*) meat (PSYV: 2.64 mg/mL) [66] and grass carp (*Ctenopharyngodon idella*) skin (VGGRP: 2.06 mg/mL) [67]. This finding suggests that MSP1, MSP2, MSP7, MSP8 and MSP13 have a strong ability to scavenge HO· and can reduce the damage to the body caused by HO·.

O_2^-· reacts with metal ions in the Fenton reaction to form HO· that triggers lipid peroxidation and causes oxidative damage to cells. MSP1, MSP2, MSP8, MSP10 and MSP13 have a strong ability to scavenge O_2^-·. A review of the literature revealed that the EC_{50} values of MSP1, MSP2, MSP8, MSP10 and MSP13 on O_2^-· were significantly lower than those of marine APs from monkfish muscle (EDIVCW: 0.76 mg/mL; YWDAW: 0.48 mg/mL) [18] and skin (GPY: 3.98 mg/mL; YGPM: 0.73 mg/mL) [67], tuna cardiac arterial bulbs (GEQSN: 1.857 mg/mL; GEGQR: 2.143 mg/mL) [50], seaweed (YLL: 1.61 mg/mL; FYKA: 1.91 mg/mL) [31] and Antarctic krill (VEKT: 0.86 mg/mL; IDSQ: 1.45 mg/mL) [29]. This result indicates that MSP1, MSP2, MSP8, MSP10 and MSP13 have good antioxidant activity similar to that of SOD against O_2^-· and can be used as O_2^-· scavengers in living cells.

$ABTS^+$· is a single oxygen ion radical with an absorption peak at 734 nm, which can be reduced by antioxidants leading to a decrease in absorbance. The EC_{50} values of MSP1, MSP2 and MSP13 were significantly lower than those of the other fifteen isolated peptides. However, through consulting the literature, it is found that the EC_{50} values of MSP1, MSP2, and MSP13 were significantly higher than those of marine APs from red stingray (*Dasyatis akajei*) cartilages (VPR: 0.15 mg/mL; IEEEQ: 0.18 mg/mL) [11], monkfish skin (GPY: 2.12 mg/mL; YGPM: 0.82 mg/mL) [62], scalloped hammerhead sharks muscle (WDR: 0.34 mg/mL; SAP: 0.19 mg/mL; PYFK: 0.12 mg/mL) [63,64], tuna milt (GHHAAA: 1.12 mg/mL; SMDV: 1.16 mg/mL) [68], tuna roes (GHHAAA: 1.12 mg/mL; SMDV: 1.16 mg/mL) [65] and tuna cardiac arterial bulbs (GEGQR: 1.218 mg/mL; GLN: 1.641 mg/mL) [50].

3.3. Structure–Activity Relationship of MSP1, MSP2, MSP7, MSP8, MSP10 and MSP13

Presently, numerous APs derived from a variety of proteins and their bioactivity has been investigated using in vitro and in vivo methods. In general, MW, AA composition and sequence, and spatial structure are generally regarded as critical factors for their activities [61,69,70]. In the study, MSP1, MSP2, MSP7, MSP8, MSP10 and MSP13 belong to tripeptides, tetrapeptides and pentapeptides with MWs of 574.54, 539.49, 417.46, 431.49, 490.47 and 503.54 Da, respectively. Therefore, smaller molecule size is very conducive to the binding of MSP1, MSP2, MSP7, MSP8, MSP10 and MSP13 and targets to play their functions [71–73].

The roles of AA composition, especially hydrophobic/aromatic AAs, are often discussed in previous literature [3,12,28]. Hydrophobic/aromatic AAs can facilitate the binding between the peptides and ROS by improving the peptides' solubility in the reactive solution [21,70]. Ala residue should play an important role in the antioxidant activity of MSP8 (ARW) and MSP13 (YPAGP). Aromatic AAs contain a benzene ring structure, which can provide hydrogen ions to convert ROS into more stable phenoxy radicals and control the peroxide domino effects mediated by ROS [10,20,74]. Sheng et al. reported that Tyr and Phe residues in GEYGFE and Phe residue in IELFPGLP exerted key roles in their antioxidant activities [20]. Therefore, Tyr residue in MSP1 (YDYD), MSP2 (QDYD) and MSP13 (YPAGP) and Trp residue in MSP7 (GRW) and MSP8 (ARW) could positively affect their activity. In addition, Pro residue could improve the flexibility of peptides and act as proton/hydrogen donors to remove ROS directly [24,31,75]. Therefore, Pro residue should be important for the activity of MSP13 (YPAGP).

Hydrophilic AA residues also are necessary for the activity of APs. Acidic (Asp, Glu, Asn and Gln) and basic (Lys and Arg) AA residues have been proven as excellent chelating agents of metal-ions because the excessive electrons in their carboxylic group could improve electrostatic and ionic with metal-ion to play their excellent metal-chelating function [10,76]. Therefore, basic (Arg and Lys) and acidic (Glu and Asp) AA residues were frequently found in APs, such as LKPGN [29], VPR, IEPH, LEEEE and IEEEQ [11], LDEPDPLI and NTDGSTDYGILQINSR [77], PHPR, VRDQY [54] and AEDKKLIQ [78]. Therefore, Asp residue in MSP1 (YDYD), Gln and Asp residues in MSP2 (QDYD), Arg residue in MSP7 (GRW) and MSP8 (ARW) and Asp and Lys residues in MSP10 (DDGGK) must be a great help to their antioxidant ability. Gly residue is often found in collagen peptides with antioxidant activity, such as GFRGTIGLVG, GPAGPAG, GFPSG [13], FTGMD, GFEPY, GFYAA, GIEWA [79], PFGPD, PYGAKG and YGPM [50] because it can maintain the high flexibility of peptide chain and act as a single hydrogen donor to neutralize ROS. Then, Gly residue presented in MSP7 (GRW), MSP10 (DDGGK) and MSP13 (YPAGP) are helpful for their activity.

4. Materials and Methods

4.1. Materials and Chemical Reagents

Monkfish (*L. litulon*) swim bladders were kindly provided by Zhejiang Hailisheng Group Co., Ltd. (Zhoushan, China). The voucher specimen (No. DC046) was authenticated by Prof. Sheng-long Zhao (Zhejiang Ocean University, Zhoushan, China) and has been deposited in the School of Food and Pharmacy, Zhejiang Ocean University. Acetonitrile of LC grade and trifluoroacetic acid (TFA) were purchased from Thermo Fisher Scientific Co., Ltd. (Shanghai, China). Glutathione (GSH, PHR1359), 2,2-Diphenyl-1-picrylhydrazyl (DPPH, D9132) and 2,2′-Azino-bis(3-ethylbenzothiazoline-6-sulfonic acid) diammonium salt (ABTS, 11557-1G) were bought from Sigma-Aldrich (Shanghai, China) Trading Co., Ltd. Papain, alcalase, trypsin, and pepsin was purchased from Beijing Genthold Biotechnology Co., Ltd. (Beijing, China). Sephadex G-15 were purchased from Shanghai Source Poly Biological Technology Co., Ltd. (Shanghai, China). Peptides of MSP1 to MSP18 (>98%) were synthesized by Shanghai Apeptide Co., Ltd. (Shanghai, China). Human hepatocarcinoma cell lines (HepG2) were purchased from the Shanghai Cell Bank of the Chinese Academy of Sciences.

4.2. Preparation of MSBH

4.2.1. Screening of Enzyme Species

The monkfish swim bladders were homogenated and defatted using isopropanol [79]. After that, the defatted powder of monkfish swim bladders was dispersed in a buffer solution to prepare 5% (w/v) protein slurry and hydrolyzed, respectively using pepsin (pH 2.0, 37 °C), trypsin (pH 7.8, 37 °C), alcalase (pH 9.0, 50 °C), papain (pH 7.0, 55 °C), flavourzyme (pH 7.0, 50 °C) with enzyme dose 2.0%. After 4 h, the monkfish swim bladder hydrolysates were placed in boiling water for 20 min, and the inactivated hydrolysates were centrifuged at 4000× g for 25 min. The resulting supernatant was freeze-dried and kept at −20 °C. The monkfish swim bladder hydrolysate produced using papain showed the highest DPPH· scavenging activity.

4.2.2. Optimization of Hydrolysis Conditions of Papain

A single-factor experiment was used to optimize the hydrolysis conditions of papain. Hydrolysis temperature (55, 60, 65, 70, and 75 °C), time (3, 4, 5, 6 and 7 h), pH (6.0, 6.5, 7.0, 7.5 and 8.0) and enzyme dose (1.0, 1.5, 2.0, 2.5 and 3%) were chosen for the following procedure.

According to the above results, the orthogonal experiment was applied to evaluate the effects of hydrolysis conditions (temperature (A), time (B), pH (C) and enzyme dose (D)) on DPPH· scavenging activity of hydrolysates. Three levels (A: 60, 65 and 70 °C; B: 7.0, 7.5 and 8.0; C: 1.5, 2.0 and 2.5%; D: 3, 4 and 5 h) were identified for evaluating the influencing of hydrolysis conditions on DPPH· scavenging rate of hydrolysates. In addition, the monkfish swim bladder hydrolysate produced under the optimized conditions of papain was referred to as MSBH.

4.3. Preparation of APs from MSBH

4.3.1. Ultrafiltration of MSBH

MSBH was fractionated using cut-off membranes with MWs of 1, 3.5 and 10 kDa and four peptide fractions of MSBH-I (MW < 1.0 kDa), MSBH-II (1.0 < MW < 3.5 kDa), MSBH-III (3.5 < MW < 10 kDa) and MSBH-IV (MW > 10 kDa) were prepared [80]. MSBH-I showed the highest radical scavenging activity.

4.3.2. Purification of APs from MSBH-I by Chromatography Methods

MSBH-I solutions (5 mL, 50.0 mg/mL) were loaded into the Sephadex G-15 column (2.0 × 120 cm) and eluted using ultrapure water at a flow rate of 0.8 mL/min. The eluent was collected each 2 min, and three fractions (MSBH-Ia, MSBH-Ib and MSBH-Ic) were collected according to the chromatographic diagram at 220 nm.

MSBH-Ib was further isolated using a Zorbax, SB C-18 column (4.6 × 250 mm, 5 μm) in the HPLC system. The Zorbax column was eluted by a linear gradient of acetonitrile (0–50% in 0–30 min) in 0.1% TFA. The eluent at a flow rate of 1.0 mL/min was detected at 214 and 254 nm. Finally, sixteen peaks (P1 to P16) were prepared on the HPLC chromatograms at 214 and 254 nm and freeze-dried.

4.4. Identification of Eighteen Isolated APs (MSP1-MSP18)

The AA sequences of eighteen peptides (MSP1-MSP18) from monkfish swim bladders were determined by a 494-protein sequencer of Applied Biosystems (Perkin Elmer Co., Ltd. Foster City, CA, USA). The MWs of eighteen peptides (MSP1-MSP18) were determined by a Q-TOF mass spectrometer with an ESI source (Micromass, Waters, Milford, MA, USA) [81,82].

4.5. Antioxidant Activity of MSP1 to MSP18

4.5.1. HO· Scavenging Activity

First, 1.0 mL of 1, 10-phenanthroline solution (1.87 mM) and 2.0 mL of the sample solution were added to a screw-capped tube and mixed. Then, 1.0 mL of a $FeSO_4 \cdot 7H_2O$ solution (1.87 mM) was added to the mixture. The reaction was initiated by adding 1.0 mL of H_2O_2 (0.03%, v/v). After incubating at 37 °C for 60 min, the absorbance of the reaction mixture was measured at 536 nm against a reagent blank. The reaction mixture without any antioxidants was used as the negative control, and a mixture without H_2O_2 was used as the blank. The HO· scavenging activity was calculated using the following formula:

$$\text{HO· scavenging activity (\%)} = [(A_s - A_n)/(A_b - A_n)] \times 100\%,$$

where A_s, A_n and A_b are the absorbance values determined at 536 nm of the sample, the negative control and the blank after the reaction, respectively.

4.5.2. DPPH· Scavenging Activity

A total of 2.0 mL of sample solution consisting of distilled water and different concentrations of the analytes was added in cuvettes, and 500 μL of an ethanolic solution of DPPH (0.02%) and 1.0 mL of ethanol were added. A control sample containing the DPPH solution without the sample was also prepared. In the blank, the DPPH solution was substituted with ethanol. The antioxidant activity of the sample was evaluated using the inhibition percentage of the DPPH· with the following equation:

$$\text{DPPH· scavenging activity (\%)} = (A_c + A_b - A_s)/A_c \times 100\%,$$

where A_s is the absorbance rate of the sample, A_c is the control group absorbance and A_b is the blank absorbance.

4.5.3. $O_2^-\cdot$ Scavenging Activity

Superoxide anions were generated in 1 mL of nitrotetrazolium blue chloride (NBT) (2.52 mM), 1 mL of NADH (624 mM) and 1 mL of different sample concentrations. The reaction was initiated by adding 1 mL of phenazine methosulphate (PMS) solution (120 μM) to the reaction mixture. The absorbance was measured at 560 nm against the corresponding blank after incubation for 5 min at 25 °C. The scavenging capacity of the $O_2^-\cdot$ was calculated using the following equation:

$$O_2^-\cdot\text{scavengingactivity}(\%) = [(A_c - A_s)/A_c] \times 100\%,$$

where A_c is the absorbance without the sample and A_s is the absorbance with the sample.

4.5.4. $ABTS^+\cdot$ Scavenging Activity

The $ABTS^+\cdot$ was generated by mixing ABTS stock solution (7 mM) with potassium persulphate (2.45 mM). The mixture was left in the dark at room temperature for 16 h. The $ABTS^+\cdot$ solution was diluted in 5 mM phosphate buffered saline (PBS) pH 7.4, to an absorbance of 0.70 ± 0.02 at 734 nm. One milliliter of diluted $ABTS^+\cdot$ solution was mixed with one milliliter of different concentrations of samples. Ten minutes later, the absorbance was measured at 734 nm against the corresponding blank. The $ABTS^+\cdot$ scavenging activity of samples was calculated using the following equation:

$$ABTS^+\cdot\text{ scavenging activity (\%)} = [(A_c - A_s)/A_c] \times 100\%,$$

where A_c was the absorbance without the sample and A_s was the absorbance with the sample.

4.5.5. Determination of Reducing Power

Generally, 2.0 mL of each sample dissolved in distilled water was mixed with 2.5 mL of 1% aqueous potassium hexacyanoferrate [$K_3Fe(CN)_6$] solution. After 30 min incubation at 50 °C, 1.5 mL of 10% trichloroacetic acid was added. Finally, 2.0 mL of the upper layer was mixed with 2.0 mL of distilled water and 0.5 mL of 0.1% aqueous $FeCl_3$ and the absorbance was recorded at 700 nm. The higher absorbance of the reaction mixture indicated the stronger reducing power.

4.5.6. Lipid Peroxidation Inhibition Assay

Briefly, a sample (5.0 mg) was dissolved in 10 mL of 50 mM PBS (pH 7.0) and added to 0.13 mL of a solution of linoleic acid and 10 mL of 99.5% ethanol. Then, the total volume was adjusted to 25 mL with deionized water. The mixture was incubated in a conical flask with a screw cap at 40 °C in a dark room, and the degree of oxidation was evaluated by measuring ferric thiocyanate values. The reaction solution (100 μL) incubated in the linoleic acid model system was mixed with 4.7 mL of 75% ethanol, 0.1 mL of 30% ammonium thiocyanate, and 0.1 mL of 20 mM ferrous chloride solution in 3.5% HCl. After 3 min, the thiocyanate value was measured at 500 nm following color development with $FeCl_2$ and thiocyanate at different intervals during the incubation period at 40 °C. The higher absorbance of the solution means lower lipid peroxidation inhibition capacity.

4.5.7. Protective Functions on Plasmid DNA of MSP1, MSP2, MSP7, MSP8, MSP10 and MSP13

The protective functions of MSP1, MSP2, MSP7, MSP8, MSP10 and MSP13 on plasmid DNA (pBR322) were determined using the previous method [83]. In short, peptide (MSP1, MSP2, MSP7, MSP8, MSP10 or MSP13, respectively) were added to the test tubes containing $FeSO_4$ (2 μL, 1.0 mM), pBR322 (1 μL, 0.5 μg) and H_2O_2 (2 μL, 1.0 mM). A total of 15 μL of the manufactured reaction solution was incubated at 37 °C. After 30 min, 2 μL of loading buffer was added to the solution. Then, the solution was subsequently electrophoresed on 1% agarose gel containing 0.5 μg/mL EtBr at 60 V for 50 min. Finally, the DNA in the agarose gel was photographed and recorded under ultraviolet light.

4.5.8. Cytoprotection of MSP1, MSP2, MSP7, MSP8, MSP10 and MSP13 on H_2O_2-Damaged HepG2 Cells

H_2O_2 (300 μM) was used for establishing the oxidative damage model of HepG2 cells according to the previous methods [84–86]. Briefly, the HepG2 cells were incubated in a 96-well plate for 24 h. The supernatant in a 96-well plate was aspirated, and peptide solution (100 μL, 100.0 μM) was added into the sample groups and incubated for 8 h. After removing peptides, H_2O_2 was added to the sample, GSH and model groups. After 24 h, the 96-wells were rinsed twice with PBS and used MTT method to determine the cell viability:

$$\text{Cell viability} = (OD_{sample}/OD_{control}) \times 100\%.$$

4.6. Stability of MSP1, MSP2, MSP7, MSP8, MSP10 and MSP13

The stability of MSP1, MSP2, MSP7, MSP8, MSP10 and MSP13 was determined according to the previous method with a light modification [87–89]. The $O_2^- \cdot$ scavenging activity (%) of MSP1, MSP2, MSP7, MSP8, MSP10 and MSP13 at 5.0 mg/mL were measured to evaluate their stability.

The thermostability of MSP1, MSP2, MSP7, MSP8, MSP10 and MSP13 was analyzed in a water bath for 2 h with temperatures of 25, 37, 60, 80 or 100 °C, respectively.

The pH values (3, 5, 7, 9 and 11) were set to evaluate the acid and alkali stability properties of MSP1, MSP2, MSP7, MSP8, MSP10 and MSP13 at 25 °C, and the incubating time with different pH solutions was set to 2 h.

Two-stage simulated GI digestion model (2 h of pepsin digestion followed by 2 h of trypsin digestion) was designed to evaluate the influence of simulated GI digestion on the stability of MSP1, MSP2, MSP7, MSP8, MSP10 and MSP13.

4.7. Statistical Analysis

All the data are expressed as the mean ± SD (n = 3). The experimental data were analyzed by an ANOVA test using SPSS 19.0. Significant differences were determined by Duncan's multiple range test ($p < 0.05$, 0.01, and 0.001).

5. Conclusions

In conclusion, the conditions of papain for hydrolyzing the protein of monkfish (*L. litulon*) swim bladders were optimized as hydrolysis temperature 65 °C, pH 7.5, enzyme dose 2.5% and time 5 h through single factor and orthogonal experiments, and eighteen APs (MSP1 to MSP18) were purified from the monkfish swim bladder hydrolysate and identified as YDYD, QDYD, AGPAS, GPGPHGPSGP, GPK, HRE, GRW, ARW, GPTE, DDGGK, IGPAS, AKPAT, YPAGP, DPT, FPGPT, GPGPT, GPT and DPAGP, respectively. In general, YDYD, ARW and DDGGK exhibited high ability on radical scavenging, lipid peroxidation inhibition, Ferric reducing antioxidant power, and protective function on oxidation-damaged Plasmid DNA and HepG2 cells. The antioxidant activity of eighteen isolated peptides (MSP1 to MSP18) was highly stable under high temperatures, but remarkably influenced by different pH and simulated GI digestion. In brief, the present finding provides a good perspective for monkfish processing byproducts-swim bladders as the high-quality biological resources to produce BPs, and the generated peptides could serve as antioxidative ingredients applied in health-promoting products. Moreover, the antioxidant mechanism of peptides (MSP1, MSP2, MSP7, MSP8, MSP10 and MSP13) and the therapeutic effects of these peptides on HepG2 cells and mice after oxidative damage will be systematically researched in our follow-up study.

Author Contributions: Y.S., W.-Y.W. and M.-F.W.: Conceptualization, Data curation, Formal analysis, Investigation, Methodology and Validation. Y.-M.W. and W.-Y.Z.: Data curation, Investigation, Methodology, Validation and Writing—Original draft. W.-Y.Z.: Investigation, Methodology, and Writing—Original draft. C.-F.C.: Funding acquisition, Resources, Supervision, Writing—Review and editing. B.W.: Conceptualization, Funding acquisition, Resources, Supervision, Writing—Review and editing. All authors have read and agreed to the published version of the manuscript.

Funding: This work was funded by the National Natural Science Foundation of China (No. 82073764) and the Ten-thousand Talents Plan of Zhejiang Province (No. 2019R52026).

Institutional Review Board Statement: Not applicable.

Informed Consent Statement: Not applicable.

Data Availability Statement: Data are contained within the article.

Conflicts of Interest: The authors declare no conflict of interest.

Abbreviations

DPPH: 2,2-diphenyl-1-picrylhydrazyl; HO·, hydroxyl radical; O_2^-·, superoxide anion radical; ABTS, 2,2′-Azinobis-(3-ethylbenzthiazoline-6-sulphonate; MTT, 3-(4,5)-dimethylthiahiazo (-z-y1)-3,5-di- phenytetrazoliumromide; BP, bioactive peptide; AA, amino acid; MW, molecular weight; ROS, reactive oxygen species; NCD, chronic non-communicable diseases; WHO, World Health Organization; AP, antioxidant peptide; AMPK, AMP-activated protein kinase; TG, triglyceride; TC, total cholesterol; Nrf2, NF-E2-related factor 2; ARE, antioxidant response element; Keap1, Kelch Like ECH-Associated Protein 1; NF-κB, nuclear factor kappa-light-chain-enhancer of activated B cells; PI3K, phosphoinositide 3-kinases; MafK, Maf bZIP transcription factor K; NAFLD, non-alcoholic fatty liver disease; NLRP3, NLR family pyrin domain containing 3; MSBH, protein hydrolysate of monkfish swim bladders; MSP, peptide of monkfish swim bladders; FRAP, Ferric reducing antioxidant power; GSH, glutathione; SC, supercoiled; LIN, linear; OC, open circular; GI, gastrointestinal; Q-TOF, Quadrupole time-of-flight.

References

1. Ahmed, M.; Verma, A.K.; Patel, R. Collagen extraction and recent biological activities of collagen peptides derived from sea-food waste: A review. *Sustain. Chem. Pharm.* **2020**, *18*, 100315. [CrossRef]
2. Zhang, L.; Zhao, G.-X.; Zhao, Y.-Q.; Qiu, Y.-T.; Chi, C.-F.; Wang, B. Identification and Active Evaluation of Antioxidant Peptides from Protein Hydrolysates of Skipjack Tuna (*Katsuwonus pelamis*) Head. *Antioxidants* **2019**, *8*, 318. [CrossRef] [PubMed]

3. Wen, C.; Zhang, J.; Zhang, H.; Duan, Y.; Ma, H. Plant protein-derived antioxidant peptides: Isolation, identification, mechanism of action and application in food systems: A review. *Trends Food Sci. Technol.* **2020**, *105*, 308–322. [CrossRef]
4. Chakrabarti, S.; Guha, S.; Majumder, K. Food-Derived Bioactive Peptides in Human Health: Challenges and Opportunities. *Nutrients* **2018**, *10*, 1738. [CrossRef]
5. Zhang, S.-Y.; Zhao, Y.-Q.; Wang, Y.-M.; Yang, X.-R.; Chi, C.-F.; Wang, B. Gelatins and antioxidant peptides from Skipjack tuna (*Katsuwonus pelamis*) skins: Purification, characterization, and cytoprotection on ultraviolet—A injured human skin fibroblasts. *Food Biosci.* **2022**, *50*, 102138. [CrossRef]
6. Qiao, Q.-Q.; Luo, Q.-B.; Suo, S.-K.; Zhao, Y.-Q.; Chi, C.-F.; Wang, B. Preparation, Characterization, and Cytoprotective Effects on HUVECs of Fourteen Novel Angiotensin-I-Converting Enzyme Inhibitory Peptides From Protein Hydrolysate of Tuna Processing By-Products. *Front. Nutr.* **2022**, *9*, 868671. [CrossRef]
7. Admassu, H.; Gasmalla, M.A.A.; Yang, R.; Zhao, W. Bioactive Peptides Derived from Seaweed Protein and Their Health Benefits: Antihypertensive, Antioxidant, and Antidiabetic Properties. *J. Food Sci.* **2018**, *83*, 6–16. [CrossRef] [PubMed]
8. Abdelhedi, O.; Nasri, M. Basic and recent advances in marine antihypertensive peptides: Production, structure-activity relationship and bioavailability. *Trends Food Sci. Technol.* **2019**, *88*, 543–557. [CrossRef]
9. Mardani, M.; Badakné, K.; Farmani, J.; Aluko, R.E. Antioxidant peptides: Overview of production, properties, and applications in food systems. *Compr. Rev. Food Sci. Food Saf.* **2023**, *22*, 46–106. [CrossRef] [PubMed]
10. Ren, L.-K.; Yang, Y.; Ma, C.-M.; Fan, J.; Bian, X.; Liu, B.-X.; Wang, D.-F.; Zhu, P.-Y.; Fu, Y.; Zhang, N. Identification and in silico analysis of novel antioxidant peptides in broken rice protein hydrolysate and its cytoprotective effect against H_2O_2-induced 2BS cell model. *Food Res. Int.* **2022**, *162*, 112108. [CrossRef]
11. Pan, X.-Y.; Wang, Y.-M.; Li, L.; Chi, C.-F.; Wang, B. Four Antioxidant Peptides from Protein Hydrolysate of Red Stingray (*Dasyatis akajei*) Cartilages: Isolation, Identification, and In Vitro Activity Evaluation. *Mar. Drugs* **2019**, *17*, 263. [CrossRef]
12. Xiang, Z.; Xue, Q.; Gao, P.; Yu, H.; Wu, M.; Zhao, Z.; Li, Y.; Wang, S.; Zhang, J.; Dai, L. Antioxidant peptides from edible aquatic animals: Preparation method, mechanism of action, and structure-activity relationships. *Food Chem.* **2023**, *404*, 134701. [CrossRef] [PubMed]
13. Wang, B.; Wang, Y.-M.; Chi, C.-F.; Luo, H.-Y.; Deng, S.-G.; Ma, J.-Y. Isolation and Characterization of Collagen and Antioxidant Collagen Peptides from Scales of Croceine Croaker (*Pseudosciaena crocea*). *Mar. Drugs* **2013**, *11*, 4641–4661. [CrossRef]
14. Zhu, L.; Xiong, H.; Huang, X.; Guyonnet, V.; Ma, M.; Chen, X.; Zheng, Y.; Wang, L.; Hu, G. Identification and molecular mechanisms of novel antioxidant peptides from two sources of eggshell membrane hydrolysates showing cytoprotection against oxidative stress: A combined in silico and in vitro study. *Food Res. Int.* **2022**, *157*, 111266. [CrossRef] [PubMed]
15. Dresen, E.; Pimiento, J.M.; Patel, J.J.; Heyland, D.K.; Rice, T.W.; Stoppe, C. Overview of oxidative stress and the role of micronutrients in critical illness. *J. Parenter. Enter. Nutr.* **2022**, *47*, S38–S39. [CrossRef] [PubMed]
16. García, N.; Zazueta, C.; Aguilera-Aguirre, L. Oxidative Stress and Inflammation in Cardiovascular Disease. *Oxid. Med. Cell. Longev.* **2017**, *2017*, 5853238. [CrossRef] [PubMed]
17. Park, Y.R.; Park, C.-I.; Soh, Y. Antioxidant and Anti-Inflammatory Effects of NCW Peptide from Clam Worm (*Marphysa sanguinea*). *J. Microbiol. Biotechnol.* **2020**, *30*, 1387–1394. [CrossRef]
18. Hu, X.-M.; Wang, Y.-M.; Zhao, Y.-Q.; Chi, C.-F.; Wang, B. Antioxidant Peptides from the Protein Hydrolysate of Monkfish (*Lophius litulon*) Muscle: Purification, Identification, and Cytoprotective Function on HepG2 Cells Damage by H_2O_2. *Mar. Drugs* **2020**, *18*, 153. [CrossRef]
19. Forman, H.J.; Zhang, H. Targeting oxidative stress in disease: Promise and limitations of antioxidant therapy. *Nat. Rev. Drug Discov.* **2021**, *20*, 689–709. [CrossRef]
20. Sheng, Y.; Qiu, Y.T.; Wang, Y.M.; Chi, C.F.; Wang, B. Novel antioxidant collagen peptides of siberian sturgeon (*Acipenser baerii*) cartilages: The preparation, characterization, and cytoprotection of H_2O_2-damaged human umbilical vein endothelial cells (HUVECs). *Mar. Drugs* **2022**, *20*, 325. [CrossRef]
21. Kong, J.; Hu, X.-M.; Cai, W.-W.; Wang, Y.-M.; Chi, C.-F.; Wang, B. Bioactive Peptides from Skipjack Tuna Cardiac Arterial Bulbs (II): Protective Function on UVB-Irradiated HaCaT Cells through Antioxidant and Anti-Apoptotic Mechanisms. *Mar. Drugs* **2023**, *20*, 105. [CrossRef] [PubMed]
22. Gao, J.; Li, T.; Chen, D.; Gu, H.; Mao, X. Identification and molecular docking of antioxidant peptides from hemp seed protein hydrolysates. *LWT* **2021**, *147*, 111453. [CrossRef]
23. Wong, F.-C.; Xiao, J.; Wang, S.; Ee, K.-Y.; Chai, T.-T. Advances on the antioxidant peptides from edible plant sources. *Trends Food Sci. Technol.* **2020**, *99*, 44–57. [CrossRef]
24. Wang, Y.-Z.; Wang, Y.-M.; Pan, X.; Chi, C.-F.; Wang, B. Antioxidant Mechanisms of the Oligopeptides (FWKVV and FMPLH) from Muscle Hydrolysate of Miiuy Croaker against Oxidative Damage of HUVECs. *Oxid. Med. Cell. Longev.* **2021**, *2021*, 9987844. [CrossRef] [PubMed]
25. Sila, A.; Bougatef, A. Antioxidant peptides from marine by-products: Isolation, identification and application in food systems. A review. *J. Funct. Foods* **2016**, *21*, 10–26. [CrossRef]
26. Wang, Y.-Z.; Zhao, Y.-Q.; Wang, Y.-M.; Zhao, W.-H.; Wang, P.; Chi, C.-F.; Wang, B. Antioxidant peptides from Antarctic Krill (*Euphausia superba*) hydrolysate: Preparation, identification and cytoprotection on H_2O_2-induced oxidative stress. *J. Funct. Foods* **2021**, *86*, 104701. [CrossRef]

27. Achar, J.C.; Nam, G.; Jung, J.; Klammler, H.; Mohamed, M.M. Microbubble ozonation of the antioxidant butylated hydroxytoluene: Degradation kinetics and toxicity reduction. *Environ. Res.* **2020**, *186*, 109496. [CrossRef]
28. Liang, X.; Zhao, Y.; Liu, W.; Li, Z.; Souders, C.L.; Martyniuk, C.J. Butylated hydroxytoluene induces hyperactivity and alters dopamine-related gene expression in larval zebrafish (*Danio rerio*). *Environ. Pollut.* **2020**, *257*, 113624. [CrossRef]
29. Eskandani, M.; Hamishehkar, H.; Dolatabadi, J.E.N. Cytotoxicity and DNA damage properties of tert-butylhydroquinone (TBHQ) food additive. *Food Chem.* **2014**, *153*, 315–320. [CrossRef]
30. Botterweck, A.; Verhagen, H.; Goldbohm, R.; Kleinjans, J.; Brandt, P.V.D. Intake of butylated hydroxyanisole and butylated hydroxytoluene and stomach cancer risk: Results from analyses in the Netherlands Cohort Study. *Food Chem. Toxicol.* **2000**, *38*, 599–605. [CrossRef]
31. Sun, K.-L.; Gao, M.; Wang, Y.-Z.; Li, X.-R.; Wang, P.; Wang, B. Antioxidant Peptides From Protein Hydrolysate of Marine Red Algae *Eucheuma cottonii*: Preparation, Identification, and Cytoprotective Mechanisms on H_2O_2 Oxidative Damaged HUVECs. *Front. Microbiol.* **2022**, *13*, 791248. [CrossRef]
32. Ahn, C.-B.; Je, J.-Y.; Cho, Y.-S. Antioxidant and anti-inflammatory peptide fraction from salmon byproduct protein hydrolysates by peptic hydrolysis. *Food Res. Int.* **2012**, *49*, 92–98. [CrossRef]
33. Senphan, T.; Benjakul, S. Antioxidative activities of hydrolysates from seabass skin prepared using protease from hepatopancreas of Pacific white shrimp. *J. Funct. Foods* **2014**, *6*, 147–156. [CrossRef]
34. Chi, C.-F.; Wang, B.; Hu, F.-Y.; Wang, Y.-M.; Zhang, B.; Deng, S.-G.; Wu, C.-W. Purification and identification of three novel antioxidant peptides from protein hydrolysate of bluefin leatherjacket (*Navodon septentrionalis*) skin. *Food Res. Int.* **2015**, *73*, 124–129. [CrossRef]
35. Leo, E.E.M.; Fernández, J.J.A.; Campos, M.R.S. Biopeptides with antioxidant and anti-inflammatory potential in the prevention and treatment of diabesity disease. *Biomed. Pharmacother.* **2016**, *83*, 816–826. [CrossRef]
36. Landim, A.P.M.; Tiburski, J.H.; Mellinger, C.G.; Juliano, P.; Rosenthal, A. Potential Application of High Hydrostatic Pressure on the Production of Hydrolyzed Proteins with Antioxidant and Antihypertensive Properties and Low Allergenicity: A Review. *Foods* **2023**, *12*, 630. [CrossRef]
37. Wang, Y.-M.; Pan, X.; He, Y.; Chi, C.-F.; Wang, B. Hypolipidemic Activities of Two Pentapeptides (VIAPW and IRWWW) from Miiuy Croaker (*Miichthys miiuy*) Muscle on Lipid Accumulation in HepG2 Cells through Regulation of AMPK Pathway. *Appl. Sci.* **2020**, *10*, 817. [CrossRef]
38. Ma, R.; Chen, Q.; Dai, Y.; Huang, Y.; Hou, Q.; Huang, Y.; Zhong, K.; Huang, Y.; Gao, H.; Bu, Q. Identification of novel antioxidant peptides from sea squirt (*Halocynthia roretzi*) and its neuroprotective effect in 6-OHDA-induced neurotoxicity. *Food Funct.* **2022**, *13*, 6008–6021. [CrossRef] [PubMed]
39. Wang, X.; Yu, H.; Xing, R.; Li, P. Hepatoprotective Effect of Oyster Peptide on Alcohol-Induced Liver Disease in Mice. *Int. J. Mol. Sci.* **2022**, *23*, 8081. [CrossRef]
40. Jiang, Y.; Wang, R.; Yin, Z.; Sun, J.; Wang, B.; Zhao, D.; Zeng, X.A.; Li, H.; Huang, M.; Sun, B. Optimization of Jiuzao protein hydrolysis conditions and antioxidant activity in vivo of Jiuzao tetrapeptide Asp-Arg-Glu-Leu by elevating the Nrf2/Keap1-p38/PI3K-MafK signaling pathway. *Food Funct.* **2021**, *12*, 4808–4824. [CrossRef]
41. Chi, C.-F.; Wang, B.; Deng, Y.-Y.; Wang, Y.-M.; Deng, S.-G.; Ma, J.-Y. Isolation and characterization of three antioxidant pentapeptides from protein hydrolysate of monkfish (*Lophius litulon*) muscle. *Food Res. Int.* **2014**, *55*, 222–228. [CrossRef]
42. Tian, X.; Zheng, J.; Xu, B.; Ye, J.; Yang, Z.; Yuan, F. Optimization of extraction of bioactive peptides from monkfish (*Lophius litulon*) and characterization of their role in H_2O_2-Induced Lesion. *Mar. Drugs* **2020**, *18*, 468. [CrossRef] [PubMed]
43. Ye, J.; Tian, X.; Wang, Q.; Zheng, J.; Yang, Y.; Xu, B.; Zhang, S.; Yuan, F.; Yang, Z. Monkfish Peptides Mitigate High Fat Diet-Induced Hepatic Steatosis in Mice. *Mar. Drugs* **2022**, *20*, 312. [CrossRef] [PubMed]
44. Ren, X.; Miao, B.; Cao, H.; Tian, X.; Shen, L.; Yang, Z.; Yuan, F.; Ding, Y. Monkfish (*Lophius litulon*) Peptides Ameliorate High-Fat-Diet-Induced Nephrotoxicity by Reducing Oxidative Stress and Inflammation via Regulation of Intestinal Flora. *Molecules* **2022**, *28*, 245. [CrossRef]
45. Ren, Z.; Yang, F.; Yao, S.; Bi, L.; Jiang, G.; Huang, J.; Tang, Y. Effects of low molecular weight peptides from monkfish (*Lophius litulon*) roe on immune response in immunosuppressed mice. *Front. Nutr.* **2022**, *9*, 929105. [CrossRef]
46. Miao, B.; Zheng, J.; Zheng, G.; Tian, X.; Zhang, W.; Yuan, F.; Yang, Z. Using Collagen Peptides From the Skin of Monkfish (*Lophius litulon*) to Ameliorate Kidney Damage in High-Fat Diet Fed Mice by Regulating the Nrf2 Pathway and NLRP3 Signaling. *Front. Nutr.* **2022**, *9*, 798708. [CrossRef]
47. Zhang, S.Y.; Zhao, G.X.; Suo, S.K.; Wang, Y.M.; Chi, C.F.; Wang, B. Purification, identification, activity evaluation, and stability of antioxidant peptides from Alcalase hydrolysate of Antarctic Krill (*Euphausia superba*) proteins. *Mar. Drugs* **2021**, *19*, 347. [CrossRef]
48. Khammuang, S.; Sarnthima, R.; Sanachai, K. Purification and identification of novel antioxidant peptides from silkworm pupae (*Bombyx mori*) protein hydrolysate and molecular docking study. *Biocatal. Agric. Biotechnol.* **2022**, *42*, 102367. [CrossRef]
49. Zhang, J.B.; Zhao, Y.Q.; Wang, Y.M.; Chi, C.F.; Wang, B. Eight peptides from collagen hydrolysate fraction of Spanish mackerel (*Scomberomorous niphonius*) skin: Isolation, identification, and antioxidant activity in vitro. *Mar. Drugs* **2019**, *17*, 224. [CrossRef]
50. Ahn, C.-B.; Lee, K.-H.; Je, J.-Y. Enzymatic production of bioactive protein hydrolysates from tuna liver: Effects of enzymes and molecular weight on bioactivity. *Int. J. Food Sci. Technol.* **2010**, *45*, 562–568. [CrossRef]

51. Jang, H.L.; Shin, S.R.; Yoon, K.Y. Hydrolysis conditions for antioxidant peptides derived from enzymatic hydrolysates of sandfish (*Arctoscopus japonicus*). *Food Sci. Biotechnol.* **2017**, *26*, 1191–1197. [CrossRef] [PubMed]
52. Chi, C.-F.; Wang, B.; Wang, Y.-M.; Zhang, B.; Deng, S.-G. Isolation and characterization of three antioxidant peptides from protein hydrolysate of bluefin leatherjacket (*Navodon septentrionalis*) heads. *J. Funct. Foods* **2015**, *12*, 1–10. [CrossRef]
53. Kim, H.-S.; Je, J.-G.; Ryu, B.; Kang, N.; Fernando, I.P.S.; Jayawardena, T.U.; Sanjeewa, K.K.A.; Oh, J.-Y.; Lee, T.-G.; Jeon, Y.-J. Antioxidant and angiotensin-I converting enzyme inhibitory peptides from *Hippocampus abdominalis*. *Eur. Food Res. Technol.* **2019**, *245*, 479–487. [CrossRef]
54. Xia, Z.; Miao, J.; Chen, B.; Guo, J.; Ou, Y.; Liang, X.; Yin, Y.; Tong, X.; Cao, Y. Purification, identification, and antioxidative mechanism of three novel selenium-enriched oyster antioxidant peptides. *Food Res. Int.* **2022**, *157*, 111359. [CrossRef]
55. Wang, B.; Li, Z.-R.; Chi, C.-F.; Zhang, Q.-H.; Luo, H.-Y. Preparation and evaluation of antioxidant peptides from ethanol-soluble proteins hydrolysate of *Sphyrna lewini* muscle. *Peptides* **2012**, *36*, 240–250. [CrossRef]
56. Luo, H.-Y.; Wang, B.; Li, Z.-R.; Chi, C.-F.; Zhang, Q.-H.; He, G.-Y. Preparation and evaluation of antioxidant peptide from papain hydrolysate of *Sphyrna lewini* muscle protein. *LWT Food Sci. Technol.* **2013**, *51*, 281–288. [CrossRef]
57. Cai, W.-W.; Hu, X.-M.; Wang, Y.-M.; Chi, C.-F.; Wang, B. Bioactive Peptides from Skipjack Tuna Cardiac Arterial Bulbs: Preparation, Identification, Antioxidant Activity, and Stability against Thermal, pH, and Simulated Gastrointestinal Digestion Treatments. *Mar. Drugs* **2022**, *20*, 626. [CrossRef]
58. Wang, J.; Wang, Y.-M.; Li, L.-Y.; Chi, C.-F.; Wang, B. Twelve Antioxidant Peptides From Protein Hydrolysate of Skipjack Tuna (*Katsuwonus pelamis*) Roe Prepared by Flavourzyme: Purification, Sequence Identification, and Activity Evaluation. *Front. Nutr.* **2022**, *8*, 813780. [CrossRef] [PubMed]
59. You, L.; Zhao, M.; Regenstein, J.M.; Ren, J. Purification and identification of antioxidative peptides from loach (*Misgurnus anguillicaudatus*) protein hydrolysate by consecutive chromatography and electrospray ionization-mass spectrometry. *Food Res. Int.* **2010**, *43*, 1167–1173. [CrossRef]
60. Cai, L.; Wu, X.; Zhang, Y.; Li, X.; Ma, S.; Li, J. Purification and characterization of three antioxidant peptides from protein hydrolysate of grass carp (*Ctenopharyngodon idella*) skin. *J. Funct. Foods* **2015**, *16*, 234–242. [CrossRef]
61. Wang, Y.-M.; Li, X.-Y.; Wang, J.; He, Y.; Chi, C.-F.; Wang, B. Antioxidant peptides from protein hydrolysate of skipjack tuna milt: Purification, identification, and cytoprotection on H_2O_2 damaged human umbilical vein endothelial cells. *Process Biochem.* **2022**, *113*, 258–269. [CrossRef]
62. Ayala, A.; Muñoz, M.F.; Argüelles, S. Lipid peroxidation: Production, metabolism, and signaling mechanisms of malondialdehyde and 4-hydroxy-2-nonenal. *Oxid. Med. Cell. Longev.* **2014**, *2014*, 360438. [CrossRef] [PubMed]
63. Li, Z.; Wang, B.; Chi, C.; Luo, H.; Gong, Y.; Ding, G. Influence of average molecular weight on antioxidant and functional properties of collagen hydrolysates from *Sphyrna lewini*, *Dasyatis akjei* and *Raja porosa*. *Food Res. Int.* **2013**, *51*, 283–293. [CrossRef]
64. He, Y.; Pan, X.; Chi, C.-F.; Sun, K.-L.; Wang, B. Ten new pentapeptides from protein hydrolysate of miiuy croaker (*Miichthys miiuy*) muscle: Preparation, identification, and antioxidant activity evaluation. *LWT* **2019**, *105*, 1–8. [CrossRef]
65. Yang, X.-R.; Zhao, Y.-Q.; Qiu, Y.-T.; Chi, C.-F.; Wang, B. Preparation and Characterization of Gelatin and Antioxidant Peptides from Gelatin Hydrolysate of Skipjack Tuna (*Katsuwonus pelamis*) Bone Stimulated by in vitro Gastrointestinal Digestion. *Mar. Drugs* **2019**, *17*, 78. [CrossRef]
66. Ktari, N.; Fakhfakh, N.; Balti, R.; Ben Khaled, H.; Nasri, M.; Bougatef, A. Effect of Degree of Hydrolysis and Protease Type on the Antioxidant Activity of Protein Hydrolysates From Cuttlefish (*Sepia officinalis*) By-Products. *J. Aquat. Food Prod. Technol.* **2013**, *22*, 436–448. [CrossRef]
67. Wang, B.; Li, L.; Chi, C.F.; Ma, J.H.; Luo, H.Y.; Xu, Y.F. Purification and characterization of a novel antioxidant peptide derived from blue mussel (*Mytilus edulis*) protein hydrolysate. *Food Chem.* **2013**, *138*, 1713–1719. [CrossRef]
68. Bougatef, A.; Hajji, M.; Balti, R.; Lassoued, I.; Triki-Ellouz, Y.; Nasri, M. Antioxidant and free radical-scavenging activities of smooth hound (*Mustelus mustelus*) muscle protein hydrolysates obtained by gastrointestinal proteases. *Food Chem.* **2009**, *114*, 1198–1205. [CrossRef]
69. Zou, T.-B.; He, T.-P.; Li, H.-B.; Tang, H.-W.; Xia, E.-Q. The Structure-Activity Relationship of the Antioxidant Peptides from Natural Proteins. *Molecules* **2016**, *21*, 72. [CrossRef]
70. Rahman, M.S.; Hee, C.Y.; Seok, C.Y.; Alam, M.B.; Han, L.S.; Cheol, Y.J. A novel antioxidant peptide, purified from Bacillus amyloliquefaciens, showed strong antioxidant potential via Nrf-2 mediated heme oxygenase-1 expression. *Food Chem.* **2018**, *239*, 502–510. [CrossRef]
71. Tonolo, F.; Moretto, L.; Grinzato, A.; Fiorese, F.; Folda, A.; Scalcon, V.; Ferro, S.; Arrigoni, G.; Bellamio, M.; Feller, E.; et al. Fermented soy-derived bioactive peptides selected by a molecular docking approach show antioxidant properties involving the Keap1/Nrf2 Pathway. *Antioxidants* **2020**, *9*, 1306. [CrossRef]
72. Sanjukta, S.; Padhi, S.; Sarkar, P.; Singh, S.P.; Sahoo, D.; Rai, A.K. Production, characterization and molecular docking of antioxidant peptides from peptidome of kinema fermented with proteolytic *Bacillus* spp. *Food Res. Int.* **2021**, *141*, 110161. [CrossRef]
73. Zhu, Y.; Lao, F.; Pan, X.; Wu, J. Food Protein-Derived Antioxidant Peptides: Molecular Mechanism, Stability and Bioavailability. *Biomolecules* **2022**, *12*, 1622. [CrossRef]
74. Sheih, I.-C.; Wu, T.-K.; Fang, T.J. Antioxidant properties of a new antioxidative peptide from algae protein waste hydrolysate in different oxidation systems. *Bioresour. Technol.* **2009**, *100*, 3419–3425. [CrossRef]

75. Chang, O.K.; Ha, G.E.; Han, G.-S.; Seol, K.-H.; Kim, H.W.; Jeong, S.-G.; Oh, M.-H.; Park, B.-Y.; Ham, J.-S. Novel Antioxidant Peptide Derived from the Ultrafiltrate of Ovomucin Hydrolysate. *J. Agric. Food Chem.* **2013**, *61*, 7294–7300. [CrossRef]
76. Phongthai, S.; D'Amico, S.; Schoenlechner, R.; Homthawornchoo, W.; Rawdkuen, S. Fractionation and antioxidant properties of rice bran protein hydrolysates stimulated by in vitro gastrointestinal digestion. *Food Chem.* **2018**, *240*, 156–164. [CrossRef]
77. Memarpoor-Yazdi, M.; Asoodeh, A.; Chamani, J. A novel antioxidant and antimicrobial peptide from hen egg white lysozyme hydrolysates. *J. Funct. Foods* **2012**, *4*, 278–286. [CrossRef]
78. Zheng, Z.; Si, D.; Ahmad, B.; Li, Z.; Zhang, R. A novel antioxidative peptide derived from chicken blood corpuscle hydrolysate. *Food Res. Int.* **2018**, *106*, 410–419. [CrossRef] [PubMed]
79. Zhao, W.-H.; Luo, Q.-B.; Pan, X.; Chi, C.-F.; Sun, K.-L.; Wang, B. Preparation, identification, and activity evaluation of ten antioxidant peptides from protein hydrolysate of swim bladders of miiuy croaker (*Miichthys miiuy*). *J. Funct. Foods* **2018**, *47*, 503–511. [CrossRef]
80. Suo, S.K.; Zhao, Y.Q.; Wang, Y.M.; Pan, X.Y.; Chi, C.F.; Wang, B. Seventeen novel angiotensin converting enzyme (ACE) inhibitory peptides from protein hydrolysate of *Mytilus edulis*: Isolation, identification, molecular docking study, and protective function on HUVECs. *Food Funct.* **2022**, *13*, 7831–7846. [CrossRef] [PubMed]
81. Suo, S.K.; Zheng, S.L.; Chi, C.F.; Luo, H.Y.; Wang, B. Novel ACE inhibitory peptides from tuna byproducts-milts: Preparation, characterization, molecular docking study and antioxidant function on H_2O_2-damaged HUVECs. *Front. Nutr.* **2022**, *9*, 957778. [CrossRef]
82. Zheng, S.-L.; Luo, Q.-B.; Suo, S.-K.; Zhao, Y.-Q.; Chi, C.-F.; Wang, B. Preparation, identification, molecular docking study and protective function on HUVECs of novel ACE inhibitory peptides from protein hydrolysate of Skipjack tuna muscle. *Mar. Drugs* **2022**, *20*, 176. [CrossRef] [PubMed]
83. Zhang, C.; Liu, Y.; Zhang, T.; Lv, C.; Zang, J.; Zhao, G. Structural comparison between the DNA-protective ability of scallop and shrimp ferritin from iron-induced oxidative damage. *Food Chem.* **2022**, *386*, 132827. [CrossRef] [PubMed]
84. Sahoo, S.; Rath, D.; Kar, D.M.; Pattanaik, S. Hepatoprotective potency of *Litsea glutinosa* (L.) C.B. Rob. leaf methanol extract on H_2O_2-induced toxicity in HepG2 cells. *J. Ethnopharmacol.* **2023**, *304*, 116076. [CrossRef]
85. Salla, S.; Sunkara, R.; Ogutu, S.; Walker, L.T.; Verghese, M. Antioxidant activity of papaya seed extracts against H_2O_2 induced oxidative stress in HepG2 cells. *LWT* **2016**, *66*, 293–297. [CrossRef]
86. Wang, W.-Y.; Zhao, Y.-Q.; Zhao, G.-X.; Chi, C.-F.; Wang, B. Antioxidant peptides from collagen hydrolysate of Redlip croaker (*Pseudosciaena polyactis*) scales: Preparation, characterization, and cytoprotective effects on H_2O_2-damaged HepG2 cells. *Mar. Drugs* **2020**, *18*, 156. [CrossRef] [PubMed]
87. Wang, K.; Luo, Q.; Hong, H.; Liu, H.; Luo, Y. Novel antioxidant and ACE inhibitory peptide identified from Arthrospira platensis protein and stability against thermal/pH treatments and simulated gastrointestinal digestion. *Food Res. Int.* **2020**, *139*, 109908. [CrossRef]
88. Wong, F.-C.; Xiao, J.; Ong, M.G.-L.; Pang, M.-J.; Wong, S.-J.; Teh, L.K.; Chai, T.-T. Identification and characterization of antioxidant peptides from hydrolysate of blue-spotted stingray and their stability against thermal, pH and simulated gastrointestinal digestion treatments. *Food Chem.* **2019**, *271*, 614–622. [CrossRef]
89. Zhao, G.-X.; Yang, X.-R.; Wang, Y.-M.; Zhao, Y.-Q.; Chi, C.-F.; Wang, B. Antioxidant peptides from the protein hydrolysate of spanish mackerel (*Scomberomorous niphonius*) muscle by in vitro gastrointestinal digestion and their in vitro activities. *Mar. Drugs* **2019**, *17*, 531. [CrossRef]

marine drugs

MDPI

Article

Bioactive Peptides from Skipjack Tuna Cardiac Arterial Bulbs (II): Protective Function on UVB-Irradiated HaCaT Cells through Antioxidant and Anti-Apoptotic Mechanisms

Jing Kong [1], Xiao-Meng Hu [2], Wei-Wei Cai [1], Yu-Mei Wang [1], Chang-Feng Chi [2,*] and Bin Wang [1,*]

[1] Zhejiang Provincial Engineering Technology Research Center of Marine Biomedical Products, School of Food and Pharmacy, Zhejiang Ocean University, Zhoushan 316022, China

[2] National and Provincial Joint Laboratory of Exploration, Utilization of Marine Aquatic Genetic Resources, National Engineering Research Center of Marine Facilities Aquaculture, School of Marine Science and Technology, Zhejiang Ocean University, Zhoushan 316022, China

* Correspondence: chichangfeng@hotmail.com (C.-F.C.); wangbin@zjou.edu.cn (B.W.); Tel./Fax: +86-580-255-4818 (C.-F.C.); +86-580-255-4781 (B.W.)

Abstract: The aim of this study was to investigate the protective function and mechanism of TCP3 (PKK), TCP6 (YEGGD) and TCP9 (GPGLM) from skipjack tuna cardiac arterial bulbs on skin photoaging using UVB-irradiated HaCaT cell model. The present results indicated that TCP3 (PKK), TCP6 (YEGGD) and TCP9 (GPGLM) had significant cytoprotective effect on UVB-irradiated HaCaT cells ($p < 0.001$). Hoechst 33342 staining showed that apoptosis of UV-irradiated HaCaT cells could be significantly reduced by the treatment of TCP3 (PKK), TCP6 (YEGGD) and TCP9 (GPGLM); JC-1 staining showed that TCP3 (PKK), TCP6 (YEGGD) and TCP9 (GPGLM) could protect HaCaT cells from apoptosis by restoring mitochondrial membrane potential (MMP); Furthermore, TCP3 (PKK), TCP6 (YEGGD) and TCP9 (GPGLM) could significantly down-regulate the ratio of Bax/Bcl-2 and reduce the expression level of the apoptosis-executing protein Caspase-3 by decreasing the expression of protein Caspase-8 and Caspase-9 ($p < 0.05$). The action mechanism indicated that TCP3 (PKK), TCP6 (YEGGD) and TCP9 (GPGLM) could up-regulate the expression levels of Nrf2, NQO1 and HO-1 ($p < 0.05$), which further increased the activity of downstream proteases (SOD, CAT and GSH-Px), and scavenged reactive oxygen species (ROS) and decreased the intracellular levels of malondialdehyde (MDA). In addition, molecular docking indicated that TCP3 (PKK) and TCP6 (YEGGD) could competitively inhibit the Nrf2 binding site because they can occupy the connection site of Nrf2 by binding to the Kelch domain of Keap1 protein. TCP9 (GPGLM) was inferred to be non-competitive inhibition because it could not bind to the active site of the Kelch domain of Keap1 protein. In summary, the antioxidant peptides TCP3 (PKK), TCP6 (YEGGD) and TCP9 (GPGLM) from cardiac arterial bulbs of skipjack tuna can effectively protect HaCaT cells from UVB-irradiated damage and can be used in the development of healthy and cosmetic products to treat diseases caused by UV radiation.

Keywords: skipjack tuna (*Katsuwonus pelamis*); antioxidant peptide; skin photoaging; ultraviolet radiation; protective function; anti-apoptosis

Citation: Kong, J.; Hu, X.-M.; Cai, W.-W.; Wang, Y.-M.; Chi, C.-F.; Wang, B. Bioactive Peptides from Skipjack Tuna Cardiac Arterial Bulbs (II): Protective Function on UVB-Irradiated HaCaT Cells through Antioxidant and Anti-Apoptotic Mechanisms. *Mar. Drugs* **2023**, *21*, 105. https://doi.org/10.3390/md21020105

Academic Editor: Claudiu T. Supuran

Received: 29 December 2022
Revised: 30 January 2023
Accepted: 30 January 2023
Published: 1 February 2023

1. Introduction

Skin aging is a complicated bio-process that occurs over time as a result of intrinsic or genetically programmed aging, as well as external aging induced by environment aspect [1,2]. Except for the internal aging process, the sun-exposed body surface including the dorsum of hands, neck, forearms, and face meets with additional destructive effects, mainly because of exposure to ultraviolet light (UV). Photoaging is defined as the influences of prolonged UV radiation and sunshine injury superposed on inherently aged skin [2]. According to the wavelength, ultraviolet radiation can be divided into: UVA, UVB, and UVC with the UV wavelengths of 315–400, 280–315 and 200–280 nm, respectively [3].

Experiments have proved that ozone in the atmosphere can absorb UVC and avoid its damage to human body. Among the UV radiation irradiated to the earth surface, UVB only accounts for 5%, but UVB causes 800–1000 times more damage to the skins than the same dose of UVA. Keratinocytes, as UVB target cells, can receive 95% of the radiation and thus induce photoaging [4]. UVB has stronger mutagenicity and carcinogenicity compared with UVA [5]. UVB radiation directly damages DNA and produces large amounts of reactive oxygen species (ROS) in skin organism [6]. With the overproduction of ROS, the oxidation–reduction dynamic balance in the body is destroyed, and proteins and lipids are oxidized, thus causing oxidative stress with a series of clinical symptoms, including pigmentation disorders, cutis laxa, wrinkles, rough skin surface, inflammation, cell apoptosis, and skin malignant tumor [2,7]. In addition, some skin functions declining with age present a stepped-up trend of decline in photoaging skins [2]. Therefore, the large increase in the aging population and the psychosocial impact of aging skin have created a great demand for effective intervention methods and drugs.

Enzymatic and non-enzymatic cutaneous antioxidants in the skin tissues can protect cells against oxidative stress damage under normal physiological condition [8,9]. However, the body's antioxidant system cannot remove excess ROS and cells are damaged when the damage degree is beyond the adaptive regulation range of cells [10–12]. Then, exogenous antioxidants, such as acorbate, flavonoids, carotenoids, and phenols, can scavenge ROS via stimulating specific signaling pathways in cells to improve the antioxidant ability of cells, which has become a potential method to control UV damage [13,14]. Therefore, UV-irradiated injury and antioxidant constituents have been researched extensively in the areas of food, cosmetic products and medicines.

Recently, bioactive peptides were found in a variety of marine organisms, and many of them have exhibited great potential for adjuvant treatment and prevention of skin photoaging due to their outstanding antioxidant function and anti-apoptosis [10,15,16]. For example, gelatin hydrolysate (AMW 873 Da) from salmon skins could ameliorate UV-induced pathologic alteration of the surface structure and morphology of the skin through inhibiting the depletion of hydroxyproline, decreasing malonaldehyde (MDA) content, improving the levels of antioxidant enzymes and glutathione (GSH), and enhancing the immune regulatory system in photoaging skins [17]. The collagen oligopeptides from chum salmon fish skins could maintain moisture, play antioxidant function, and promote the production of collagen and elastin in UVB-irradiated skin tissue of ICR rats. [18]. ATPGDEG from boiled abalone by-products could protect type I pro collagen and DNA in UVB-induced HaCaT cells via reducing the generation of intercellular ROS, decreasing activities of matrix metalloproteinase-1 (MMP-1), MMP-9, and mitogen-activating the MAPKs and NF-κB signaling [19]. It is very similar that YGDEY from tilapia skin has a therapeutic effectiveness in prevention of UVB-induced cellular damage by mitogen-activating the signaling pathways of MAPK and NF-κB, decreasing ROS level, and increasing intracellular antioxidants [20]. Therefore, marine-derived peptides showed great application value in treating skin photoaging in the future.

Skipjack tuna is the most important raw material for canned aquatic products because of its high catch and low value [21–23]. It is worth paying attention that many bioactive peptides were prepared from skipjack tuna and its canning processing by-products [18,24–26]. These peptides have shown great application potential in functional food, cosmetics and drugs because of their significant bioactivity, such as ACE inhibitory activity [23,27], radical scavenging activity [12,28,29], and cytoprotective ability on H_2O_2-damaged cells [8,18,21]. Elastin hydrolysate of tuna cardiac arterial bulbs was usually used in daily cosmetics. Then, eleven antioxidant peptides, including QGD (TCP1), GEQSN (TCP2), PKK (TCP3), GPQ (TCP4), GEEGD (TCP5), YEGGD (TCP6), GEGER (TCP7), GEGQR (TCP8), GPGLM (TCP9), GLN (TCP10), and GDRGD (TCP11), were purified and identified from its hydrolysate in our previous research, and TCP3 (PKK), TCP6 (YEGGD) and TCP9 (GPGLM) were found to have significantly radical scavenging ability and protective function on H_2O_2-damaged DNA and HepG2 cells [30]. Therefore, the objectives of the study were to systematic research the cytoprotective function of TCP3 (PKK), TCP6 (YEGGD) and TCP9 (GPGLM) on UVB-irradiated HaCaT Cells through antioxidant and anti-apoptotic mechanisms.

2. Results

2.1. Cytoprotection of TCP3 (PKK), TCP6 (YEGGD) and TCP9 (GPGLM) on UVB-Irradiated HaCaT Cells

2.1.1. Establishment of UVB-Irradiated Model of HaCaT Cells

As shown in Figure 1, HaCaT cells were irradiated with different doses of UVB (0, 5, 8, 10, 12 and 15 mJ/cm^2), and the cell viability was diminished gradually when the doses of UVB were increased from 0 to 15 mJ/cm^2. The cell viability was 52.52 ± 1.13% at the UVB radiation dose of 8 mJ/cm^2. As reported by Chen et al. (2016) [19] and Xiao et al. (2019) [20], the optimal radiation dose for establishing UVB injured cell model was decided based on the median lethal radiation intensity. Therefore, 8 mJ/cm^2 was chosen to the optimal radiation dose for establishing the UVB-irradiated model of HaCaT cells.

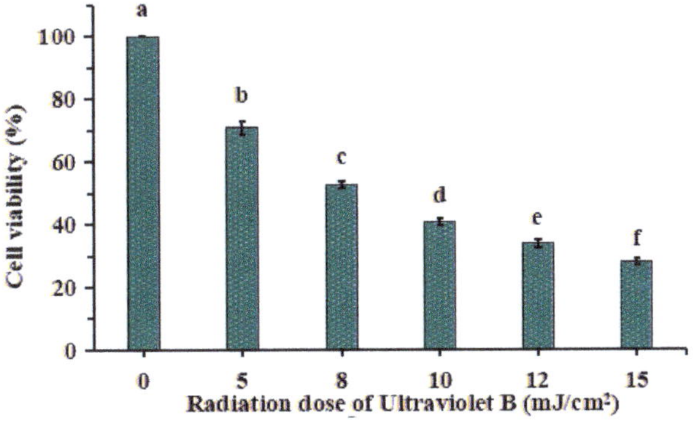

Figure 1. Effects of different ultraviolet B (UVB) radiation doses on the viability of HaCaT cells. a–f Values with same letters indicate no significant difference ($p > 0.05$).

2.1.2. Effects of Antioxidant Peptides TCP1-TCP11 on the Viability of UVB-Irradiated Cell Model

After incubated with 200 μM of TCP1-TCP11 and irradiated with 8 mJ/cm^2 of UVB for 24 h, the cell viability was measured and showed in Figure 2. The results indicated that the cell viability in the model group was 52.82 ± 0.67%, which was significantly lower than that in the blank group ($p < 0.001$). The cell viability of TCP3 (PKK), TCP6 (YEGGD) and TCP9 (GPGLM) groups were 70.15 ± 3.98%, 66.17 ± 5.04% and 65.20 ± 1.66%, respectively, which was significantly higher than those of the model group and other eight peptide groups ($p < 0.001$), suggesting that they could significantly alleviate the oxidative stress damage of HaCaT cells caused by UVB radiation. This finding was in agreement with the previous results that TCP3 (PKK), TCP6 (YEGGD) and TCP9 (GPGLM) exhibited higher antioxidant ability among 11 antioxidant peptides (TCP1-TCP11) [30]. Therefore, the protective function and mechanism of TCP3 (PKK), TCP6 (YEGGD) and TCP9 (GPGLM) on the UVB-irradiated HaCaT cell model will be further discussed.

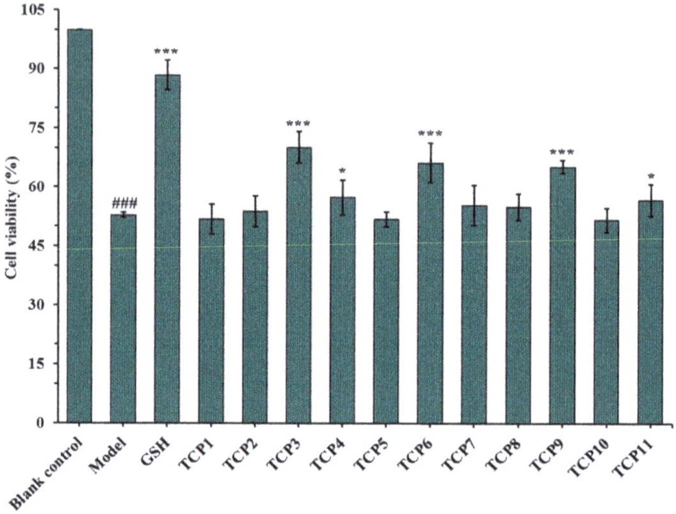

Figure 2. Effects of antioxidant peptides TCP1-TCP11 on the viability of UVB-irradiated cell model. Glutathione (GSH) at 200 μM was served as the positive control. All data are presented as the mean ± SD of triplicate results. ### $p < 0.001$ vs. blank control group; *** $p < 0.001$ and * $p < 0.05$ vs. model group.

2.1.3. Effects of TCP3 (PKK), TCP6 (YEGGD) and TCP9 (GPGLM) on the Viability of HaCaT Cells

Figure 3 indicated that the viability of HaCaT cells in all determined group was ranged from 98.04 ± 3.94% to 104.32 ± 1.27%. In addition, TCP3 (PKK), TCP6 (YEGGD) and TCP9 (GPGLM) could increase the viability of HaCaT cells at 100-400 μM, but the cell viability was lowered when the peptide concentration exceeded 400 μM. However, no significant difference was found at different concentration ($p > 0.05$). Then, the concentrations of 100, 200, and 400 μM were chosen for further experiment.

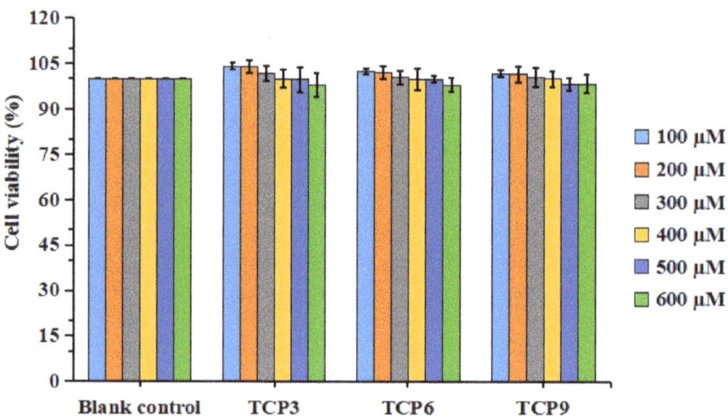

Figure 3. Effects of different concentrations (100–600 μM) of TCP3 (PKK), TCP6 (YEGGD) and TCP9 (GPGLM) on the viability of HaCaT cells. All data are presented as the mean ± SD of triplicate results.

2.1.4. Effects of Different Concentrations of TCP3 (PKK), TCP6 (YEGGD) and TCP9 (GPGLM) on the Viability of UVB-Irradiated HaCaT Cell Model

Figure 4 showed that the cell viability in TCP3 (PKK), TCP6 (YEGGD) and TCP9 (GPGLM) groups increased steadily when the peptide concentration raised from 100 μM to

400 μM. At 400 μM, the cell viability in TCP3 (PKK), TCP6 (YEGGD) and TCP9 (GPGLM) groups was 76.17 ± 3.87%, 70.81 ± 3.86%, and 69.32 ± 3.32%, respectively, which was significantly higher than that of model group (52.20 ± 3.12%)($p < 0.001$). The data indicated that TCP3 (PKK), TCP6 (YEGGD) and TCP9 (GPGLM) could dose-dependently protect HaCaT cells from UVB damage.

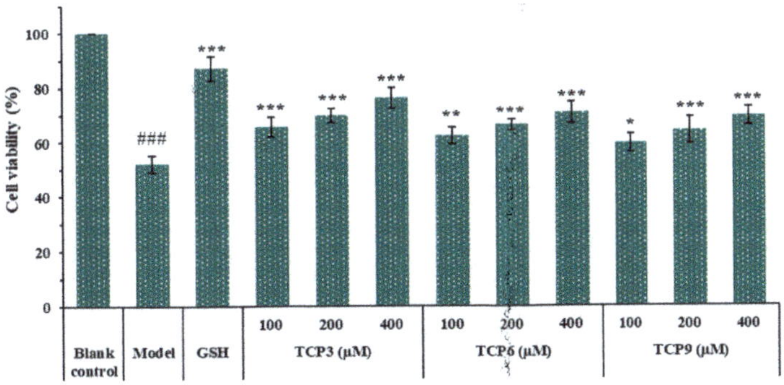

Figure 4. Effects of different concentrations (100, 200, and 400 μM) of TCP3 (PKK), TCP6 (YEGGD) and TCP9 (GPGLM) on the viability of UVB-irradiated cell model. Glutathione (GSH) at 200 μM was served as the positive control. All data are presented as the mean ± SD of triplicate results. ### $p < 0.001$ vs. blank control group; *** $p < 0.001$, ** $p < 0.01$ and * $p < 0.05$ vs. model group.

2.1.5. Effects of TCP3 (PKK), TCP6 (YEGGD) and TCP9 (GPGLM) on the ROS Levels of UVB-Irradiated Cell Model

The influence of TCP3 (PKK), TCP6 (YEGGD) and TCP9 (GPGLM) on the ROS levels in the UVB-damaged model of HaCaT cells was presented in Figures 5 and 6. After DCFH-DA staining, fluorescence intensity and fluorescence area in model group (B) were increased compared with blank group (A), indicating a significant increase in intracellular ROS content. Fluorescence area and intensity of TCP3 (PKK), TCP6 (YEGGD) and TCP9 (GPGLM) groups decreased with the increase of antioxidant peptide concentration compared with the model group, indicating a significant decrease in intracellular ROS content. Figure 6 accurately quantified the influence of TCP3 (PKK), TCP6 (YEGGD) and TCP9 (GPGLM) on ROS levels in the UVB-irradiated HaCaT cells. The ROS levels of TCP3 group at 100, 200 and 400 μM were decreased from 338 ± 8% to 265 ± 10%, 230 ± 14%, and 190 ± 21% of the control group, respectively. The ROS levels of TCP6 group at 100, 200 and 400 μM were decreased from 338 ± 8% to 293 ± 15%, 242 ± 15%, and 214 ± 14% of the control group, respectively. The ROS levels of TCP9 group at 100, 200 and 400 μM were decreased from 338 ± 8% to 301 ± 17%, 249 ± 11%, and 222 ± 13% of the control group, respectively. Therefore, ROS levels were significantly decreased by TCP3 (PKK), TCP6 (YEGGD) and TCP9 (GPGLM) pretreatment at designed concentrations compared with the model group ($p < 0.001$).

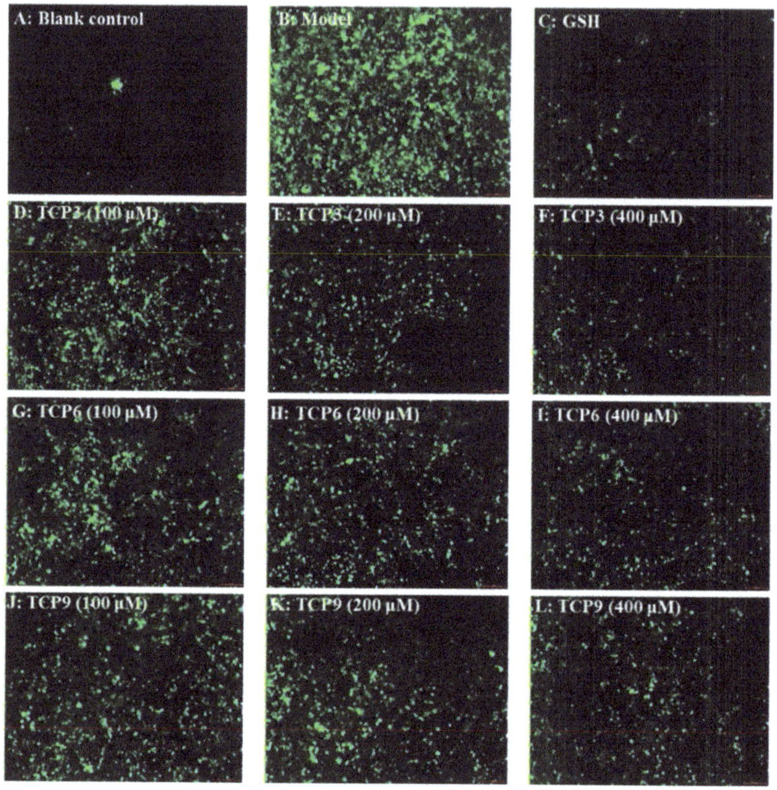

Figure 5. Determination of ROS content in cells by DCFH-DA staining. Glutathione (GSH) at 200 μM served as the positive control. (**A**) Control; (**B**) UVB-irradiated HaCaT cell model; (**C**) GSH; (**D–F**) TCP3 with 100, 200, and 400 μM, respectively; (**G–I**) TCP6 with 100, 200, and 400 μM, respectively; (**J–L**) TCP9 with 100, 200, and 400 μM, respectively.

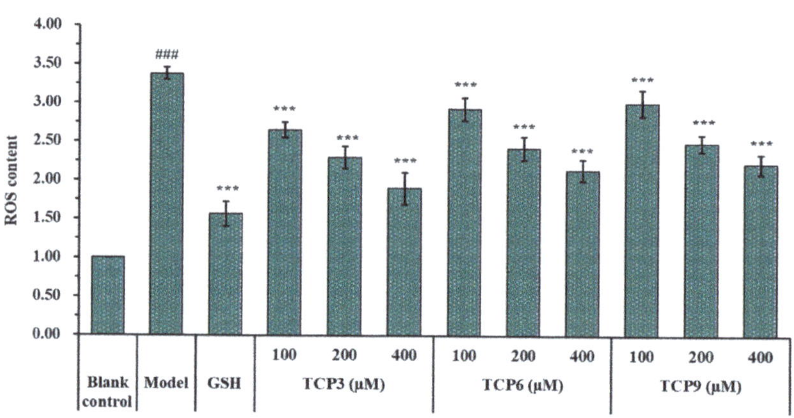

Figure 6. Effects of different concentrations (100, 200, and 400 μM) of TCP3 (PKK), TCP6 (YEGGD) and TCP9 (GPGLM) on ROS levels of UVB-irradiated HaCaT cell model. Glutathione (GSH) at 200 μM was served as the positive control. All data are presented as the mean ± SD of triplicate results. ### $p < 0.001$ vs. blank control group; *** $p < 0.001$ vs. model group.

2.1.6. Effects of TCP3 (PKK), TCP6 (YEGGD) and TCP9 (GPGLM) on the Intracellular Oxidases and Oxide Levels of UVB-Irradiated HaCaT Cell Model

As shown in Figure 7, the levels of antioxidases (SOD, CAT and GSH-Px) in UVB-irradiated HaCaT cells incubated with TCP3 (PKK), TCP6 (YEGGD) and TCP9 (GPGLM) were gradually increased when the peptide concentrations increased from 100 μM to 400 μM. At 400 μM, the SOD activity in TCP3 (PKK), TCP6 (YEGGD) and TCP9 (GPGLM) groups were 143.82 ± 13.04, 130.43 ± 5.63, and 117.38 ± 10.23 U/mg prot, respectively; the CAT activity in TCP3 (PKK), TCP6 (YEGGD) and TCP9 (GPGLM) groups were 143.82 ± 13.04, 130.43 ± 5.63, and 117.38 ± 10.23 U/mg prot, respectively; the GSH-Px levels in TCP3 (PKK), TCP6 (YEGGD) and TCP9 (GPGLM) groups were 81.28 ± 2.26, 79.77 ± 3.58, and 76.00 ± 1.25 U/mg prot, respectively. The activity of antioxidases in TCP3 (PKK), TCP6 (YEGGD) and TCP9 (GPGLM) groups were significantly higher than those of the model group ($p < 0.001$). Figure 5D showed that the MDA levels of TCP3 (PKK), TCP6 (YEGGD) and TCP9 (GPGLM) groups were decreased dose-dependently with the concentrations of TCP3 (PKK), TCP6 (YEGGD) and TCP9 (GPGLM) increased from 100 μM to 400 μM. At 400 μM, The MDA levels of TCP3 (PKK), TCP6 (YEGGD) and TCP9 (GPGLM) groups decreased to 3.42 ± 0.60, 4.06 ± 0.52, and 4.15 ± 0.39 nmol/mg prot, respectively, which were significantly lower than that of the model group (7.24 ± 0.47 nmol/mg prot) ($p < 0.001$).

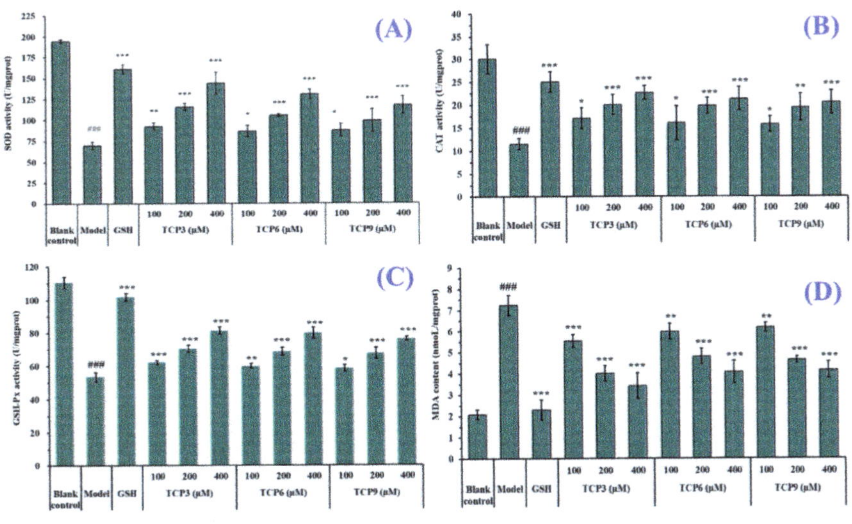

Figure 7. Effects of different concentrations (100, 200, and 400 μM) of TCP3 (PKK), TCP6 (YEGGD) and TCP9 (GPGLM) on the levels of SOD (**A**), CAT (**B**), GSH-Px (**C**), and MDA (**D**) in UVB-irradiated HaCaT cell model. Glutathione (GSH) at 200 μM was served as the positive control. All data are presented as the mean ± SD of triplicate results. ### $p < 0.001$ vs. blank control group; *** $p < 0.001$, ** $p < 0.01$, and * $p < 0.05$ vs. model group.

2.2. *Effects of TCP3 (PKK), TCP6 (YEGGD) and TCP9 (GPGLM) on the Apoptosis Rates of UVB-Irradiated HaCaT Cell Model*

2.2.1. Effects of TCP3 (PKK), TCP6 (YEGGD) and TCP9 (GPGLM) on the Apoptosis Rates of UVB-Irradiated HaCaT Cell Model

Hoechst 33342 is a solution used to stain the nuclei of living cells and often applied to detect apoptosis. After staining, the nuclei of apoptotic cells were densely or fragmented densely stained. Figure 8A showed that HaCaT cells in the blank group were uniform in size, full in shape, and less burst blue light, but HaCaT cells in the model group (Figure 8B) showed a large amount of blue fluorescence and were in a densely stained state, which indicated a large number of HaCaT cells were damaged by UVB radiation and in an apoptosis state. However, the fluorescence area and intensity of the peptide group gradually decreased with the increase of TCP3, TCP6 and TCP concentrations (Figure 8D–L). In addition, TCP3 showed stronger inhibition than TCP6 and TCP9 on UVB-irradiated HaCaT cell apoptosis. These results illustrated that TCP3 (PKK), TCP6 (YEGGD) and TCP9 (GPGLM) could significantly reduce the apoptosis to protect UVB-irradiated HaCaT cells, which was in agreement with the results in Figures 2 and 4.

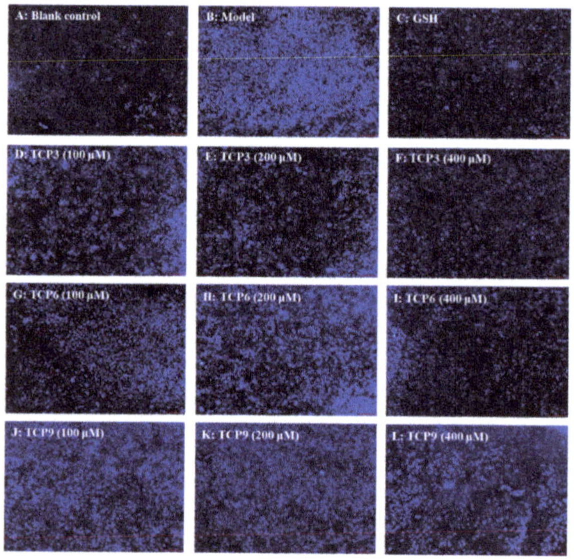

Figure 8. Apoptosis analysis of TCP3 (PKK), TCP6 (YEGGD) and TCP9 (GPGLM) on UVB-irradiated HaCaT cell model by Hoechst 33342. Glutathione (GSH) at 200 μM served as the positive control. (**A**) Control; (**B**) UVB-irradiated HaCaT cell model; (**C**) GSH; (**D–F**) TCP3 with 100, 200, and 400 μM, respectively; (**G–I**) TCP6 with 100, 200, and 400 μM, respectively; (**J–L**) TCP9 with 100, 200, and 400 μM, respectively.

2.2.2. Effects of TCP3 (PKK), TCP6 (YEGGD) and TCP9 (GPGLM) on Mitochondrial Membrane Potential (MMP) of UVB-Irradiated HaCaT Cell Model

Mitochondria are the main energy supply units of cells and mitochondrial alterations are one of the most important mechanisms controlling cell apoptosis [31]. MMP is the most reliable indicator of mitochondrial function and can reflect the functional activity of cells, and mitochondrial function can be assessed through monitoring changes in MMP [11,32]. Moreover, the fluorescence intensity of JC-1 can reflect the change degree of MMP (Figure 9). Mitochondria showed red fluorescence at high membrane potential. The reverse is green. The MMP tended to decrease when cells entered the early stage of apoptosis. That is to say, the red fluorescence gradually converted to green fluorescence [33].

Compared with the blank group (Figure 9A), the red fluorescence in model group (Figure 9B) decreased, the green fluorescence increased, and the MMP decreased significantly ($p < 0.001$). In addition, the JC-1 fluorescence intensity (red/green) of the model group was 5.51% of the blank group (Figure 9G). These data indicated that UVB irradiation caused the cells in model group to enter the early stage of apoptosis. The decrease of MMP induced by UVB was concentration-dependently restrained when the HaCaT cells were incubated with TCP3 (PKK), TCP6 (YEGGD) and TCP9 (GPGLM) at 100-400 μM ($p < 0.01$) (Figure 9D–F). At 400 μM, the JC-1 fluorescence intensity (red/green) of TCP3 (PKK), TCP6 (YEGGD) and TCP9 (GPGLM) groups was 140.75, 130.30, and 116.42-fold of model group, and TCP3 showed a better increasing function in MMP, which agreed with the results of

Figure 8. These finding confirmed that TCP3 (PKK), TCP6 (YEGGD) and TCP9 (GPGLM) could reduce the apoptosis induced by UVB through controlling the decrease of MMP.

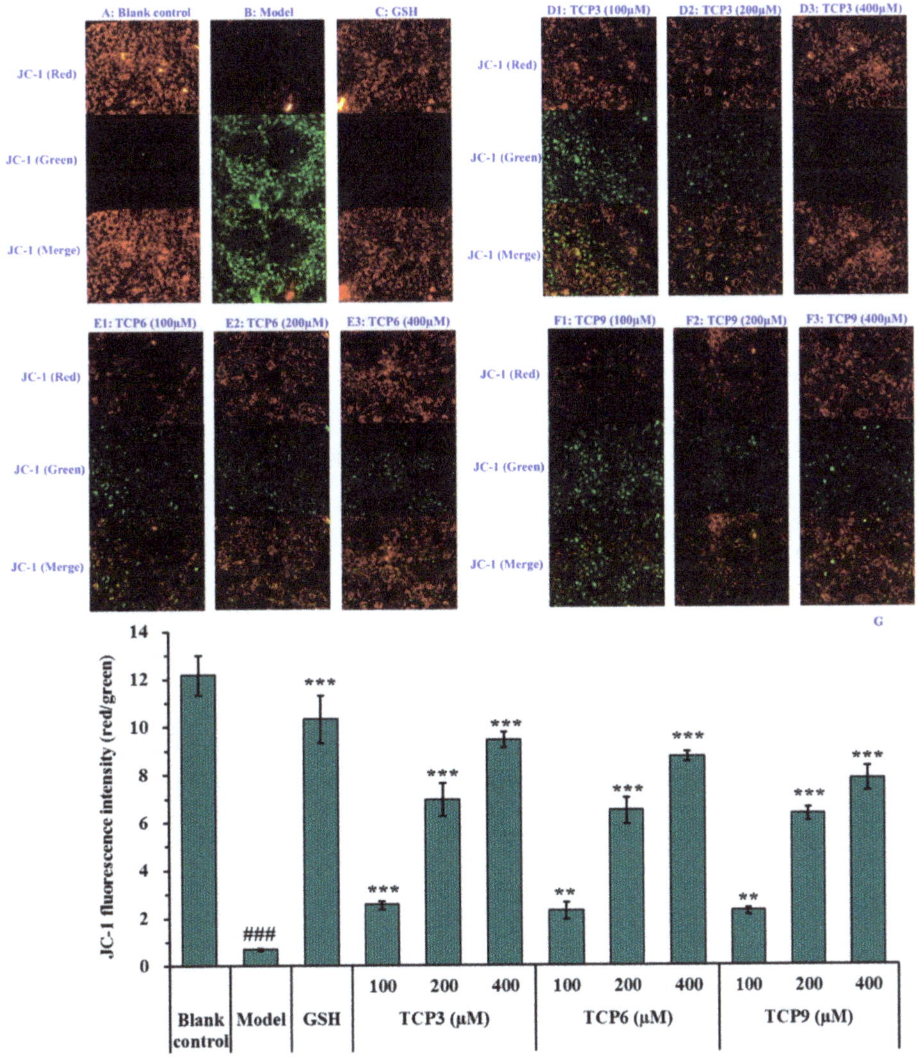

Figure 9. Effects of TCP3 (PKK), TCP6 (YEGGD) and TCP9 (GPGLM) on the mitochondrial membrane potential (MMP) of UVB-irradiated HaCaT cell model. Glutathione (GSH) at 200 μM served as the positive control. (**A**) Control; (**B**) UVB-irradiated HaCaT cell model; (**C**) GSH; (**D1–D3**) TCP3 with 100, 200, and 400 μM, respectively; (**E1–E3**) TCP6 with 100, 200, and 400 μM, respectively; (**F1–F3**) TCP6 with 100, 200, and 400 μM, respectively; (**G**) JC-Fluorescence intensity (red/green). All data are presented as the mean ± SD of triplicate results. ### $p < 0.001$ vs Control group; *** $p < 0.001$, ** $p < 0.01$ vs UVB-irradiated HaCaT cell model.

2.3. Effects of TCP3 (PKK), TCP6 (YEGGD) and TCP9 (GPGLM) on the Expression of Antioxidant and Apoptotic Proteins in UVB-Irradiated HaCaT Cell Model

2.3.1. Expression of Antioxidant-linked Proteins in UVB-Irradiated HaCaT Cell Model

The expression of antioxidant-linked proteins including Nrf2, HO-1, and NQO1 were investigated to determine the protective function of TCP3 (PKK), TCP6 (YEGGD) and TCP9 (GPGLM) in the UVB-irradiated HaCaT cell model (Figure 10A). As a transcription factor, Nrf2 can regulate the cellular defense system against oxidative insults by the expression of genes sucked up into oxidative stress response [34–36]. As shown in Figure 10B, the protein expression of Nrf2 in the model group was significantly lowered. However, the protein expression level of Nrf2 was apparently recovered after incubating with 100 and 400 μM of TCP3 (PKK), TCP6 (YEGGD) and TCP9 (GPGLM), respectively ($p < 0.01$). At 400 μM, the protein expression level of Nrf2 in TCP3 (PKK), TCP6 (YEGGD) and TCP9 (GPGLM) groups was 1.96-, 1.69-, and 1.79-fold of the model group. It was indicated that TCP3 (PKK), TCP6 (YEGGD) and TCP9 (GPGLM) could activate the Nrf2 pathway, regulating downstream antioxidant enzymes to reduce the UVB damage to HaCaT cells. The finding was verified by the Figure 7A–C that the activity of intracellular antioxidases (SOD, CAT and GSH-Px) in UVB-irradiated HaCaT cells incubated with TCP3 (PKK), TCP6 (YEGGD) and TCP9 (GPGLM) were gradually increased.

HO-1 presents protective effects by metabolizing heme groups to prevent group oxidation or removing ROS by biliverdin and reduced bilirubin. The level of HO-1 is a key indicator to evaluate the antioxidant, anti-inflammatory and anti-apoptosis of drugs [37,38]. As shown in Figure 10C, HO-1 protein expression in the model group was significantly reduced ($p < 0.001$), but the protein expression level of HO-1 was significantly increased with the addition of TCP3 (PKK), TCP6 (YEGGD) and TCP9 (GPGLM) ($p < 0.001$). At 400 μM, the protein expression level of HO-1 in TCP3 (PKK), TCP6 (YEGGD) and TCP9 (GPGLM) groups was 1.72-, 1.65-, and 1.58-fold of the model group. The result proved that TCP3 (PKK), TCP6 (YEGGD) and TCP9 (GPGLM) could protect HaCaT cells against UVB damage by increasing the level of HO-1.

NQO1 is a cytosolic homodimeric flavoprotein that catalyses the two-electron reduction of quinones to reduce the chance of generating reactive oxygen intermediates through the REDOX cycle. NQO1 also maintains α-tocopherol and coenzyme Q10 in a reduced state and protect endogenous antioxidants [39,40]. Figure 10D indicated that the protein expression of NQO1 in the model group was significantly reduced, but the protein expression level of NQO1 in the peptide groups was significantly increased after incubating with TCP3 (PKK), TCP6 (YEGGD) and TCP9 (GPGLM) ($p < 0.01$). At 400 μM, the protein expression level of NQO1 in TCP3 (PKK), TCP6 (YEGGD) and TCP9 (GPGLM) groups was 1.71-, 1.68-, and 1.55-fold of the model group. It was demonstrated that TCP3 (PKK), TCP6 (YEGGD) and TCP9 (GPGLM) could reduce the oxidative damage of HaCaT induced by UV radiation by increasing the expression level of NQO1 protein.

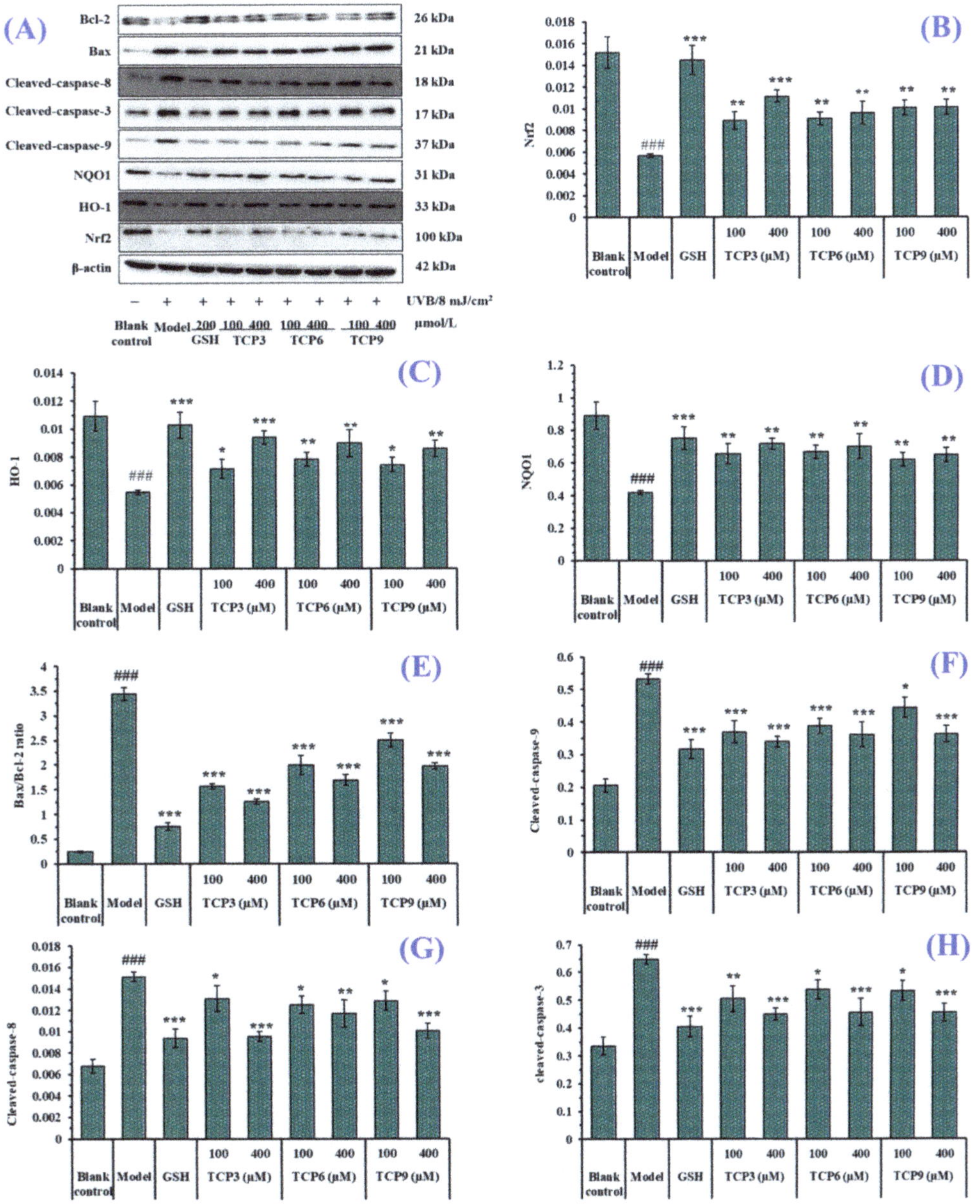

Figure 10. Effect of TCP3 (PKK), TCP6 (YEGGD) and TCP9 (GPGLM) on expression of antioxidant and apoptosis related proteins in UVB-irradiated HaCaT cell model. Glutathione (GSH) at 200 μM was served as the positive control. (**A**) Western-Blot; (**B**) the protein expression of Nrf2; (**C**) the protein expression of HO-1; (**D**) the protein expression of NQO1; (**E**) Bax/Bcl-2 ratio; (**F**) the protein expression of Cleaved-caspase-9; (**G**) the protein expression of Cleaved-caspase-8; (**H**) the protein expression of Cleaved-caspase-3. All data are presented as the mean ± SD of triplicate results. ### $p < 0.001$ vs. control group; * $p < 0.05$, ** $p < 0.01$, and *** $p < 0.001$ vs. UVB-irradiated HaCaT cell model.

2.3.2. Expression of Apoptosis-linked Proteins in UVB-Irradiated HaCaT Cell Model

The expression of apoptosis-linked proteins including Bax, Bcl-2, caspase 3, caspase 8, and caspase 9 were investigated to determine the protective function of TCP3 (PKK), TCP6 (YEGGD) and TCP9 (GPGLM) in the UVB-irradiated HaCaT cell model (Figure 10A). In the mitochondrial apoptosis pathway, two members of the Bcl protein family (Bax and Bcl-2) play an important role in inhibiting or promoting apoptosis. Mitochondria are the main source of ROS production in keratinocytes exposed to UVB [41]. When ROS content is excessive in mitochondria, the ion concentration on both sides of mitochondrial membrane changes, causing cytochrome C to flow into cytoplasm and form apoptotic bodies with promoter Caspase-9, which then activates apoptotic executive protein Caspase-3, leading to cell apoptosis [42]. In addition, the exogenous pathway is initiated by activation of the death receptor, which is dependent on the protein caspase-8. In the UVB-treated HaCaT cells, the anti-apoptotic Bcl-2 expression was decreased, while the apoptotic Bax expression was increased compared with the control cells (Figure 10A,E). In addition, expression of the cleaved caspase 3, caspase 8, and caspase 9 was highly measured in the UVB-irradiated HaCaT cells (Figure 10A,F–H). However, the expressions of the apoptosis-linked proteins (Bax, Bcl-2, caspase 3, caspase 8, and caspase 9) in TCP3 (PKK), TCP6 (YEGGD) and TCP9 (GPGLM) treated HaCaT cells were reversed, suggesting that TCP3 (PKK), TCP6 (YEGGD) and TCP9 (GPGLM) could promote the expression of Bcl-2/Bax anti-apoptosis protein and down-regulate the expression of cleaved caspase 3, caspase 8, and caspase 9 apoptosis proteins, thus playing their protective role in photoaging HaCaT cells caused by UVB.

2.4. Molecular Docking Model of TCP3 (PKK), TCP6 (YEGGD) and TCP9 (GPGLM) with Keap1 Protein

Under normal condition, Nrf2 exists in cytoplasm coupled with Keap1 protein. When ROS are excessive, cysteine residues of Keap1 exposed to ROS are modified, leading to ubiquitination of the Keap1 protein, which interferes with Nrf2 ubiquitination and dissociates Nrf2 from Keap1. In addition, some antioxidant peptides can occupy the binding site of Keap1 and Nrf2, resulting in the dissociation of Nrf2 and Keap1, increasing the amount of free Nrf2 entering the nucleus, and initiating the transcription and translation of downstream antioxidant genes after binding with ARE [43,44].

In Figure 10B, TCP3 (PKK), TCP6 (YEGGD) and TCP9 (GPGLM) can increase the expression level of Nrf2 protein in the nucleus. In order to illustrate the mechanism of TCP3 (PKK), TCP6 (YEGGD) and TCP9 (GPGLM) in the Keap1/Nrf2 pathway, molecular docking method was used to simulate and predict the interactions between TCP3 (PKK), TCP6 (YEGGD) and TCP9 (GPGLM) with Keap1.

Keap1 (MW 70 kDa) is a cysteine-rich protein and consists of more than 625 amino acid residues, including 27 cysteine residues. The Kelch domain of Keap1 is combined with the Neh2 domain of Nrf2 [45,46]. The binding sites of Keap1 in the Kelch domain can be divided into five sub-pockets, namely P1 (Arg415, Ile461, Gly462, Phe478, Arg483 and Ser508), P2 (Ser363, Arg380, Asn382 and Asn414), P3 (Gly509, Ser555, Ala556, Gly571, Ser602 and Gly603), P4 (Tyr525, Gln530 and Tyr572), and P5 (Tyr334 and Phe577) [45,46]. Bioactive peptides bind to other macromolecular substances mainly through hydrogen bond force, van der Waals force and electrostatic interaction force, among which hydrogen bond force is the most important [27,47]. The molecular docking analysis indicated that the affinity of TCP3 with the middle cavity and bottom of Kelch domain was −7.4 kcal/mol and −6.6 kcal/mol, which was similar to those of TCP6 (−8.9 kcal/mol) and TCP9 (−8.5 kcal/mol) interacted with the middle cavity of Kelch domain. These data indicated that TCP3 (PKK), TCP6 (YEGGD) and TCP9 (GPGLM) could bind to Keap1 protein. Figure 11A,B indicated TCP3 (PKK) formed hydrogen bonds with Val418, Val465, Val512, Ala510, Leu557, Gly364, Leu365, Ile416, Val606, Gly367, and Gly464 residues when TCP3 (PKK) interacted at the middle cavity of the Kelch domain and interacted with Arg415 residues of Kelch domain by electrostatic force. In addition, TCP3 (PKK) formed hydrogen bonds with Ser508 and Arg380 residues when TCP3 (PKK) interacted at the middle cavity of the Kelch domain and interacted with Phe478 residues of Kelch domain by electrostatic force (Figure 11C,D). Figure 11E,F showed that TCP6 (YEGGD) formed hydrogen bonds with Cys513, Val465, Val512, and Ala556 residues, interacted with Val420 and Cys368 residues through hydrophobic effect, and acted with Arg415 residue by electrostatic force when it interacted at the middle cavity of the Kelch domain. Figure 11G,H showed that TCP9 (YEGDP) formed three hydrogen bonds with Val418, Val604, and Gly419 residues, and interacted with Ala466, Cys513, Val514, Val512 and Val465 residues through hydrophobic effect when it interacted at the middle cavity of the Kelch domain. In summary, TCP3 (PKK) and TCP6 (YEGGD) occupy the amino acid residues Arg380, Arg415 and Arg415 Ala556 that have an impact on Keap1-Nrf2 interaction, respectively, so it could be concluded that TCP3 and TCP6 can competitively inhibit Nrf2 binding. However, TCP9 (GPGLM) could not bind to the active site of the Kelch domain of Keap1 protein, which was inferred to be non-competitive inhibition.

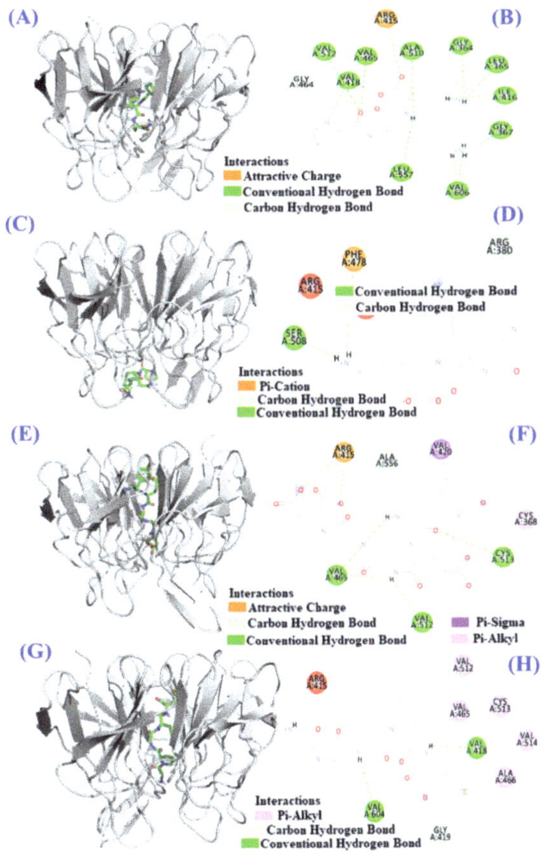

Figure 11. Molecular docking models of TCP3, TCP6, and TCP9 with Keap1 protein. (**A**) 3D details of the middle cavity of the Kelch domain and TCP3 interaction. (**B**) 2D details of the middle cavity of the Kelch domain and TCP3 interaction. (**C**) 3D details of the bottom of the Kelch domain and TCP3 interaction. (**D**) 2D details of the bottom of the Kelch domain and TCP3 interaction. (**E**) 3D details of the middle cavity of the Kelch domain and TCP6 interaction. (**F**) 2D details of the middle cavity of the Kelch domain and TCP6 interaction. (**G**) 3D details of the middle cavity of the Kelch domain and TCP9 interaction. (**H**) 2D details of the middle cavity of the Kelch domain and TCP9 interaction.

3. Discussion

UV radiation is one of the important environmental factors that causes skin photoaging, which accounts for about 80% of skin aging [48–50]. Prolonged skin exposure to UV radiation can induce detrimental intracellular physiological effects and produce superfluous ROS, which can injury intracellular bioactive molecules, such as DNA, enzymes and proteins, and membrane lipids, and further cause oxidative stress and promote cell apoptosis [51–53]. Then, inhibiting photoaging induced by UVB can delay skin aging and provides a reasonable basis for studying cosmetic products to treat diseases caused by UV radiation [48]. Therefore, this paper also discusses the protective effects of TCP3 (PKK), TCP6 (YEGGD) and TCP9 (GPGLM) on the cells damaged by UV oxidation from two aspects of antioxidant and apoptosis inhibition.

Induced by UVB, HaCaT cells produce excessive ROS, which destroy the oxidation-reduction dynamic equilibrium system, and decrease the activities of antioxidant enzymes [54]. With the accumulation of ROS and oxidative metabolites, lipid peroxidation occurs in cells. As one of the end products of lipid peroxidation, MDA can damage the structural and functional integrity of cell membranes [48,53]. The intervention of antioxidant therapy is identified as a potential approach to constrain oxidative stress and improve skin cell function by alleviating ROS damage [50,55]. Therefore, the activity of intracellular antioxidant enzymes and the content of lipid peroxides (MDA) were firstly explored to evaluate the protective effect of TCP3 (PKK), TCP6 (YEGGD) and TCP9 (GPGLM) on the oxidative damage of HaCaT cells after UVB irradiation. The results showed that TCP3 (PKK), TCP6 (YEGGD) and TCP9 (GPGLM) could dose-dependently increase the activity of SOD, CAT and GSH-Px, and reduce the level of MDA in UVB-irradiated HaCaT cells. The results indicated that TCP3 (PKK), TCP6 (YEGGD) and TCP9 (GPGLM) had strong protective effects on UVB-irradiated cells.

The literature indicated that an increase the level of ROS in cells could negatively affect the Keap1/Nrf2 signaling pathway, thereby bringing down the expression of antioxidant/phase II detoxifying enzymes and leading to oxidative injury and cell apoptosis [31,56]. Protective mechanism indicated that TCP3 (PKK), TCP6 (YEGGD) and TCP9 (GPGLM) could reverse these negative effects by activating Nrf2 pathway to up-regulate the protein expression of Nrf2, HO-1 and NQO1. Oxidative stress can motivate the separation of Nrf2 and Keap1 and accelerate the entry of Nrf2 into the nucleus to bind to the antioxidant response element ARE. Thus, it can promote the expression of antioxidant genes and facilitate the cell REDOX balance [56]. A molecular docking experiment showed that TCP3 and TCP6 occupied the active sites Arg380 and Arg415 of Nrf2 in the Kelch domain of Keap1 protein, while TCP9 did not bind to the active site of Keap1. Therefore, we conclude that TCP3 and TCP6 inhibit Keap1-NrF2 coupling by occupying the active sites of Nrf2 and Keap1 and allow Nrf2 to enter the nucleus and activate pathways to protect cells from oxidative stress.

Apoptosis is an active reaction of cells after external stimulation, and this process is a form of programmed death regulated by related genes [52,54]. UVB irradiation can cause excessive accumulation of ROS in cells, damage mitochondrial structure and change the permeability of mitochondrial membrane, and mitochondrial alterations are one of the critical paths for manipulating apoptosis [31]. The results of Hoechst 33342 fluorescence staining showed that TCP3 (PKK), TCP6 (YEGGD) and TCP9 (GPGLM) showed inhibitory effects on UVB-induced HaCaT apoptosis. In addition, TCP3 (PKK), TCP6 (YEGGD) and TCP9 (GPGLM) could dose-dependently inhibit the decline of MMP to alleviate cell apoptosis in JC-1 fluorescence double staining assay. In apoptosis, the high Bax/Bcl-2 ratio is a key index in controlling the breakdown of permeability and function of mitochondrial membrane [31,57]. Mechanism of TCP3 (PKK), TCP6 (YEGGD) and TCP9 (GPGLM) inhibiting HaCaT apoptosis suggested that TCP3 (PKK), TCP6 (YEGGD) and TCP9 (GPGLM) could reduce the proportion of Bax/Bcl-2, down-regulate the protein expression levels of caspase 3, caspase 8 and caspase 9, and reverse apoptosis.

Presently, some marine bioactive peptides showed significant protective effect on UV radiation-induced photoaging. Fu et al. reported that collagen peptides from skins and bones of bigeye tuna could reduce the UVB-induced photoaging through regulating MAPK and TGF-β signaling pathways [55]. Peptide fraction from *Pinctada martensii* meat containing oligopeptides FH, AL, MY, AGF, and IYP showed the anti-photoaging activity by increase cell viability, reduced the interstitial MMP-1 and MMP-3 contents, and downregulated the expression of p38, EKR, JNK, MMP-1, and MMP-3 in UVB-induced HaCaT cells [58]. Heptapeptide DAPTMGY from *Isochrysis zhanjiangensis* showed protective effects on HaCaT cells against UVB-induced damage through regulating anti-apoptosis and MAPK/AP-1/MMP pathway [59]. Hydrolysate (TCH) from *Theragra chalcogramma* was rich in GLPYT and could alleviates photoaging via controlling the deposition of collagen fibers and recovery of extracellular component matrix in SD rats [60]. WNLNP from oyster protein hydrolysate had great potential to prevent skin photoaging because it exerted a remarkable antiphotoaging effect on the UVB-irradiated HaCaT cells by regulating MAPK/NF-κB signaling pathway and expression of bax and bcl-2 in UVB-irradiated HaCaT cells [61]. In the study, TCP3 (PKK), TCP6 (YEGGD) and TCP9 (GPGLM) showed a significantly protective function on UVB-damaged HaCaT cells through activating Nrf2 signaling pathways and reducing cell apoptosis.

4. Materials and Methods

4.1. Materials and Chemical Reagents

Glutathione (GSP), penicillin–streptomycin solution, phosphate buffered saline (PBS), RPMI modified medium (RPMI-1640), fetal bovine serum, Tris, MTT, and trypsin-EDTA were purchased from Beijing Solabao Technology Co., Ltd. (Beijing, China). Assay kits for determination of the activities of SOD, CAT, and GSH-Px and contents of BCA, ROS and MDA were purchased from Nanjing Jiancheng Bioengineering Institute (Nanjing, China). QGD (TCP1), GEQSN (TCP2), PKK (TCP3), GPQ (TCP4), GEEGD (TCP5), YEGGD (TCP6), GEGER (TCP7), GEGQR (TCP8), GPGLM (TCP9), GLN (TCP10), and GDRGD (TCP11) were synthesized by Shanghai Apeptide Co., Ltd. (Shanghai, China) and their purities were higher than 98%.

4.2. HaCaT Cell Culture and Establishment of UV-Irradiated Cell Model

HaCaT cells were bought from the Chinese Academy of Sciences (Shanghai, China) and plated in DMEM supplemented with 12% FBS, streptomycin (100 mg/mL)/penicillin (100 U/mL) at 37 °C in a humidified incubator with 5% CO_2 [62].

HaCaT cells with the density of 3×10^4 cells/well were seeded into a 96-well plate containing 100 μL of culture media. After 24 h, the culture media was discarded and HaCaT Cells were washed with PBS buffer 3 times. Then, the resulting HaCaT cells were covered with a thin layer PBS and irradiated with different doses of UVB (0, 5, 8, 10, 12, and 15 mJ/cm^2, respectively) using a UVB (313 nm) light source (Shenzhen Guanya Photoelectric Technology Co., Ltd., Shenzhen, China) with a UVB blocking filter.

$$\text{Radiation dosage (mJ/cm}^2\text{)} = \text{Radiation intensity (mw/cm}^2\text{)} \times \text{Time (s)}$$

After radiation, HaCaT cells were washed three times with PBS and cultured in new culture media for 24 h. After that, the wells were washed with PBS and MTT was added for an additional 4h. Then, DMSO was added to dissolve the formazan crystals formed by active cells. After that, the absorbance was measured at 570 nm [35,63]. Cell viability was calculated according to the following formula:

$$\text{Cell viability (\%)} = (\text{OD}_{\text{sample}}/\text{OD}_{\text{control}}) \times 100.$$

The cell viability was determined and the doses of UVB-induced the HaCaT cell viability of about 50% was chosen to establish the cell model [19,20,27].

4.3. Effects of Antioxidant Peptides on Cell Viability

After culturing for 24 h, HaCaT cells were treated with 20 μL of peptides (TCP1-TCP11) with the final concentration of 200 μM for 24 h. Then, HaCaT cells were exposed to UVB radiation (8 mJ/cm^2). After the serum-free medium was incubated for 24 h, cell viability was calculated according to the method in 4.2. The blank group was set without UVB radiation and peptide treatment. The model group was irradiated by UVB without peptide treatment.

In order to research the effects of TCP3 (PKK), TCP6 (YEGGD) and TCP9 (GPGLM) on the UVB-injured cell viability, the final concentration of TCP3 (PKK), TCP6 (YEGGD) and TCP9 (GPGLM) was designed as 100, 200, and 400 μM.

4.4. Determination of Intracellular ROS, MDA, and Antioxidases

ROS level in HaCaT cells was monitored according to the previous method [35]. In brief, HaCaT cells were preincubated with peptides at 100, 200, or 400 μM for 12.0 h, and then exposed to UVB (8 mJ/cm^2). Subsequently, the cells were rinsed by PBS and treated with 10 μM DCFH2-DA in fresh culture medium for 30 min. ROS level indicated by DCF fluorescence were quantified on a BD FACS Calibur flow cytometer.

The activity of SOD, GSH-Px and CAT and content of MDA were measured using assay kits according to the manufacturer's instructions [64].

4.5. Morphological Observation of HaCaT Cells Using Hoechst 33342 Staining Assay

Hoechst 33342 staining assay was performed using previous method [65]. After treating with peptides and UVB radiation, the HaCaT cells were washed, harvested, fixed, and exposed to 8 mg/mL Hoechst 33,342 solution at 37 °C and 5% CO_2 atmosphere for 30 min. After clearing away the Hoechst 33,342 solution and rinsing three times with serum-free DMEM, the morphology of HaCaT cells was observed using a fluorescence microscope (LSM710; Carl Zeiss Microscopy GmbH, Jena, Germany).

4.6. Determination of MMP

MMP was determined using previous method [66]. After treating with peptide and UVB radiation, 100 μL fresh medium and 100 μL JC-1 working medium were added in sequence in the 96-well plate of HaCaT cells. After 40 min, cells were cleaned with PBS and an invertedfluorescence microscopy was employed to capture the fluorescence intensity of HaCaT cells. The intensities of green fluorescence and fluorescence were determined at Ex/Em: 490/530 nm and Ex/Em: 525/590 nm, respectively

4.7. Determination of Protein Expression

Western blot was used to measure the protein expression of Bax, Bcl-2, Nrf2, HO-1, NQO1, β-actin, caspase-3, caspase-8, and caspase-9 in HaCaT cells according to our previous method [67]. Total proteins were extracted with a RIPA buffer. After separation of protein with SDS-PAGE, the proteins were transferred into a polyvinylidene difluoride (PVDF) membrane, and the PVDF membrane was blocked with 10% non-immune serum for 2 h. PVDF membranes were incubated with primary antibodies for 12 h at 4 °C and horseradish peroxidaseconjugated secondary antibodies for 2 h at 37 °C. The intensity of the specific immunoreactive bands was determined using enhanced chemiluminescence, quantified by densitometry, and expressed as a ratio to β-actin.

4.8. Molecular Docking Experiment of TCP3 (PKK), TCP6 (YEGGD) and TCP9 (GPGLM)

This assay of TCP3 (PKK), TCP6 (YEGGD) and TCP9 (GPGLM) was commissioned to Shanghai NovoPro Biotechnology Co., Ltd. (Shanghai, china). The crystal structure of Keap1 (PDB ID: 2FLU) was acquired from the PDB database. To investigate the possible binding mode of TCP3 (PKK), TCP6 (YEGGD) and TCP9 (GPGLM) to Keap1, the small ligand-binding C-terminal kelch domain of the human Keap1) was selected according to the previous studies [68–70]. Molecular docking analysis of TCP3 (PKK), TCP6 (YEGGD) and TCP9 (GPGLM) were carried out in the kelch pockets of Keap1 using AutoDock vina.

4.9. Statistical Analysis

All the results are expressed as the mean ± SD ($n = 3$) and analyzed by an ANOVA test using SPSS 19.0. Significant differences between the means of parameters were analyzed by Duncan's multiple range test ($p < 0.05$).

5. Conclusions

In summary, the cytoprotective effects of TCP3 (PKK), TCP6 (YEGGD) and TCP9 (GPGLM) were evaluated against UVB-irradiated HaCaT cells. The cytoprotective mechanisms for TCP3 (PKK), TCP6 (YEGGD) and TCP9 (GPGLM) were the increase in cellular antioxidant capacity through activating Nrf2 signaling pathway and the suppression of cell apoptosis through downregulating Bax-dependent mitochondrial apoptosis. This work laid a theoretical foundation for employing TCP3 (PKK), TCP6 (YEGGD) and TCP9 (GPGLM) to attenuate UVB-irradiated photoaging. In addition, more scientific studies are needed to verify the function of TCP3 (PKK), TCP6 (YEGGD) and TCP9 (GPGLM) in animals to serve as nutraceuticals or functional ingredients in healthy food and cosmetics.

Author Contributions: J.K. and X.-M.H.: Conceptualization, data curation, formal analysis, investigation, methodology, and validation; W.-W.C. and Y.-M.W.: investigation, methodology, validation, and writing—original draft; C.-F.C.: resources, supervision, writing—review and editing; B.W.: conceptualization, funding acquisition, resources, supervision, writing—review and editing. All authors have read and agreed to the published version of the manuscript.

Funding: This work was funded by the National Natural Science Foundation of China (No. 82073764) and the Ten-thousand Talents Plan of Zhejiang Province (No. 2019R52026).

Institutional Review Board Statement: Not applicable.

Informed Consent Statement: Not applicable.

Data Availability Statement: Data are contained within the article.

Conflicts of Interest: The authors declare no conflict of interest.

Abbreviations

UV: ultraviolet; ROS, reactive oxygen species; NF-κB, nuclear factor kappa-light chain enhancer of B cells; HaCaT cells, human immortal keratinocyte cell line; Nrf2, nuclear factor erythroid-2-related factor 2; HO-1, heme oxygenase-1; NQO1, nicotinamide quinone oxidore-ductase 1; MTT, methylthiazolyldiphenyl-tetrazolium bromide; GSP, glutathione; SOD, superoxide dismutase; CAT, catalase; GSH-Px, glutathione peroxidase; MDA, malondialdehyde; MAPKs, mitogen-activate protein kinases; DNA, deoxyribonucleic acid; MMP, mitochondrial membrane potential; ACE, angiotensin-I-converting enzyme; DCFH-DA, 2′,7′-Dichlorodihydrofluorescein diacetate; Bax, Bcl-2-associated X-protein; Bcl-2, Proteins of the B-cell lymphoma-2; Keap1, Kelch-like ECH associated protein 1; ARE, antioxidant response elements; TGF-β, Transforming growth factor-β; MMP-1, matrix metalloproteinase-1; MMP-9, matrix metalloproteinase-9; LDH, lactate dehydrogenase; MMP-3, matrix lysing enzyme; MTT, 3-(4, 5-dimethylthiazol-2-yl)-2,5-diphenyltetrazo lium bromide; PVDF: polyvinylidene difluoride.

References

1. McCullough, J.L.; Kelly, K.M. Prevention and treatment of skin aging. *Anne. N. Y. Acad. Sci.* **2006**, *1067*, 323–331. [CrossRef] [PubMed]
2. Rabe, J.H.; Mamelak, A.J.; McElgunn, P.J.; Morison, W.L.; Sauder, D.N. Photoaging: Mechanisms and repair. *J. Am. Acad. Dermatol.* **2006**, *55*, 1–19. [CrossRef] [PubMed]
3. Nichols, J.A.; Katiyar, S.K. Skin Photoprotection by natural polyphenols: Anti-Inflammatory, antioxidant and DNA repair mechanisms. *Arch. Dermatol. Res.* **2010**, *302*, 71–83. [CrossRef] [PubMed]

4. Krutmann, J.; Schalka, S.; Watson, R.E.B.; Wei, L.; Morita, A. Daily photoprotection to prevent photoaging. *Photodermatol. Photoimmunol. Photomed.* **2021**, *37*, 482–489. [CrossRef]
5. Marabini, L.; Melzi, G.; Lolli, F.; Dell'Agli, M.; Piazza, S.; Sangiovanni, E.; Marinovich, M. Effects of *Vitis vinifera* L. leaves extract on UV radiation damage in human keratinocytes (HaCaT). *J. Photochem. Photobiol. B* **2020**, *204*, 111810. [CrossRef]
6. Elias, P.M. The skin barrier as an innate immune element. *Semin. Immunopathol.* **2007**, *29*, 3–14. [CrossRef]
7. Wang, W.Y.; Zhao, Y.Q.; Zhao, G.X.; Chi, C.F.; Wang, B. Antioxidant peptides from collagen hydrolysate of redlip croaker (*Pseudosciaena polyactis*) scales: Preparation, characterization, and cytoprotective effects on H_2O_2-damaged HepG2 cells. *Mar. Drugs* **2020**, *18*, 156. [CrossRef]
8. Wang, Y.M.; Li, X.Y.; Wang, J.; He, Y.; Chi, C.F.; Wang, B. Antioxidant peptides from protein hydrolysate of skipjack tuna milt: Purification, identification, and cytoprotection on H_2O_2 damaged human umbilical vein endothelial cells. *Process Biochem.* **2022**, *113*, 258–269. [CrossRef]
9. Li, H.; Li, Z.; Peng, L.; Jiang, N.; Liu, Q.; Zhang, E.; Liang, B.; Li, R.; Zhu, H. *Lycium barbarum* polysaccharide protects human keratinocytes against UVB-induced photo-damage. *Free Radic. Res.* **2017**, *51*, 200–210. [CrossRef]
10. Sila, A.; Bougatef, A. Antioxidant peptides from marine by-products: Isolation, identification and application in food systems. *J. Funct. Foods* **2016**, *21*, 10–26. [CrossRef]
11. Wang, Y.Z.; Zhao, Y.Q.; Wang, Y.M.; Zhao, W.H.; Wang, P.; Chi, C.F. Antioxidant peptides from Antarctic Krill (*Euphausia superba*) hydrolysate: Preparation, identification and cytoprotection on H_2O_2-induced oxidative stress. *J. Funct. Foods* **2021**, *86*, 104701. [CrossRef]
12. Zhang, L.; Zhao, G.X.; Zhao, Y.Q.; Qiu, Y.T.; Chi, C.F.; Wang, B. Identification and active evaluation of antioxidant peptides from protein hydrolysates of skipjack tuna (*Katsuwonus pelamis*) head. *Antioxidants* **2019**, *8*, 318. [CrossRef]
13. Sheng, Y.; Qiu, Y.T.; Wang, Y.M.; Chi, C.F.; Wang, B. Novel antioxidant collagen peptides of siberian sturgeon (*Acipenser baerii*) cartilages: The preparation, characterization, and cytoprotection of H_2O_2-damaged human umbilical vein endothelial cells (HUVECs). *Mar. Drugs* **2022**, *20*, 325. [CrossRef]
14. Yoshikawa, M.; Mizutani, T.; Okano, Y.; Masaki, H. An extract of young olive fruit residues attenuates oxidative stress in HaCaT keratinocytes through the ativation of Nrf2 signaling. *J. Oleo. Sci.* **2020**, *69*, 719–726. [CrossRef] [PubMed]
15. Al, N.S.; Dayah, A.A.; Hasan, I.; Daghmash, R. Cosmetic, biomedical and pharmaceutical applications of fish gelatin/hydrolysates. *Mar. Drugs* **2021**, *19*, 145.
16. Siahaan, E.A.; Agusman; Pangestuti, R.; Shin, K.H.; Kim, S.K. Potential cosmetic active ingredients derived from marine by-products. *Mar. Drugs* **2022**, *20*, 734. [CrossRef] [PubMed]
17. Chen, T.; Hou, H.; Lu, J.; Zhang, K.; Li, B. Protective effect of gelatin and gelatin hydrolysate from salmon skin on UV irradiation-induced photoaging of mice skin. *J. Ocean Univ. China* **2016**, *15*, 711–718. [CrossRef]
18. Qin, X.Y.; Xu, Y.; Wei, Y.; Zhang, R.X.; Fang, L.; Zhang, H.X.; Bi, Y.; Gu, R.Z. Effects of topical application of different molecular weight marine fish skin collagen oligopeptides on UVB-induced photoaging rat skin. *J. Cosmet. Dermatol.* **2022**, *21*, 2205–2214. [CrossRef]
19. Chen, J.; Liang, P.; Xiao, Z.; Chen, M.F.; Gong, F.; Li, C.; Zhou, C.; Hong, P.; Jung, W.K.; Qian, Z.J. Antiphotoaging effect of boiled abalone residual peptide ATPGDEG on UVB-induced keratinocyte HaCaT cells. *Food Nutr. Res.* **2019**, *8*, 63. [CrossRef]
20. Xiao, Z.; Liang, P.; Chen, J.; Chen, M.F.; Gong, F.; Li, C.; Zhou, C.; Hong, P.; Yang, P.; Qian, Z.J. A peptide YGDEY from tilapia gelatin hydrolysates inhibits UVB-mediated skin photoaging by regulating MMP-1 and MMP-9 expression in HaCaT cells. *Photochem. Photobiol.* **2019**, *95*, 1424–1432. [CrossRef]
21. Suo, S.K.; Zheng, S.L.; Chi, C.F.; Luo, H.Y.; Wang, B. Novel ACE inhibitory peptides from tuna byproducts-milts: Preparation, characterization, molecular docking study and antioxidant function on H_2O_2-damaged HUVECs. *Front. Nutr.* **2022**, *9*, 957778. [CrossRef]
22. Artetxe-Arrate, I.; Fraile, I.; Marsac, F.; Farley, J.H.; Rodriguez-Ezpeleta, N.; Davies, C.R.; Clear, N.P.; Grewe, P.; Murua, H. A review of the fisheries, life history and stock structure of tropical tuna (skipjack *Katsuwonus pelamis*, yellowfin *Thunnus albacares* and bigeye *Thunnus obesus*) in the Indian ocean. *Adv. Mar. Biol.* **2021**, *88*, 39–89.
23. Qiao, Q.Q.; Luo, Q.B.; Suo, S.K.; Zhao, Y.Q.; Chi, C.F.; Wang, B. Preparation, characterization, and cytoprotective effects on HUVECs of fourteen novel angiotensin-I-converting enzyme inhibitory peptides from protein hydrolysate of tuna processing by-products. *Front. Nutr.* **2022**, *9*, 868681. [CrossRef]
24. Ding, D.; Du, B.; Zhang, C.; Zaman, F.; Huang, Y. Isolation and identification of an antioxidant collagen peptide from skipjack tuna (*Katsuwonus pelamis*) bone. *RSC Adv.* **2019**, *9*, 27032–27041. [CrossRef]
25. Seo, J.K.; Lee, M.J.; Go, H.J.; Kim, Y.J.; Park, N.G. Antimicrobial function of the GAPDH-related antimicrobial peptide in the skin of skipjack tuna, Katsuwonus pelamis. *Fish Shellfish Immunol.* **2014**, *36*, 571–581. [CrossRef] [PubMed]
26. Chi, C.F.; Hu, F.Y.; Wang, B.; Li, Z.R.; Luo, H.Y. Influence of amino acid compositions and peptide profiles on antioxidant capacities of two protein hydrolysates from skipjack tuna (*Katsuwonus pelamis*) dark muscle. *Mar. Drugs* **2015**, *13*, 2580–2601. [CrossRef] [PubMed]
27. Zheng, S.L.; Luo, Q.B.; Suo, S.K.; Zhao, Y.Q.; Chi, C.F.; Wang, B. Preparation, identification, molecular docking study and protective function on HUVECs of novel ACE inhibitory peptides from protein hydrolysate of skipjack tuna muscle. *Mar. Drugs* **2022**, *20*, 176. [CrossRef]

28. Zhang, S.Y.; Zhao, Y.Q.; Wang, Y.M.; Yang, X.R.; Chi, C.F.; Wang, B. Gelatins and antioxidant peptides from Skipjack tuna (*Katsuwonus pelamis*) skins: Purification, characterization, and cytoprotection on ultraviolet-A injured human skin fibroblasts. *Food Biosci.* **2022**, *50*, 102138. [CrossRef]
29. Wang, J.; Wang, Y.M.; Li, L.Y.; Chi, C.F.; Wang, B. Twelve antioxidant peptides from protein hydrolysate of Skipjack tuna (*Katsuwonus pelamis*) roe prepared by flavourzyme: Purification, sequence identification, and activity evaluation. *Front. Nutr.* **2022**, *8*, 813780. [CrossRef]
30. Cai, W.W.; Hu, X.-M.; Wang, Y.M.; Chi, C.F.; Wang, B. Bioactive peptides from skipjack tuna cardiac arterial bulbs: Preparation, identification, antioxidant activity and stability against thermal, pH and simulated gastrointestinal digestion treatments. *Mar. Drugs* **2022**, *20*, 626. [CrossRef] [PubMed]
31. Oh, Y.; Jung, W.K.; Je, J.Y. Protective effect of multifunctional peptides PIISVYWK and FSVVPSPK on oxidative stress-mediated HUVEC injury through antioxidant and anti-apoptotic action. *Process Biochem.* **2023**, *125*, 121–129. [CrossRef]
32. Sakamuru, S.; Zhao, J.; Attene-Ramos, M.S.; Xia, M. Mitochondrial membrane potential assay. *Methods Mol. Biol.* **2022**, *2474*, 11–19. [PubMed]
33. Xin, Z.; Meiyan, F.; Kunbo, W.; Shi, Y.; Xie, X.; Pan, W.; Hu, B.; Wang, Y.; Wen, H.; Wang, K.; et al. Anti-damage effect of theaflavin-3′-gallate from black tea on UVB-irradiated HaCaT cells by photoprotection and maintaining cell homeostasis. *J. Photochem. Photobiol. B* **2021**, *224*, 112304.
34. Lohakul, J.; Chaiprasongsuk, A.; Jeayeng, S.; Saelim, M.; Muanjumpon, P.; Thanachaiphiwat, S.; Tripatara, P.; Soontrapa, K.; Lumlerdkij, N.; Akarasereenont, P.; et al. The protective effect of polyherbal formulation, harak formula, on UVA-induced photoaging of human dermal fibroblasts and mouse skin via promoting Nrf2-regulated antioxidant defense. *Front. Pharmacol.* **2021**, *12*, 649820. [CrossRef] [PubMed]
35. Cai, S.Y.; Wang, Y.M.; Zhao, Y.Q.; Chi, C.F.; Wang, B. Cytoprotective effect of antioxidant pentapeptides from the protein hydrolysate of swim bladders of miiuy croaker (*Miichthys miiuy*) against H_2O_2-mediated human umbilical vein endothelial cell (HUVEC) injury. *Int. J. Mol. Sci.* **2019**, *20*, 5425. [CrossRef] [PubMed]
36. He, F.; Ru, X.; Wen, T. NRF2, a transcription factor for stress response and beyond. *Int. J. Mol. Sci.* **2020**, *21*, 4777. [CrossRef]
37. Bellner, L.; Lebovics, N.B.; Rubinstein, R.; Buchen, Y.D.; Sinatra, E.; Sinatra, G.; Abraham, N.G.; McClung, J.A.; Thompson, E.A. Heme oxygenase-1 upregulation: A novel approach in the treatment of cardiovascular disease. *Antioxid. Redox Signal.* **2020**, *32*, 1045–1060. [CrossRef]
38. Consoli, V.; Sorrenti, V.; Grosso, S.; Vanella, L. Heme oxygenase-1 signaling and redox homeostasis in physiopathological conditions. *Biomolecules* **2021**, *11*, 589. [CrossRef]
39. Chhetri, J.; King, A.E.; Gueven, N. Alzheimer's disease and NQO1: Is there a link? *Curr. Alzheimer Res.* **2018**, *15*, 56–66. [CrossRef]
40. Preethi, S.; Arthiga, K.; Patil, A.B.; Spandana, A.; Jain, V. Review on NAD(P)H dehydrogenase quinone 1 (NQO1) pathway. *Mol. Biol. Rep.* **2022**, *49*, 8907–8924. [CrossRef]
41. Choi, Y.H. Activation of the Nrf2/HO-1 signaling pathway contributes to the protective effects of coptisine against oxidative stress-induced DNA damage and apoptosis in HaCaT keratinocytes. *Gen. Physiol. Biophys.* **2019**, *38*, 281–294. [CrossRef]
42. Tamura, R.; Takada, M.; Sakaue, M.; Yoshida, A.; Ohi, S.; Hirano, K.; Hayakawa, T.; Hirohashi, N.; Yura, K.; Chiba, K. Starfish Apaf-1 activates effector caspase-3/9 upon apoptosis of aged eggs. *Sci. Rep.* **2018**, *8*, 1611. [CrossRef]
43. Wells, G. Peptide and small molecule inhibitors of the Keap1-Nrf2 protein-protein interaction. *Biochem. Soc. Trans.* **2015**, *43*, 674–679. [CrossRef] [PubMed]
44. Aparici, M.; Bravo, M.; Calama, E.; García-González, V.; Domènech, T.; Córdoba, M.; Roger, I.; Cortijo, J.; Góngora-Benítez, M.; Paradís-Bas, M.; et al. Pharmacological characterization of a novel peptide inhibitor of the Keap1-Nrf2 protein-protein interaction. *Biochem. Pharmacol.* **2022**, *204*, 115226. [CrossRef] [PubMed]
45. Padmanabhan, B.; Tong, K.I.; Ohta, T.; Nakamura, Y.; Scharlock, M.; Ohtsuji, M.; Kang, M.I.; Kobayashi, A.; Yokoyama, S.; Yamamoto, M. Structural basis for defects of Keap1 activity provoked by its point mutations in lung cancer. *Mol. Cell.* **2006**, *21*, 689–700. [CrossRef]
46. Lo, S.C.; Li, X.; Henzl, M.T.; Beamer, L.J.; Hannink, M. Structure of the Keap1: Nrf2 interface provides mechanistic insight into Nrf2 signaling. *EMBO J.* **2006**, *25*, 3605–3617. [CrossRef]
47. Suo, S.K.; Zhao, Y.Q.; Wang, Y.M.; Pan, X.Y.; Chi, C.F.; Wang, B. Seventeen novel angiotensin converting enzyme (ACE) inhibitory peptides from protein hydrolysate of *Mytilus edulis*: Isolation, identification, molecular docking study, and protective function on HUVECs. *Food Funct.* **2022**, *13*, 7831–7846. [CrossRef]
48. Zhou, F.; Huang, X.; Pan, Y.; Cao, D.; Liu, C.; Liu, Y.; Chen, A. Resveratrol protects HaCaT cells from ultraviolet B-induced photoaging via upregulation of HSP27 and modulation of mitochondrial caspase-dependent apoptotic pathway. *Biochem. Biophys. Res. Commun.* **2018**, *499*, 662–668. [CrossRef]
49. Kammeyer, A.; Luiten, R.M. Oxidation events and skin aging. *Ageing Res. Rev.* **2015**, *21*, 16–29. [CrossRef] [PubMed]
50. Cui, B.; Wang, Y.; Jin, J.; Yang, Z.; Guo, R.; Li, X.; Yang, L.; Li, Z. Resveratrol treats UVB-induced photoaging by anti-MMP expression, through anti-inflammatory, antioxidant, and antiapoptotic properties, and treats photoaging by upregulating VEGF-B expression. *Oxid. Med. Cell. Longev.* **2022**, *2022*, 6037303. [CrossRef]
51. Zhao, P.; Alam, M.B.; Lee, S.H. Protection of UVB-induced photoaging by Fuzhuan-Brick tea aqueous extract via MAPKs/Nrf2-mediated down-regulation of MMP-1. *Nutrients* **2018**, *11*, 60. [CrossRef] [PubMed]

52. Mostafa, D.K.; Nayel, O.A.; Abdulmalek, S.; Abdelbarym, A.A.; Ismailm, C.A. Modulation of autophagy, apoptosis and oxidative stress: A clue for repurposing metformin in photoaging. *Inflammopharmacology* **2022**, *30*, 2521–2535. [CrossRef] [PubMed]
53. Liu, T.; Xia, Q.; Lv, Y.; Wang, Z.; Zhu, S.; Qin, W.; Yang, Y.; Liu, T.; Wang, X.; Zhao, Z.; et al. ErZhiFormula prevents UV-induced skin photoaging by Nrf2/HO-1/NQO1 signaling: An in vitro and in vivo studies. *J. Ethnopharmacol.* **2022**, 115935, *in press*. [CrossRef]
54. Souto, E.B.; Zielinska, A.; Souto, S.B.; Durazzo, A.; Lucarini, M.; Santini, A.; Silva, A.M.; Atanasov, A.G.; Marques, C.; Andrade, L.N.; et al. (+)-limonene 1,2-epoxide-loaded SLNs: Evaluation of drug release, antioxidant activity, and cytotoxicity in an HaCaT cell line. *Int. J. Mol. Sci.* **2020**, *21*, 1449. [CrossRef] [PubMed]
55. Fu, Y.; Li, C.; Wang, Q.; Gao, R.; Cai, X.; Wang, S.; Zhang, Y. The protective effect of collagen peptides from bigeye tuna (*Thunnus obesus*) skin and bone to attenuate UVB-induced photoaging via MAPK and TGF-β signaling pathways. *J. Funct. Foods* **2022**, *93*, 105101. [CrossRef]
56. Yu, C.; Xiao, J.H. The Keap1-Nrf2 system: A mediator between oxidative stress and aging. *Oxid. Med. Cell. Longev.* **2021**, *2021*, 6635460. [CrossRef]
57. Karmakar, I.; Haldar, S.; Chakraborty, M.; Chaudhury, K.; Dewanjee, S.; Haldar, P.K. Regulation of apoptosis through bcl-2/bax proteins expression and DNA damage by *Zanthoxylum alatum*. *Pharm. Biol.* **2016**, *54*, 503–508. [CrossRef]
58. Wei, M.; Qiu, H.; Zhou, J.; Yang, C.; Chen, Y.; You, L. The anti-photoaging activity of peptides from *Pinctada martensii* meat. *Mar. Drugs* **2022**, *20*, 770. [CrossRef]
59. Zheng, Z.; Xiao, Z.; He, Y.L.; Tang, Y.; Li, L.; Zhou, C.; Hong, P.; Luo, H.; Qian, Z.J. Heptapeptide isolated from *Isochrysis zhanjiangensis* exhibited anti-Photoaging potential via MAPK/AP-1/MMP pathway and anti-apoptosis in UVB-irradiated HaCaT cells. *Mar. Drugs* **2021**, *19*, 626. [CrossRef]
60. Xu, D.; Li, C.; Zhao, M. *Theragra chalcogramma* hydrolysate, rich in Gly-Leu-Pro-Ser-Tyr-Thr, alleviates photoaging via modulating deposition of collagen fibers and restoration of extracellular components matrix in SD rats. *Mar. Drugs* **2022**, *20*, 252. [CrossRef] [PubMed]
61. Peng, Z.; Gao, J.; Su, W.; Cao, W.; Zhu, G.; Qin, X.; Zhang, C.; Qi, Y. Purification and identification of peptides from oyster (*Crassostrea hongkongensis*) protein enzymatic hydrolysates and their anti-skin photoaging effects on UVB-irradiated HaCaT cells. *Mar. Drugs* **2022**, *20*, 749. [CrossRef] [PubMed]
62. Xiao, Z.; Yang, S.; Chen, J.; Li, C.; Zhou, C.; Hong, P.; Sun, S.; Qian, Z. Trehalose against UVB-induced skin photoaging by suppressing MMP expression and enhancing procollagen I synthesis in HaCaT cells. *J. Funct. Foods* **2020**, *74*, 104198. [CrossRef]
63. Zhang, Z.; Wang, Y.M.; Qiu, Y.T.; Chi, C.F.; Luo, H.Y.; Wang, B. Gelatin from cartilage of Siberian sturgeon (Acipenser baerii): Characterization and protective function on ultraviolet-A injured human skin fibroblasts. *Front. Mar. Sci.* **2022**, *9*, 925407. [CrossRef]
64. Hu, X.M.; Wang, Y.M.; Zhao, Y.Q.; Chi, C.F.; Wang, B. Antioxidant peptides from the protein hydrolysate of monkfish (*Lophius litulon*) muscle: Purification, identification, and cytoprotective function on HepG2 cells damage by H_2O_2. *Mar. Drugs* **2020**, *18*, 153. [CrossRef] [PubMed]
65. Wang, Y.Z.; Wang, Y.M.; Pan, X.; Chi, C.F.; Wang, B. Antioxidant mechanisms of the oligopeptides (FWKVV and FMPLH) from muscle hydrolysate of miiuy croaker against oxidative damage of HUVECs. *Oxid. Med. Cell. Longev.* **2021**, *2021*, 9987844. [CrossRef] [PubMed]
66. Zhao, W.H.; Luo, Q.B.; Pan, X.; Chi, C.F.; Sun, K.L.; Wang, B. Preparation, identification, and activity evaluation of ten antioxidant peptides from protein hydrolysate of swim bladders of miiuy croaker (*Miichthys miiuy*). *J. Funct. Foods* **2018**, *47*, 503–511. [CrossRef]
67. Wang, Y.M.; Pan, X.; He, Y.; Chi, C.F.; Wang, B. Hypolipidemic activities of two pentapeptides (VIAPW and IRWWW) from miiuy croaker (*Miichthys miiuy*) muscle on lipid accumulation in HepG2 cells through regulation of AMPK pathway. *Appl. Sci.* **2020**, *10*, 817. [CrossRef]
68. Zhang, Y.; Yan, T.; Sun, D.; Xie, C.; Wang, T.; Liu, X.; Wang, J.; Wang, Q.; Luo, Y.; Wang, P.; et al. Rutaecarpine inhibits KEAP1-NRF2 interaction to activate NRF2 and ameliorate dextran sulfate sodium-induced colitis. *Free Radic. Biol. Med.* **2020**, *148*, 33–41. [CrossRef]
69. Zhu, L.; Xiong, H.; Huang, X.; Guyonnet, V.; Ma, M.; Chen, X.; Zheng, Y.; Wang, L.; Hu, G. Identification and molecular mechanisms of novel antioxidant peptides from two sources of eggshell membrane hydrolysates showing cytoprotection against oxidative stress: A combined in silico and in vitro study. *Food Res. Int.* **2022**, *157*, 111266. [CrossRef]
70. Khalaf, M.M.; Hassan, S.M.; Sayed, A.M.; Abo-Youssefm, A.M. Ameliorate impacts of scopoletin against vancomycin-induced intoxication in rat model through modulation of Keap1-Nrf2/HO-1 and IκBα-P65 NF-κB/P38 MAPK signaling pathways: Molecular study, molecular docking evidence and network pharmacology analysis. *Int. Immunopharmacol.* **2022**, *102*, 108382. [CrossRef]

marine drugs

Article

Identification of Bioactive Peptides from a *Laminaria digitata* Protein Hydrolysate Using In Silico and In Vitro Methods to Identify Angiotensin-1-Converting Enzyme (ACE-1) Inhibitory Peptides

Diane Purcell [1,2,*], Michael A. Packer [2] and Maria Hayes [1]

1 Food BioSciences Department, Teagasc Food Research Centre, Ashtown, Dublin 15, D15 DY05 Dublin, Ireland
2 Cawthron Institute, 98 Halifax Street, Nelson 7010, New Zealand
* Correspondence: dianepurcell651@gmail.com

Abstract: Bioactive peptides range in size from 2–30 amino acids and may be derived from any protein-containing biomass using hydrolysis, fermentation or high-pressure processing. Pro-peptides or cryptides result in shorter peptide sequences following digestion and may have enhanced bioactivity. Previously, we identified a protein hydrolysate generated from *Laminaria digitata* that inhibited ACE-1 in vitro and had an ACE-1 IC_{50} value of 590 μg/mL compared to an ACE-1 IC_{50} value of 500 μg/mL (~2.3 μM) observed for the anti-hypertensive drug Captopril©. A number of peptide sequences (130 in total) were identified using mass spectrometry from a 3 kDa permeate of this hydrolysate. Predicted bioactivities for these peptides were determined using an in silico strategy previously published by this group utilizing available databases including Expasy peptide cutter, BIOPEP and Peptide Ranker. Peptide sequences YIGNNPAKGGLF and IGNNPAKGGLF had Peptide Ranker scores of 0.81 and 0.80, respectively, and were chemically synthesized. Synthesized peptides were evaluated for ACE-1 inhibitory activity in vitro and were found to inhibit ACE-1 by 80 ± 8% and 91 ± 16%, respectively. The observed ACE-1 IC_{50} values for IGNNPAKGGLF and YIGNNPAKGGLF were determined as 174.4 μg/mL and 133.1 μg/mL. Both peptides produced sequences following simulated digestion with the potential to inhibit Dipeptidyl peptidase IV (DPP-IV).

Keywords: *Laminaria digitata*; ACE-1 inhibition; bioactive peptides; protein hydrolysate; brown seaweed; in silico analysis

Citation: Purcell, D.; Packer, M.A.; Hayes, M. Identification of Bioactive Peptides from a *Laminaria digitata* Protein Hydrolysate Using In Silico and In Vitro Methods to Identify Angiotensin-1-Converting Enzyme (ACE-1) Inhibitory Peptides. *Mar. Drugs* **2023**, *21*, 90. https://doi.org/10.3390/md21020090

Academic Editors: Chang-Feng Chi and Bin Wang

Received: 12 December 2022
Revised: 16 January 2023
Accepted: 17 January 2023
Published: 27 January 2023

1. Introduction

Bioactive peptides are sequences of amino acids ranging in size from 2–30 in length providing health benefits beyond basic nutrition when consumed [1]. Health benefits associated with bioactive peptides are extensive and include the reduction of hypertension and associated illnesses such as stroke and heart attack. The bioactive peptide activity pathway is thought to occur through the inhibition of enzymes within the Renin-Angiotensin-Aldosterone-System (RAAS) including Angiotensin-Converting-Enzyme-1 (ACE-1; EC3.4.15.1) and Renin (EC 3.4.23.15) [2–5]. In addition, other potential health benefits associated with bioactive peptides include anti-microbial and anti-inflammatory benefits, prevention of type 2 diabetes (T2D) through inhibition of alpha amylase (EC 3.2.1.1) and dipeptidyl peptidase IV (DPP-IV; EC 3.4.14.5) and inhibition of enzymes such as Prolyloligopeptidase (POP; EC 3.4.21.26) and BACE-1 that may result in mental health benefits. These peptides can be derived from any protein source including non-food sources such as natural protein produced in the gastrointestinal tract, but the most well-recognized sources are dairy, meat and fish [6,7].

Recently, we utilized enzymatic hydrolysis combining the enzymes Viscozyme® and Alcalase® as a method to extract protein from the brown seaweed *Laminaria digitata* [8].

Hydrolysis is a well-known strategy for the generation of bioactive peptides. Hydrolysis may increase the health benefits of protein hydrolysates. Several ACE-1 inhibitory peptides were identified to date from products including cheese, milk and yoghurt. ACE-1 is a zinc metallic protease, which converts Angiotensin I to the potent vasoconstrictor Angiotensin II, and enhances the degradation of the vasodilator Bradykinin [9]. Arterial Hypertension (AHT) is treated using drugs that inhibit the Angiotensin I-Converting Enzyme (ACE-1; EC 3.4.15.1) such as Enalapril® or Captopril© [10–13]. However, side effects associated with these drugs have prompted research for natural remedies that may also treat or prevent the development of high blood pressure [14–17]. Previous studies have shown the ACE-1 and anti-hypertensive activities of the brown seaweeds *Undaria pinnatifida, Sargassum siliquosum and Sargassum polycystum*, [18,19].

In silico analysis is a valuable technique for predicting the potential bioactivities of peptides [3,20–22]. In silico analysis was used recently to identify anti-thrombotic [23–25] peptides from a variety of sources including dairy, mealworms, plants, peas, canola, maize and, more recently, seaweeds [20,26–28]. This approach has not, to the best of the authors' knowledge, been applied to the brown seaweed *Laminaria digitata*.

This paper details the identification of peptides generated through hydrolysis of *Laminaria digitata* protein using enzymes and the characterisation of peptide sequences using mass spectrometry (MS). Subsequently, identified peptide sequences were ranked for potential bioactivities using an in silico approach described herein. One hundred and thirty peptides were identified from the *L. digitata permeates* and two peptides were synthesized. The ACE-1 IC_{50} values of these peptides were subsequently determined.

2. Results

2.1. Identification of Peptides Using Mass Spectrophometery and In Silico Analysis of Sequenced Peptides

A total of 130 peptides were identified from the 3-kDa permeate fraction using mass spectrometry (MS) as shown in Table 1 (n = 3). The identified peptide sequences had a >95% confidence level as being derived from the identified proteins listed in Table 2 and homology was confirmed using UniProt (https://www.uniprot.org/, accessed on 10 December 2022) [29]. Peptides had amino acid sequence homology with proteins from red seaweeds including *Neopyriopia yezoensis, Porphyra umbilicalis* and *Sporolithon durum*, and from the brown seaweeds including *Laminaria digitata; Colpomenia wynnei; Dictyopteris divaricate; Fucus vesiculosus, Ascophyllum nodosum; Sargassum horneri; Ectocarpus siliculosus; Carpomitra costata; Coccophora langsdorfii, Asterocladon rhodochortonoides; Choristocarpus tenellus; Asteronema ferruginea, Cladosiphon okamuranus and Tilopteris* mertensii as well as the red microalga *Porphyridium purpureum*, a marine bacterium *Tamlana fucoidanivorans* and the alpha proteobacteria *Pseudooceanicola algae*. The software programme Peptide Ranker (http://distilldeep.ucd.ie/PeptideRanker/, accessed on 10 December 2022) [30] identified peptides with potential bioactivities. Ten peptides including peptide IGNNPAKGGLF corresponding to amino acid peptide sequence f(315–326) of protein with accession number UniProtKB_Q1XDG4 (PBSS_NCOYE) derived from *Neopyriopia yezoensis* and peptide YIGNNPAKGGLF corresponding to f(314–326) of a protein with accession number UniProtKB_P51322 (PSBB_PORPU) from *Porphyra purpurea* were identified. Peptide DAALDFGPAL derived from the protein OX = 1537215 UniProt KB-A0A4185KT7_9RHOB and peptide AFYDYIGNNPAKGGLF from protein UniProtKB-Q1XDG4 (PSBB_NEOYE), and following peptides, SDGKIFDPL (UniProtKB_A0A6H5TY18 (A0A6H5J418_9PHAE); QGRVPGDIGFDPL (UniProtKB-A0A6HSJUW7_9PHAE); SMSGHPGAPM (UniProtKB_10A6H5L712_9PHAE); SEFIGFPIK (Uni-ProtKB-A0H6H5L026_9PHAE); and the final peptide GDFGNKDGKLTF (Uni-ProtKB-D8LG03) are all listed in Table 1, were identified. Identified peptides varied in length from 9–16 amino acids and had Peptide Ranker scores ranging from 0.64–0.82 (Table 1).

Table 1. Identified peptide sequences from a *Laminaria digitata* protein hydrolysate 3 kDa permeate fraction. These were identified using MS, and the Peptide Ranker score indicates potential bioactivity (a score closer to 1 is indicative of bioactivity).

Cleaved Peptide Sequence	Peptide Ranker Value (Accessed on 10 December 2022), (#)
IGNNPAKGGLF	0.82
YIGNNPAKGGLF	0.81
DAALDFGPAL	0.78
AFYDYIGNNPAKGGLF	0.78
SDGKIFDPL	0.74
YDYIGNNPAKGGLF	0.73
QGRVPGDIGFDPL	0.67
SMSGHPGAPM	0.65
SEFIGFPIK	0.64
GDFGNKDGKLTF	0.64

universal mathematical symbol for a number.

2.1.1. Peptide Ranker

Peptide Ranker (http://distilldeep.ucd.ie/PeptideRanker/, accessed on 24 November 2022) is an open source software resource, which can be used to predict the potential bioactivity of peptides based on a novel N-to-1 neural network. Any user can submit peptides to Peptide Ranker, which will be returned to the user ranked by the probability that the peptide will be bioactive. It is important to note that this is not a prediction of the probability that the peptide has bioactivity [30].

Identified peptide IGNNPAKGGLF had a Peptide Ranker score of 0.82 which was the highest value obtained for any peptide identified using MS from the *L. digitata* 3 kDa permeate. This indicates that this peptide likely has bioactivity. Acceptable probability values for bioactivity are between 1.0–0.5. The peptide YIGNNPAKGGLF had a Peptide Ranker score of 0.81, indicating high potential bioactivity (Table 1). Peptides DAALDFGPAL and AFYDYIGNNPAKGGLF had Peptide ranker scores of 0.78. Peptide SDGKIFDPL had a score of 0.74 (Table 1).

Table 2. Identified peptide sequences and potential bioactivities associated with a *Laminaria digitata* protein hydrolysate 3 kDa permeate fraction identified using MS and in silico analysis.

Parent Protein Name and UniProt Accession Number	Peptide Single Amino Acid Sequence	f(X–X) of Parent Protein	Peptide Ranker Value [1]	Novelty (Found in BIOPEP [2] Database)	Observed Bioactivity	Simulated Digestion Using PeptideCutter [3]/ Peptide Digestion Fragments	Associated Predicted Bioactivities	References
Neopyriopia yezoensis NCBI Taxonomy ID 2788 Photosystem II CP47 reaction centre protein UniProtKB_Q1XDG4 (PBSS_NCOYE)	IGNNPAKGGLF	f(315–326)	0.82	Novel	ACE-1 inhibition	IGNNPAK; GGL; F	(GGL) Antimicrobial activity; Alpha-glucosidase inhibition	[31]
Porphyra purpurea NCBI Taxonomy ID P51322 Photosystem II CP47 reaction centre protein UniProtKB_P51322 (PSBB_PORPU)	YIGNNPAKGGLF	f(314–326)	0.81	Novel	ACE-1 inhibition	Y; IGNNPAK; GGL; F	Antimicrobial; Alpha-glucosidase inhibition	[31]
Pseudooceanicola algae OX = 1537215 UniProt KB-A0A4185KT7_9RHOB	DAALDFGPAL	f(53–62)	0.78	Novel	ACE-1 inhibition	DAA; L; D; F; GPAL	Antimicrobial	[32]
Neopyropia yezoensis (Susabi-nori) (*Pyropia yezoensis*) UniProtKB-Q1XDG4 (PSBB_NEOYE) Photosystem II CP47 reaction centre protein	AFYDYIGNNPAKGGLF	f(310–325)	0.78	Novel	ACE-1 inhibition	A; F; Y; DY; IGNNPAK; GGL; F	Antimicrobial; Alpha-glucosidase inhibition; ACE inhibitor	[33,34]
Ectocarpus species CCAP UniProtKB_A0A6H5TY18 (A0A6H5J418_9PHAE) LHCP protein	SDGKIFDPL	f(57–65)	0.74	Novel	ACE-1 inhibition	SDGK; I; F; DP; L	Dipeptidyl peptidase IV inhibitor; ACE inhibitor	[35,36]
Neopyropia yezoensis Photosystem II CP47 reaction centre protein PSbB UniProtKB_Q1XDG4	YDYIGNNPAKGGLF	f(312–325)	0.73	Novel	ACE-1 inhibition	Y; DY; IGNNPAK; GGL; F	Alpha glucosidase inhibition; ACE inhibitor; Antimicrobial	[31,34]
Ectocarpus sp. CCAP 1310/34 Uncharacterised protein UniProtKB-A0A6HSJUW7_9PHAE	QGRVPGDIGFDPL	f(151–163)	0.67	Novel	ACE-1 inhibition	QGR; VPGDIG; F; D; PL	Antimicrobial (QGR); ACE inhibitor; (PL) ACE inhibitor	[37–39]

Table 2. *Cont.*

Parent Protein Name and UniProt Accession Number	Peptide Single Amino Acid Sequence	f(X–X) of Parent Protein	Peptide Ranker Value [1]	Novelty (Found in BIOPEP [2] Database)	Observed Bioactivity	Simulated Digestion Using PeptideCutter [3]/ Peptide Digestion Fragments	Associated Predicted Bioactivities	References
Ectocarpus sp. CCAP 131-/34 Transketolase_1_domain containing protein UniProtKB_10A6H5L712_9PHAE	SMSGHPGAPM	f(37–46)	0.65	Novel	ACE-1 inhibition	SM; SGHPGAPM	DPP-III inhibitor (SM)	[40]
Ectocarpus sp. CCAP 131/34 HSP90 protein UniProtKB-A0H6H5L026_9PHAE	SEFIGFPIK	f(208–216)	0.64	Novel	ACE-1 inhibition	SE; F; IGF; PIK	Anti-inflammatory (IGF); Antimicrobial (PIK); Stimulating vasoactive substance release (SE)	[41,42]
Ectocarpus siliculosus (Brown algae) Manganese stabilising protein UniProtKB-D8LG03	GDFGNKDGKLTF	f(161–172)	0.64	Novel	ACE-1 inhibition	GD; F; GNK; DGK; L; TF	ACE inhibitor (GD); Fibrinogen interaction inhibitor (GNK-part of a peptide called Arietin); ACE inhibitor (TF)	[43–45]

[1] http://distilldeep.ucd.ie/PeptideRanker/, accessed on 10 December 2022, [2] https://biochemia.uwm.edu.pl/biopep-uwm/, accessed on 10 December 2022, [3] software http://web.expasy.org/peptide_cutter/, accessed on 10 December 2022.

2.1.2. BIOPEP

A search of the BIOPEP database (https://biochemia.uwm.edu.pl/biopep-uwm/, accessed on 10 December 2022) [46] determined the novelty of the peptides identified and shown in Table 1. Of the ten peptides analyzed and listed in Table 2, their amino acid sequences were not identified in previously published papers concerning seaweed proteins and bioactive peptides [31–45].

2.1.3. Simulated Digestion Using Peptide Cutter

Peptide cutter software (http://web.expasy.org/peptide_cutter/, accessed on 10 December 2022) [47] was used to determine if the identified peptides could potentially survive GI digestion. Peptides shown in Table 1 underwent simulated digestion using the GI tract enzymes, pepsin (pH 1.3), trypsin, and chymotrypsin. All peptides were cleaved into shorter peptide fragments that in some instances had known bioactivities and are found in BIOPEP (Table 2). Simulated GI digestion of the 10 peptides shown in Table 1 produced smaller peptides such as the active peptide GGL (derived following GI simulated digestion from YIGNNPAKGGLF). GGL is an active fragment, is a known anti-microbial peptide found in BIOPEP and it also has alpha-glucosidase inhibitory activities seen previously in Iberian dry-cured ham [31]. Peptides associated with other bioactivities include DPP-IV inhibition for monopeptides I, L; ACE-1 inhibition for dipeptides GD, TF, DP [35,36,43–45]. The monopeptide F, is a hydrophobic aromatic, amino acid, and it is thought, to enhance anti-oxidant activity [31]. Peptide IGNNPAKGGLF was digested into 3 peptides with sequences of IGNNPAK; GG and F. When comparing the first two peptides sequences listed in Table 2, the monopeptide Y, was one of two differing peptides. This monopeptide, Y, is hydrophobic, an aromatic amino acid, with anti-oxidant and anti-microbial bioactivity [31–33].

Several bioactive peptides also result from simulated GI digestion of the peptide DAALDFGPAL. Following simulated GI digestion the peptides DAA and GPAL result. DAA is a known antimicrobial peptide sequence found in the peptide tenecin 1, an insect defensin peptide [32]. The dipeptide DY results from simulated digestion of AFYDYIGNNPAKGGLF. This dipeptide is a known ACE-1 inhibitory peptide [34].

Simulated GI digestion of peptide SDGKIFDPL produces peptides SDGK and DP. The dipeptide DP identified previously from the dark muscle of tuna is a known ACE-1 inhibitor that also has anti-hypertensive activity shown in rat studies previously [36].

The peptide QGR occurs following simulated GI digestion of QGRVPGDIGFDPL. This tripeptide has known anti-microbial activity [37]. The peptide PL results following simulated GI digestion of YDYIGNNPAKGGLF. This tripeptide has known anti-microbial activity, and PL is also an ACE-1 inhibitor [37,38].

2.1.4. Toxicity Assessment Using In Silico Analysis

All 130 peptides identified using MS were assessed for their potential to be toxic using ToxinPred (https://webs.iiitd.edu.in/raghava/toxinpred2/batch.html, accessed on 10 December 2022) [48]. Of the 130 peptides, tested results indicate that no peptides have potential toxicity.

2.1.5. Peptide Synthesis and ACE-1 Inhibition

The peptides IGNNPAKGGLF and YIGNNPAKGGLF were synthesized and assessed in vitro for their ability to inhibit ACE-1. The peptide IGNNPAKGGLF was found to inhibit ACE-1 by 80% and YIGNNPAKGGLF inhibited ACE-1 by 91% when assayed at a concentration of 1 mg/mL compared to the control Captopril® assayed at a concentration of 0.05 mg/mL. The ACE-1 IC_{50} values determined for both peptides were 174.4 μg/mL and 133.1 μg/mL for IGNNPAKGGLF and YIGNNPAKGGLF, respectively.

3. Discussion

Ten different peptide sequences were identified from the *L. digitata* protein 3 kDa permeate using MS. The ACE-1 inhibitory activity of two of these peptides was confirmed using chemical synthesis and assessment in vitro for ACE-1 inhibition. Additionally, other bioactivities were predicted using in silico methods. The MS-sequenced peptides ranged in length from 9–15 amino acids. All identified peptides were novel based on a search of the BIOPEP database and the literature. Peptide Ranker values were obtained for all peptides and the peptides likely to have bioactivities are shown in Table 1. These peptides had Peptide Ranker values greater than 0.5.

Two peptides, with Peptide Ranker scores of 0.82 and 0.81 were selected for chemical synthesis. ACE-1 inhibition values were determined in vitro for these peptides with amino acid sequences IGNNPAKGGLF and YIGNNPAKGGLF. ACE-1 and IC_{50} results for these synthesized peptides were obtained. Peptide IGNNPAKGGLF inhibited ACE-1 by 80% and YIHNNPAKGGLF inhibited ACE-1 by 91% when assayed at 1 mg/mL. The ACE-1 IC_{50} value for IGNNPAKGGLF was 174.4 μg/mL (0.161 μM) ACE-1. Peptide YIGNNPAKGGLF had an IC_{50} value of 133.1 μg/mL (0.11 μM) compared to Captopril© with a documented ACE-1 IC_{50} value of 500 μg/mL (2.3 μM) [8]. Previous studies on marine cryptides, used Captopril© as a positive control with IC_{50} values of (1.79–15.1 nM) for ACE-1, and another drug Losartan was used as a negative control for ACE-II inhibition, and had IC_{50} values of (17.13–146 μM) [49]. The IC_{50} for Captopril© varies depending on application and extraction methods used, with an IC_{50} of 7.09 nM from visible spectrophotometric (VSP) and for high-performance liquid chromatography (HPLC), and an IC_{50} of 4.94 nM [50]. Common hypertensive drugs, using the ACE-1 mechanism of control include Captopril©, Enalapril, Tekturna and Rasilez [51].

Peptides with ACE-1 IC_{50} values ranging from 2.42–20.63 μM [52] were identified from protein hydrolysates generated from *Laminaria japonica* previously. The IC_{50} values obtained for our synthesized peptides are greater than ACE-1 IC_{50} values reported previously for peptides such as HR, extracted from a bovine hydrolysate with an ACE-1 IC_{50} of 0.19 mM [51]. The ACE-1 inhibitory activity of the synthesized peptides is greater than the value reported for the *L. digitata* hydrolysate and shows the potential of these peptides for potential use in the treatment of hypertension.

Simulated GI digestion increased the potential bioactivities of identified peptides and several peptides with alpha-glucosidase and anti-microbial activities were found. Inhibition of alpha-glucosidase reduces carbohydrate digestion, consequently decreasing carbohydrate content in blood, which improves human health outcomes regarding type 2 diabetes [31,53]. The dipeptide sequence SE, cleaved from the novel peptide SEFIGFPIK (shown in Table 2), has potential stimulating vasoactive substance release bioactivity, discovered in peptides sourced from casein and soy protein previously [43,53]. The anti-inflammatory peptide sequence IGF also results from the GI digestion of SEFIGFPIK. This tripeptide is found in the pepsin hydrolysis of hempseed protein [42]. The peptide GNK that is cleaved from sequenced peptide GDFGNKDGKLTF is found in the Arietin peptide-A known as Fibrinogen interaction inhibitor. The dipeptide TF is also cleaved from the same sequenced peptide and is a known ACE-1 inhibitor [43–45].

This work identified two novel ACE-1 inhibitory peptides with pharmaceutically relevant ACE-1 IC_{50} values. In addition, the array of bioactive peptides that result following simulated GI digestion demonstrates the potential bioactivities still to be harnessed from brown seaweed proteins in *L. digitata*.

Additional bioactivities were also identified from cryptides identified following simulated gastrointestinal (GI) digestion. These bioactivities included Dipeptidyl peptidase IV (DPP-IV) inhibition potential for peptide sequences SDGK and alpha-glucosidase inhibition potential of peptides GGL and IGNNPAK. Future work will involve the synthesis of these peptides and determination of their in vitro inhibitory activities as well as the determination of their relevant IC_{50} values. Inhibitors of DPP-IV and alpha-glucosidase enzymes are the key targets for the pharmaceutical sector for development of drugs to prevent or to control type 2 diabetes [T2D].

4. Materials and Methods

4.1. Mass Spectrophotometry (MS) Characterisation of 3kDa Permeates

Protein extraction and peptide enrichment using molecular weight cut-off (MWCO) filtration was performed prior to MS characterisation in accordance with the method outlined in [8].

Peptide fractions were prepared for MS characterisation using the Phoenix peptide clean-up kit 4X, manufactured by Peromics and following the clean-up method supplied by the manufacturer. Peptides were identified using a mass spectrometer nanoESI qQTOF (6600 plus TripleTOF, AB SCIEX, Framingham, MA, U.S.A.) using liquid chromatography and tandem mass spectrometry (LC–MS/MS). A total of 1 µL of microalgal permeate was loaded onto a trap column (3 µ C18-CL 120 Ǎ, 350 µM × 0.5 mm; Eksigent) and desalted with 0.1% TFA (trifluoroacetic acid) at 5 µL/min for 5 min. The peptides were then loaded onto an analytical column (3 µ C18-CL 120 Ǎ, 0.075 × 150 mm; Eksigent) equilibrated in 5% acetonitrile 0.1% FA (formic acid). Elution was carried out with a linear gradient from 7 to 45% B in A for 20 min, where solvent A was 0.1% FA and solvent B was ACN (acetonitrile) with 0.1% FA at a flow rate of 300 nL/min. The sample was ionized in an electrospray source Optiflow < 1 µL Nano applying 3.0 kV to the spray emitter at 200 °C. Analysis was carried out in a data-dependent mode. Survey MS1 scans were acquired from 350 to 1400 m/z for 250 ms. The quadrupole resolution was set to 'LOW' for MS2 experiments, which were acquired from 100 to 1500 m/z for 25 ms in 'high sensitivity' mode. Up to 50 ions were selected for fragmentation after each survey 400 scan. Dynamic exclusion was set to 15 s. The system sensitivity was controlled by analyz-401 ing 500 ng of K562 protein extract digest (SCIEX); in these conditions, 2260 proteins were identified (FDR < 1%) in a 45 min gradient. Peptides identified as having potential bioactivities were chemically synthesised by GenScript Biotech (Leiden, The Netherlands). GenScript also verified the purity of the peptides by analytical RP-HPLC–MS.

4.2. In Silico Analysis of MS Sequenced Peptides

Peptide Ranker was used to predict the bioactivity of peptide sequences and values of between 0.5 and 1 were taken as indicative of peptides having bioactivity.

Figure 1 shows the six steps used during in silico analysis. Of the 130 peptides identified using MS, only those with >95% confidence were selected for synthesis and in silico analysis. Selected peptides were input into the software programme Peptide Ranker (http://distilldeep.ucd.ie/PeptideRanker/, accessed on 15 December 2022). A value indicative of potential bioactivity was obtained for each peptide. Only peptides with Peptide Ranker scores greater than 0.5 were used in further analysis. Ten peptide sequences were identified as having potential bioactivities. The novelty of these peptides was determined following a search in the peptide database BIOPEP (http://www.uwm.edu.pl/biochemia/index.php/pl/biopep, accessed on 12 December 2022). Active peptides were further assessed for their ability to survive simulated GI digestion using Expasy peptide cutter (http://web.expasy.org/peptide_cutter/, accessed on 10 December 2022). The UniProt database was used to identify proteins containing the peptide sequences. Additionally, the potential toxicity of identified peptides was assessed using the software programme ToxinPred (https://webs.iiitd.edu.in/raghava/toxinpred2/batch.html, accessed on 10 December 2022).

I **Analysis of peptide sequences with >95% confidence intervals:**
To select the most suitable, potentially bioactive peptides of the total 130 generated from the original protein hydrolysate only those that fall with >95% confidence intervals were selected for *in silico* analysis.

II **Assess the peptide sequence in Peptide Ranker:**
http://distilldeep.ucd.ie/PeptideRanker/
The selected peptides are then inputted into the Peptide Ranker software, which enables an initial bioranker score to be generated. Bioranker scores of >0.5 generated are considered to have potential bioactivity which requires then further analysis.

III **Input peptide sequences ranked in Peptide Ranker in BIOPEP to determine if sequences are novel:**
http://www.uwm.edu.pl/biochemia/index.php/pl/biopep
The purpose of using this uwm database is, it allows comparisons to be made with known and unknown sequences which have previously shown bioactivity. This database allows, a list of potential bioactivities is generated for each peptide sequence analysed.

IV **Insert peptide sequences into Expasy Peptide Cutter to determine if peptides survive GI digestion:**
http://web.expasy.org/peptide_cutter/ **then select the following enzymes pepsin; trypsin; chemotrypsin.**
The peptide cutter database enables a selected set of enzymes by the user to virtually cut the peptides where the GI system would typically act of each peptide. The creates virtually cleaved peptides from each sequence analysed

V **Assess sequences in UniProt database:**
Add sequences to UniProt: https//www.uniprot.org/ **if sequence identified within the parent protein then mark where it sits within the parent protein and will also list whether it is a novel sequence.**
The cleaved peptides as a product of the peptide cutter analysis enables a database search to be conducted of known and unknown peptides. This allows any novel peptide sequences to be identified, from the cleaved sequences inputted based on the peptide cutter analysis.

VI **Assess potential toxicity:**
Add sequence into this webpage https://webs.iiitd.edu.in/raghava/toxinpred2/batch.html
The goal of the majority of these peptides is for potential use within the food of pharmaceutical industry which will require human consumption, therefore it is vital that any possible toxicity that may be present within these peptides is tested for virtually, prior to any potential in-vivo trials takes place.

Figure 1. In silico methodology based on the method by Lafarga et al. 2014, Hayes et al., 2018, and Hayes et al., 2021 [3,6,7] was used for the identification and generation of ACE-I inhibitory peptides from *L. digitata* proteins. Information including the structure, amino acid sequence and composition of the proteins was collected. Peptide Ranker; BIOPEP; Expasy PeptideCutter Tool; UniProt and ToxinPred were used on the peptide sequences. Peptide Ranker and BIOPEP ranked the potentially most bioactive sequences and identified the bioactivities of these peptides. Expasy PeptideCutter Tool was used to predict the probable cleavage sites of selected enzymes within the top ten sequences listed in Table 1. ToxinPred was used for predicting the toxicity of peptides identified in this project.

4.3. ACE-1 Inhibitory Activity Assessment

The peptides with the highest Peptide Ranker scores IGNNPAKGGLF, with a peptide ranker value of 0.82, and YIGNNPAKGGLF, with a value of 0.81,were selected for synthesis. Once made, peptides were re-tested using in vitro screening assays. ACE-1 activity was tested using an assay kit supplied by Cambridge BioSciences (Cambridge, UK) as described previously. Captopril© (a known ACE-1 inhibitor) dissolved in distilled water was used as a positive control.

5. Conclusions

In silico and in vitro methods are useful tools for selection of enzymes to generate bioactive peptides from protein containing biomass. Moreover, they are useful to determine potential bioactivities of peptides prior to chemical synthesis and can save time and money prior to animal studies to determine potential health benefits. A combination of these methods was used previously to identify and confirm the bioactivity of peptides derived from blood proteins [51] and microalgae previously [54]. However, limitations of this approach exist and specifically include limits concerning the folding of protein, which has an impact on how enzymes cut the protein and which in turn can impact production of the resulting peptides. One of the main barriers for entering the human functional foods market is unknown and unstable peptide product qualities. It is required to have analytical methods for characterising the peptide fraction. Today, research groups are using Fourier-transform Infrared (FTIR) fingerprints to gain new insight in quality variations of peptide products. These fingerprints can be related to raw material composition and processing factors [55]. The method used in this study has advantages over in vitro only methods as it can help to predict the best enzymes to use to generate bioactive peptide containing hydrolysates and additionally can predict the most bioactive peptides and those that may be toxic before any in vitro assays are performed.

Two novel ACE-1 inhibitory peptides with amino acid sequences corresponding to IGNNPAKGGLF and YIGNNPAKGGLF were identified from a 3 kDa permeate of a protein hydrolysate generated from the brown seaweed *L. digitata*. In silico methods also predicted the potential of this seaweed as a source of novel, bioactive peptides that may impart additional health benefits to the consumer including prevention of T2D and antimicrobial activities following GI digestion. Identified, chemically synthesized peptides had ACE-1 inhibition IC_{50} values of 174.4 μg/mL (0.161 μM) for peptide IGNNPAKGGLF and 133.1 μg/mL (0.107 μM) for peptide YIGNNPAKGGLF and both peptides were similar in terms of bioactivity to other ACE-1 inhibitory peptides identified from tuna and meat muscle previously. This study highlights the potential bioactivity of this brown seaweed. However, future work is required to confirm an anti-hypertensive effect of the seaweed hydrolysate and synthesized peptides in vivo. This work will involve assessment of the *L. digitata* hydrolysate and synthesized peptides in spontaneously hypertensive rats (SHRs) to assess if the ACE-1 inhibitory peptides have an anti-hypertensive effect in vivo.

Author Contributions: Conceptualization, M.H., D.P. and M.A.P.; methodology, M.H.; software, D.P.; validation, M.H., D.P. and M.A.P.; formal analysis, D.P.; investigation, D.P.; resources, D.P.; data curation, D.P.; writing—original draft preparation, D.P.; writing—review and editing, M.H., D.P. and M.A.P.; visualization, D.P.; supervision, M.H. and M.A.P.; project administration, D.P.; funding acquisition, D.P. All authors have read and agreed to the published version of the manuscript.

Funding: Diane Purcell-Meyerink, also known as Diane Purcell, has received funding from the Teagasc Research Leaders 2025 programme co-funded by Teagasc and the European Union's Horizon 2020 research and innovation programme under the Marie Skłodowska-Curie grant agreement number 754380.

Data Availability Statement: Data are available from the corresponding author.

Acknowledgments: The author would like to acknowledge the technical support of Karen Hussey at Teagasc for her assistance in sample analysis.

Conflicts of Interest: The authors declare no conflict of interest.

References

1. Ondetti, M.F.; Cushman, D.W. Enzymes of the renin-angiotensin system and their inhibitors. *Annu. Rev. Biochem.* **1982**, *51*, 283–308. [CrossRef]
2. He, Z.; Liu, G.; Qiao, Z.; Cao, Y.; Song, M. Novel Angiotensin-I Converting Enzyme Inhibitory Peptides Isolated from Rice Wine Lees: Purification, Characterization, and Structure-Activity Relationship. *Front. Nutr.* **2021**, *8*, 746113. [CrossRef]
3. Lafarga, T.; O'Connor, P.; Hayes, M. Identification of novel dipeptidyl peptidase-IV and angiotensin-I-converting enzyme inhibitory peptides from meat proteins using in silico analysis. *Peptides* **2014**, *59*, 53–62. [CrossRef]
4. Goossens, G.H. The Renin-Angiotensin System in the Pathophysiology of Type 2 Diabetes. *Obes. Facts* **2012**, *5*, 611–624. [CrossRef]
5. Wang, Y.; Tikellis, C.; Thomas, M.C.; Golledge, J. Angiotensin converting enzyme 2 and atherosclerosis. *Atherosclerosis* **2013**, *226*, 3–8. [CrossRef]
6. Hayes, M. Food Proteins and Bioactive Peptides: New and Novel Sources, Characterisation Strategies and Applications. *Foods* **2018**, *7*, 38. [CrossRef] [PubMed]
7. Hayes, M. Bioactive Peptides in Preventative Healthcare: An Overview of Bioactivities and Suggested Methods to Assess Potential Applications. *Curr. Pharm. Des.* **2021**, *27*, 1332–1341. [CrossRef] [PubMed]
8. Purcell, D.; Packer, M.A.; Hayes, M. Angiotensin-I-Converting Enzyme Inhibitory Activity of Protein Hydrolysates Generated from the Macroalga Laminaria digitata (Hudson) JV Lamouroux 1813. *Foods* **2022**, *11*, 1792. [CrossRef] [PubMed]
9. Soffer, R.L. Angiotensin-Converting Enzyme and the Regulation of Vasoactive Peptides. *Annu. Rev. Biochem.* **1976**, *45*, 73–94. [CrossRef] [PubMed]
10. Julius, S.; Nesbitt, S.D.; Egan, B.M.; Weber, M.A.; Michelson, E.L.; Kaciroti, N.; Black, H.R.; Grimm, R.H.; Messerli, F.H.; Oparil, S.; et al. Feasibility of treating prehypertension with an angiotensin-receptor blocker. *N. Engl. J. Med.* **2006**, *354*, 1685–1697. [CrossRef]

11. Bhuyan, B.J.; Mugesh, G. Synthesis, characterization and antioxidant activity of angiotensin converting enzyme inhibitors. *Org. Biomol. Chem.* **2011**, *9*, 1356–1365. [CrossRef] [PubMed]
12. Osterziel, K.J.; Dietz, R.; Harder, K.; Kübler, W. Comparison of captopril with enalapril in the treatment of heart failure: Influence on hemodynamics and measures of renal function. *Cardiovasc. Drugs Ther.* **1992**, *6*, 173–180. [CrossRef] [PubMed]
13. Alan, S.L.A.; Yu, M.B.; Chir, B. Renovascular Hypertension and Ischemic Nephropathy. In *Brenner & Rector's the Kidney*; Chertow, G., Luyckx, V., Marsden, P., Skorecki, K., Maarten, M., Yu, A., Eds.; Elsevier, Inc.: Philadelphia, PA, USA, 2020; pp. 1580–1621.
14. Lordan, S.; Ross, R.P.; Stanton, C. Marine bioactives as functional food ingredients: Potential to reduce the incidence of chronic diseases. *Mar. Drugs* **2011**, *9*, 1056–1100. [CrossRef] [PubMed]
15. Wijesekara, I.; Kim, S.-K. Angiotensin-I-converting enzyme (ACE) inhibitors from marine resources: Prospects in the pharmaceutical industry. *Mar. Drugs* **2010**, *8*, 1080–1093. [CrossRef]
16. Seca, A.M.L.; Pinto, D.C.G.A. Overview on the Antihypertensive and Anti-Obesity Effects of Secondary Metabolites from Seaweeds. *Mar. Drugs* **2018**, *16*, 237. [CrossRef] [PubMed]
17. Pujiastuti, D.Y.; Ghoyatul Amin, M.N.; Alamsjah, M.A.; Hsu, J.-L. Marine Organisms as Potential Sources of Bioactive Peptides that Inhibit the Activity of Angiotensin I-Converting Enzyme: A Review. *Molecules* **2019**, *24*, 2541. [CrossRef]
18. Nagappan, H.; Pee, P.P.; Kee, S.H.Y.; Ow, J.T.; Yan, S.W.; Chew, L.Y.; Kong, K.W. Malaysian brown seaweeds Sargassum siliquosumnand Sargassum polycystum: Low density lipoprotein (LDL) oxidation, angiotensin converting enzyme (ACE)—Amylase, and-glucosidase inhibition activities. *Food Res. Int.* **2017**, *99 Pt 2*, 950–958. [CrossRef]
19. Hata, Y.; Nakajima, K.; Uchida, J.-I.; Hidaka, H.; Nakano, T. Clinical Effects of Brown Seaweed, *Undaria pinnatifida* (wakame) on Blood Pressure in Hypertensive Subjects. *J. Clin. Biochem. Nutr.* **2001**, *30*, 43–53. [CrossRef]
20. Vermeirssen, V.; van der Bent, A.; Van Camp, J.; van Amerongen, A.; Verstraete, W. A quantitative in silico analysis calculates the angiotensin I converting enzyme (ACE) inhibitory activity in pea and whey protein digests. *Biochimie* **2004**, *86*, 231–239. [CrossRef]
21. Udenigwe, C.C.; Gong, M.; Wu, S. In silico analysis of the large and small subunits of cereal RuBisCO as precursors of cryptic bioactive peptides. *Process Biochem.* **2013**, *48*, 1794–1799. [CrossRef]
22. Hashemi, Z.S.; Zarei, M.; Fath, M.K.; Ganji, M.; Farahani, M.S.; Afsharnouri, F.; Pourzardosht, N.; Khalesi, B.; Jahangiri, A.; Rahbar, M.R.; et al. In silico Approaches for the Design and Optimization of Interfering Peptides Against Protein–Protein Interactions. *Front. Mol. Biosci.* **2021**, *8*, 669431. [CrossRef] [PubMed]
23. Chen, F.; Jiang, H.; Lu, Y.; Chen, W.; Huang, G. Identification and in silico analysis of anti-thrombotic peptides from the enzymatic hydrolysates of Tenebrio molitor larvae. *Eur. Food Res. Technol.* **2019**, *245*, 2687–2695. [CrossRef]
24. Zengin, G.; Stefanucci, A.; Rodrigues, M.J.; Mollica, A.; Custodio, L.; Aumeeruddy, M.Z.; Mahomoodally, M.F. Scrophularia lucida L. as a valuable source of bioactive compounds for pharmaceutical applications: In vitro anti-oxidant, anti-inflammatory, enzyme inhibitory properties, in silico studies, and HPLC profiles. *J. Pharm. Biomed. Anal.* **2019**, *162*, 225–233. [CrossRef] [PubMed]
25. Hayes, M.; Stanton, C.; Slattery, H.; O'Sullivan, O.; Hill, C.; Fitzgerald, G.F.; Ross, R.P. Casein fermentate of Lactobacillus animalis DPC6134 contains a range of novel propeptide angiotensin-converting enzyme inhibitors. *Appl. Environ. Microbiol.* **2007**, *73*, 4658–4667. [CrossRef] [PubMed]
26. Cian, R.E.; Nardo, A.E.; Garzón, A.G.; Añon, M.C.; Drago, S.R. Identification and in silico study of a novel dipeptidyl peptidase IV inhibitory peptide derived from green seaweed Ulva spp. hydrolysates. *LWT* **2022**, *154*, 112738. [CrossRef]
27. Díaz-Gómez, J.L.; Neundorf, I.; López-Castillo, L.-M.; Castorena-Torres, F.; Serna-Saldívar, S.O.; García-Lara, S. In Silico Analysis and In Vitro Characterization of the Bioactive Profile of Three Novel Peptides Identified from 19 kDa α-Zein Sequences of Maize. *Molecules* **2020**, *25*, 5405. [CrossRef]
28. Duan, X.; Zhang, M.; Chen, F. Prediction and analysis of anti-microbial peptides from rapeseed protein using in silico approach. *J. Food Biochem.* **2021**, *45*, e13598. [CrossRef]
29. Consortium, T.U. UniProt: The universal protein knowledgebase in 2021. *Nucleic Acids Res.* **2020**, *49*, D480–D489. [CrossRef] [PubMed]
30. Mooney, C.; Haslam, N.J.; Pollastri, G.; Shields, D.C. Towards the Improved Discovery and Design of Functional Peptides: Common Features of Diverse Classes Permit Generalized Prediction of Bioactivity. *PLoS ONE* **2012**, *7*, e45012. [CrossRef]
31. Mora, L.; González-Rogel, D.; Heres, A.; Toldrá, F. Iberian dry-cured ham as a potential source of α-glucosidase-inhibitory peptides. *J. Funct. Foods* **2020**, *67*, 103840. [CrossRef]
32. Ren, J.; Zhao, M.; Shi, J.; Wang, J.; Jiang, Y.; Cui, C.; Kakuda, Y.; Xue, S.J. Purification and identification of anti-oxidant peptides from grass carp muscle hydrolysates by consecutive chromatography and electrospray ionization-mass spectrometry. *Food Chem.* **2008**, *108*, 727–736. [CrossRef] [PubMed]
33. Rajapakse, N.; Mendis, E.; Byun, H.-G.; Kim, S.-K. Purification and in vitro anti-oxidative effects of giant squid muscle peptides on free radical-mediated oxidative systems. *J. Nutr. Biochem.* **2005**, *16*, 562–569. [CrossRef]
34. Ziganshin, R.H.; Svieryaev, V.I.; Vas'kovskiĭ, B.V.; Mikhaleva, I.I.; Ivanov, V.T.; Kokoz, Y.M.; Alekseev, A.E.; Korystova, A.F.; Sukhova, G.S.; Emel'ianova, T.G.; et al. Biologically active peptides isolated from the brain of hibernating ground squirrels. *Bioorg. Khim.* **1994**, *20*, 899–918.
35. Wu, J.; Aluko, R.E.; Nakai, S. Structural requirements of Angiotensin I-converting enzyme inhibitory peptides: Quantitative structure-activity relationship study of di- and tripeptides. *J. Agric. Food Chem.* **2006**, *54*, 732–738. [CrossRef] [PubMed]

36. Lan, V.T.; Ito, K.; Ohno, M.; Motoyama, T.; Ito, S.; Kawarasaki, Y. Analyzing a dipeptide library to identify human dipeptidyl peptidase IV inhibitor. *Food Chem.* **2015**, *175*, 66–73. [CrossRef]
37. Qian, Z.J.; Je, J.Y.; Kim, S.K. Anti-hypertensive effect of angiotensin i converting enzyme-inhibitory peptide from hydrolysates of Bigeye tuna dark muscle, *Thunnus obesus*. *J Agric. Food Chem.* **2007**, *55*, 8398–8403. [CrossRef] [PubMed]
38. Byun, H.G.; Kim, S.K. Structure and activity of angiotensin I converting enzyme inhibitory peptides derived from Alaskan pollack skin. *J. Biochem. Mol. Biol.* **2002**, *35*, 239–243. [CrossRef]
39. Nogata, Y.; Nagamine, T.; Yanaka, M.; Ohta, H. Angiotensin I Converting Enzyme Inhibitory Peptides Produced by Autolysis Reactions from Wheat Bran. *J. Agric. Food Chem.* **2009**, *57*, 6618–6622. [CrossRef]
40. Forghani, B.; Zarei, M.; Ebrahimpour, A.; Philip, R.; Bakar, J.; Abdul Hamid, A.; Saari, N. Purification and characterization of angiotensin converting enzyme-inhibitory peptides derived from Stichopus horrens: Stability study against the ACE and inhibition kinetics. *J. Funct. Foods* **2016**, *20*, 276–290. [CrossRef]
41. Dhanda, S.; Singh, J.; Singh, H. Hydrolysis of various bioactive peptides by goat brain dipeptidylpeptidase-III homologue. *Cell Biochem. Funct.* **2008**, *26*, 339–345. [CrossRef]
42. Cruz-Chamorro, I.; Santos-Sánchez, G.; Bollati, C.; Bartolomei, M.; Li, J.; Arnoldi, A.; Lammi, C. Hempseed (*Cannabis sativa*) Peptides WVSPLAGRT and IGFLIIWV Exert Anti-inflammatory Activity in the LPS-Stimulated Human Hepatic Cell Line. *J. Agric. Food Chem.* **2022**, *70*, 577–583. [CrossRef] [PubMed]
43. Ringseis, R.; Matthes, B.; Lehmann, V.; Becker, K.; Schöps, R.; Ulbrich-Hofmann, R.; Eder, K. Peptides and hydrolysates from casein and soy protein modulate the release of vasoactive substances from human aortic endothelial cells. *Biochim. Biophys. Acta* **2005**, *1721*, 89–97. [CrossRef]
44. Cheung, H.-S.; Wang, F.-L.; Ondetti, M.A.; Sabo, E.F.; Cushman, D.W. Binding of peptide substrates and inhibitors of angiotensin-converting enzyme. Importance of the COOH-terminal dipeptide sequence. *J. Biol. Chem.* **1980**, *255*, 401–407. [PubMed]
45. Huang, T.F.; Holt, J.C.; Lukasiewicz, H.; Niewiarowski, S. A low molecular weight peptide inhibiting fibrinogen interaction with platelet receptors expressed on glycoprotein IIb-IIIa complex. *J. Biol. Chem.* **1987**, *262*, 16157–16163. [CrossRef]
46. Minkiewicz, P.; Iwaniak, A.; Darewicz, M. BIOPEP-UWM Database of Bioactive Peptides: Current Opportunities. *Int. J. Mol. Sci.* **2019**, *20*, 5978. [CrossRef]
47. Gasteiger, E.; Hoogland, C.; Gattiker, A.; Duvaud, S.E.; Wilkins, M.R.; Appel, R.D.; Bairoch, A. Protein Identification and Analysis Tools on the ExPASy Server. In *The Proteomics Protocols Handbook*; Walker, J.M., Ed.; Humana Press: Totowa, NJ, USA, 2005; pp. 571–607.
48. Gupta, S.; Kapoor, P.; Chaudhary, K.; Gautam, A.; Kumar, R.; Open Source Drug Discovery, C.; Raghava, G.P.S. In Silico Ap-proach for Predicting Toxicity of Peptides and Proteins. *PLoS ONE* **2013**, *8*, e73957. [CrossRef]
49. Henda, Y.B.; Labidi, A.; Arnaudin, I.; Bridiau, N.; Delatouche, R.; Maugard, T.; Piot, J.-M.; Sannier, F.; Thiéry, V.; Bordenave-Juchereau, S. Measuring Angiotensin-I Converting Enzyme Inhibitory Activity by Micro Plate Assays: Comparison Using Marine Cryptides and Tentative Threshold Determinations with Captopril and Losartan. *J. Agr. Food Chem.* **2013**, *61*, 10685–10690. [CrossRef]
50. Chen, J.; Wang, Y.R.; Wu, Y.; Xia, W. Comparison of analytical methods to assay inhibitors of angiotensin I-converting enzyme. *Food Chem.* **2013**, *141*, 3329–3334. [CrossRef]
51. Lafarga, T.; Rai, D.K.; O'Connor, P.; Hayes, M. Generation of Bioactive Hydrolysates and Peptides from Bovine Hemoglobin with In Vitro Renin, Angiotensin-I-Converting Enzyme and Dipeptidyl Peptidase-IV Inhibitory Activities. *J. Food Biochem.* **2016**, *40*, 673–685. [CrossRef]
52. Chen, J.-C.; Wang, J.; Zheng, B.-D.; Pang, J.; Chen, L.-J.; Lin, H.-T.; Guo, X. Simultaneous Determination of 8 Small Anti-hypertensive Peptides with Tyrosine at the C-Terminal in Laminaria japonica Hydrolysates by RP-HPLC Method. *J. Food Process. Preserv.* **2016**, *40*, 492–501. [CrossRef]
53. Annane, D.; Ouanes-Besbes, L.; de Backer, D.; Du, B.; Gordon, A.C.; Hernández, G.; Olsen, K.M.; Osborn, T.M.; Peake, S.; Russell, J.A.; et al. A global perspective on vasoactive agents in shock. *Intensive Care Med.* **2018**, *44*, 833–846. [CrossRef] [PubMed]
54. Hayes, M.; Mora, L.; Lucakova, S. Identification of Bioactive Peptides from Nannochloropsis oculata Using a Combination of Enzymatic Treatment, in Silico Analysis and Chemical Synthesis. *Biomolecules* **2022**, *12*, 1806. [CrossRef] [PubMed]
55. Måge, I.; Böcker, U.; Wubshet, S.; Lindberg, D.; Afseth, N. Fourier-transform infrared (FTIR) fingerprinting for quality assessment of protein hydrolysates. *LWT* **2021**, *152*, 112339. [CrossRef]

marine drugs

Article

Characterisation of Bioactive Peptides from Red Alga *Gracilariopsis chorda*

Martin Alain Mune Mune [1], Yoshikatsu Miyabe [2,3], Takeshi Shimizu [4], Wataru Matsui [2], Yuya Kumagai [5] and Hideki Kishimura [5,*]

1 Faculty of Science, University of Maroua, Maroua P.O. Box 814, Cameroon
2 Chair of Marine Chemical Resource Development, Graduate School of Fisheries Sciences, Hokkaido University, Hakodate 041-8611, Hokkaido, Japan
3 Aomori Prefectural Industrial Technology Research Center, Hachinohe 031-0831, Aomori, Japan
4 Hokkaido Industrial Technology Center, Department of Research and Development, Hakodate 041-0801, Hokkaido, Japan
5 Laboratory of Marine Chemical Resource Development, Faculty of Fisheries Sciences, Hokkaido University, Hakodate 041-8611, Hokkaido, Japan
* Correspondence: i-dulse@fish.hokudai.ac.jp; Tel.: +81-138-40-5519

Abstract: In this study, we studied the bioactive peptides produced by thermolysin hydrolysis of a water-soluble protein (WSP) from the red alga *Gracilariopsis chorda*, whose major components are phycobiliproteins and Ribulose-1,5-bisphosphate carboxylase-oxygenase (RuBisCo). The results showed that WSP hydrolysate exhibited significantly higher ACE inhibitory activity (92% inhibition) compared to DPP-IV inhibitory activity and DPPH scavenging activity. The phycobiliproteins and RuBisCo of *G. chorda* contain a high proportion of hydrophobic (31.0–46.5%) and aromatic (5.1–46.5%) amino acid residues, which was considered suitable for the formation of peptides with strong ACE inhibitory activity. Therefore, we searched for peptides with strong ACE inhibitory activity and identified two novel peptides (IDHY and LVVER). Then, their interaction with human ACE was evaluated by molecular docking, and IDHY was found to be a promising inhibitor. In silico analysis was then performed on the structural factors affecting ACE inhibitory peptide release, using the predicted 3D structures of phycobiliproteins and RuBisCo. The results showed that most of the ACE inhibitory peptides are located in the highly solvent accessible α-helix. Therefore, it was suggested that *G. chorda* is a good source of bioactive peptides, especially ACE-inhibitory peptides.

Keywords: red alga; *Gracilariopsis chorda*; bioactive peptides; ACE inhibitory activity; DPP-IV inhibitory activity; DPPH scavenging activity

Citation: Mune Mune, M.A.; Miyabe, Y.; Shimizu, T.; Matsui, W.; Kumagai, Y.; Kishimura, H. Characterisation of Bioactive Peptides from Red Alga *Gracilariopsis chorda*. *Mar. Drugs* **2023**, *21*, 49. https://doi.org/10.3390/md21010049

Academic Editors: Chang-Feng Chi and Bin Wang

Received: 23 December 2022
Revised: 6 January 2023
Accepted: 7 January 2023
Published: 11 January 2023

1. Introduction

Red algae are commonly used by the people near the coastal areas in Asia and Europe as a food source, to prepare many kind of dishes and soup. The consumption of red algae is actually expanding because they are a good source of essential nutrients, minerals and vitamins, and also contain bioactive compounds with attractive biological activities. The compounds found in red algae such as amino acids, proteins, polysaccharides, polyunsaturated fatty acids, sterols and polyphenols exhibited antioxidant, antimicrobial, antihelmintic, antidiabetic, antihypertensive, antiinflammatory and anticoagulant properties [1]. Applications of these bioactive compounds in the pharmaceutical industry are now very common. In this regard, bioactive metabolites found in algae are used to treat AIDS (acquired immune-deficiency syndrome), inflammation, arthritis, and microbial infections [2]. The red algae of Gracilariaceae were found particularly attractive because they presented the ability to achieve high yields and produced extracts with important industrial and biotechnological applications. In this regard, *Gracilariopsis chorda*, one of the most popular red algae of Gracilariaceae, is utilized as a functional food in Korea, and as a raw material in Europe and Asia for the production of agar [1,2]. Red alga generally contains a high quantity of proteins, mainly located on the stromal side of thylakoid membranes in the chloroplast, arranged as phycobilisomes and called phycobiliproteins, as well as ribulose-1,5-bisphosphate carboxylase-oxygenase (RuBisCo). These water-soluble proteins (WSP) particularly contain sequences of many potent bioactive peptides encrypted in their polypeptide sequence. Studies with red algae revealed the presence of peptides with Angiotensin-converting enzyme (ACE), dipeptidyl peptidase-IV (DPP-IV) inhibitory activity, as well as antioxidant properties in the sequence of phycobiliproteins, which could be released following enzymatic hydrolysis [3–8]. Therefore, it could be important to enhance utilization of *G. chorda* as a functional food by the release of potential bioactive peptides found in the sequence of WSP. Such an ingredient could find application in the prevention or treatment of diseases such as diabetes and hypertension, since synthetics drugs produce many undesirable side effects. However, to be able to optimize and predict the release of bioactive peptides from chloroplast proteins by enzymatic hydrolysis, their sequences are usually required, as well as 3D conformation.

The main WSP found in red algae are phycobiliproteins and RuBisCo. These proteins play an important role during the photosynthesis. Basically, phycobiliproteins contain phycoerythrin (PE), phycocyanin (PC) and allophycocyanin (APC), which are covalently linked to one or several chromophores at specific Cys residues. In a previous study, we analyzed the steric structure of PE from dulse (*Devaleraea inkyureii*), which is a type of red algae harvested in the cold waters of Japan. We found that its structure is an α-helix-rich $(\alpha\beta)_6$ hexamer complex with a toroidal shape [7]. It is well known that enzymatic hydrolysis of chloroplast proteins from red algae produces hydrolysates with important ACE inhibitory, DPP-IV inhibitory, and antioxidant activities. Many potent bioactive peptides have been purified from these hydrolysates. Particularly, new ACE inhibitory peptides were purified from algae WSP hydrolyzed by thermolysin [9], and inhibition mechanism was found competitive and non-competitive [9,10]. Recently, the analysis of the whole chloroplast genome from dulse was used as a tool for a wide characterization of bioactive peptides in the sequence of chloroplast proteins [3]. Presence of bioactive peptides with a wide range of bioactivities has been revealed. However, interaction between protease with chloroplast proteins also depends on the conformation of the protein in the mixture. It is well known that hydrolysis of protein secondary structures such as sheets and hairpins is more difficult than alpha helix conformation or turns [11]. Therefore, to be able to design efficient processes for the hydrolysis of chloroplast proteins to produce bioactive peptides, it is important to analyze the release of bioactive peptides from the protein matrices. The complex rod-shape structure of phycobiliproteins rich in alpha-helix secondary conformation, as well as the 3D structure of RuBisCo [12], probably affects the release of bioactive peptides encrypted in their primary sequence. Actually, bioinformatic tools are increasingly used to predict the structure of proteins as well as the release of bioactive peptides, with great accuracy. In this regard, combining information from the chloroplast protein's structure and bioactive properties of protein hydrolysates could be important to understand structural factors that influence the release of bioactive peptides from red algae chloroplast proteins. Therefore, in this study *G. chorda* soluble chloroplast proteins were hydrolyzed by thermolysin, then ACE inhibitory, DPP-IV inhibitory, and antioxidant activities of the hydrolysate were determined. Moreover, protein hydrolysate was fractionated, and the release of bioactive peptides related to ACE inhibitory effect was analysed by several in silico techniques to understand the structure–function relationship of *G. chorda* WSP.

2. Results and Discussion

2.1. Characteristics of *G. cholda* WSP

WSP from red alga usually contain a high amount of phycobiliproteins, which are composed primary of α and β subunits, each linked covalently to one or several phycobilin chromophores at specific Cys residues [13]. The linked Cys residues are usually well conserved in the primary structure of phycobiliproteins, and in *G. chorda* (Figure 1a), their linkage with phycobilin chromophore provided a characteristic red color to WSP (Figure 1b). The absorption spectrum of *G. chorda* WSP is characteristic to the chromophore composition in the mixture (Figure 1c). WSP presented high absorbance at 543, 565 and 500 nm, and low absorbance at 620 and 655 nm. Generally, PE presents maximum absorbance at λ = 490–570 nm, PC at λ = 610–625 nm and APC at λ = 650–660 nm. PE binds phycoerythrobilin and phycourobilin chromophores, PC binds phycoerythrobilin and phycocyanobilin, and APC binds phycocyanobilin. Therefore, the high absorbance at 500–565 nm of *G. chorda* soluble protein is characteristic to high content of PE in the mixture. Similar results were obtained for other red algae such as dulse [3]: i.e., we calculated the ratio of PE, PC, and APC present based on the absorbance of the visible light absorption spectrum, and the main component of the phycobiliprotein was PE (PE = 5.0 mg/mL, PC = 1.8 mg/mL, APC = 0.01 mg/mL) [14]. The electrophoresis analysis of *G. chorda* WSP provided additional information on the protein composition (Figure 1d). It was observed by SDS-PAGE analysis two major bands at approximately 20 and 55 kDa, and two minor bands at 16 and 32 kDa. The band at 55 kDa was also observed in WSP from Japanese dulse and *P. pseudolinearis* and was related to the large subunit of RuBisCo (RuBisCo-L) [3,13]. RuBisCo is a multimeric protein which plays an important role in the assimilation of CO_2 to form sugars during photosynthesis, and then one of the most abundant WSP in plants. The band at 16 kDa was probably related to the small subunit of RuBisCo (RuBisCo-S). The band at 20 kDa produced fluorescence following excitation at 490–560 nm, indicating it was phycobiliproteins linked to chromophores.

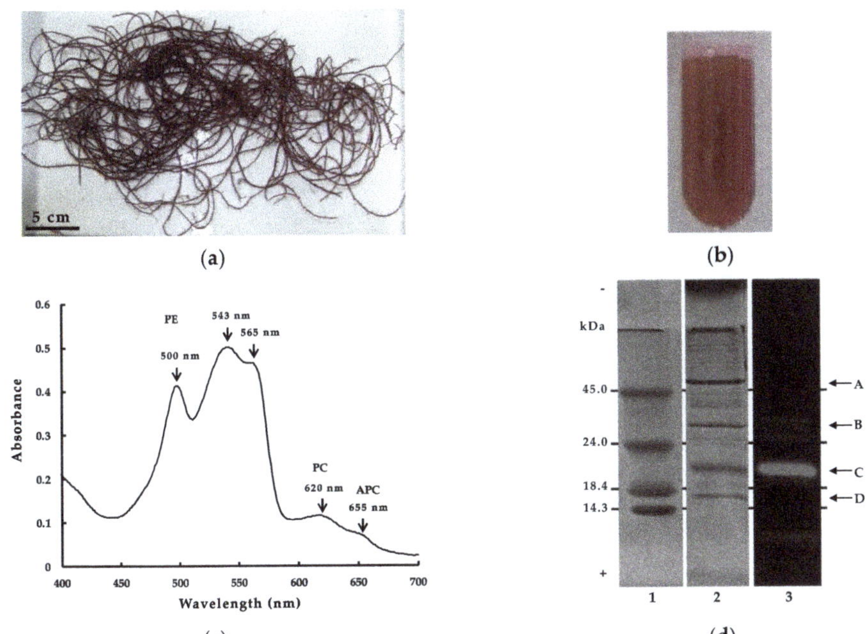

Figure 1. (**a**) Harvested *G. chorda* on the coast of Hakodate; (**b**) *G. chorda* WSP; (**c**) Visible ray absorption spectrum of *G. chorda* WSP; (**d**) SDS-PAGE electrophoresis of *G. chorda* WSP: (**1**) MW markers; (**2**) *G. chorda* WSP stained by Coomassie Brilliant Blue R-250; (**3**) *G. chorda* WSP fluorescent photography; (A) RuBisCo-L; (B) PE-γ; (C) PE-α, PE-β; (D) RuBisCo-S.

2.2. Bioactive Properties of G. chorda WSP Hydrolysate and Isolation of ACE Inhibitory Peptides

Previously, hydrolysis of red algal proteins produced peptides with several types of bioactivities [3,5–7]. In this study, *G. chorda* WSP were hydrolyzed by thermolysin, and bioactive properties of the hydrolysate were evaluated, especially ACE inhibitory activity, DPP-IV inhibitory activity, and DPPH scavenging activity (Figure 2a–c). It was observed as a significant increase in these activities in the hydrolysate compared to WSP. The particularly high ACE inhibitory activity of *G. chorda* hydrolysate (92%) compared to WSP (35%) was noteworthy. Conversely, *G. chorda* WSP thermolysin hydrolysate was a poor source of DPP-IV inhibitory (28% inhibitory activity at 5.0 mg/mL) and DPPH radical scavenging peptides (63% DPPH scavenging activity at 3.2 mg). Proteins from the red alga dulse previously showed low radical scavenging activity, probably due to low content of amino acids capable of scavenging free radicals [6]. In addition, high ACE inhibitory activity was also observed in red alga *Porphyra dioica* proteins hydrolyzed by Alcalase and Flavourzyme [15], and DPP-IV inhibitory effect was noticed in Irish dulse proteins digested by Corolase PP [16]. In a study of Japanese dulse, it was reported that the antioxidant activity of WSP (DPPH and ABTS radical scavenging activity) is relatively low and that the main antioxidant activity of WSP is derived from the chromophore of phycobiliproteins [6]. Therefore, we believe that the antioxidant activity of WSP and its hydrolysates is low, even when antioxidant activity is measured by other methods.

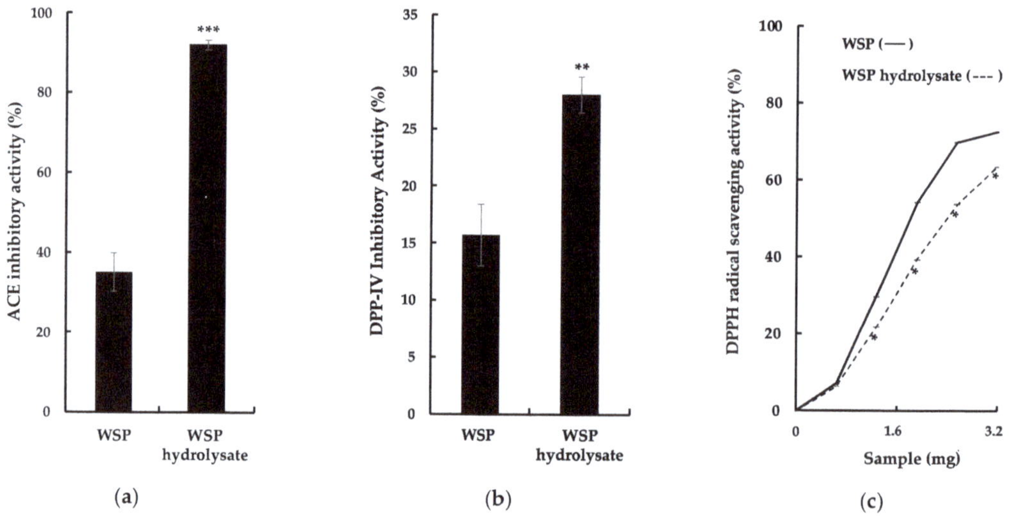

Figure 2. Bioactive properties of *G. chorda* WSP and its thermolysin hydrolysate: (**a**) ACE inhibitory activity; (**b**) DPP-IV inhibitory activity; (**c**) DPPH scavenging activity. *: $p < 0.05$; **: $p < 0.01$; ***: $p < 0.001$.

Since *G. chorda* WSP hydrolyzed by thermolysin presented interesting potential for utilization as functional food in the prevention or treatment of hypertension, and then subjected to fractionation by RP-HPLC and mass spectrometry to identify bioactive peptides (Figure 3a,b). For this purpose, four fractions (Fractions 1, 2, 7, and 8 in Figure 3) with ACE inhibitory activity > 40% were selected for peptide identification. The mass spectrometry analysis of fractions 2, 7, and 8 provided 3 peptide sequences, respectively, IDHY, LVVER, and LRY. No peak with m/z ratio > 400 was identified in fraction 1. This fraction probably contained a dipeptide with the m/z peak mixed with those representing the matrix used for MALDI during mass spectrometry. Thermolysin is an endopeptidase which recognises amino groups of a wide range of hydrophobic amino acid residues, including Ile, Leu, Val and Phe. Several potent dipeptides with hydrophobic amino acid residues at the amino terminal, such as VY, IY and IW, have been identified in plant protein hydrolysates prepared by thermolysin [17,18]. The three peptides LRY, IDHY, and LVVER were checked in the BIOPEP-UWM database (https://biochemia.uwm.edu.pl/biopep/start_biopep.php), and the result showed that IDHY and LVVER were new peptides not yet registered. The two new peptides exhibited some important characteristics for ACE inhibition such as presence of Arg and Tyr at the C-terminal residue [19]. However, IDHY was probably more potent than LVVER for the inhibition of ACE, since it showed higher score in PeptideRanker (Table 1). The peptide LRY was already found in thermolysin hydrolysates of other red algal WSP [3,20]. In the previous study we identified a novel ACE inhibitory peptide LRY from dulse [2]. The IC_{50} value of synthesized LRY against the ACE from rabbit lung was 0.044 μmol, and its effect was the same level as that of the sesame peptide LVY (IC_{50} value: 0.045 μmol) used as a Food for Specified Health Uses (FOSHU) in Japan. Then, we performed a docking simulation of LRY with human ACE and found that −9.50 kcal/mol. Since the affinity of IDHY for human ACE in this study was −9.50 kcal/mol, it was presumed that IDHY has a hypotensive effect on humans as well as LVY. We are currently planning a clinical trial on the blood pressure-lowering effects of LRY and IDHY from red algae in collaboration with a company.

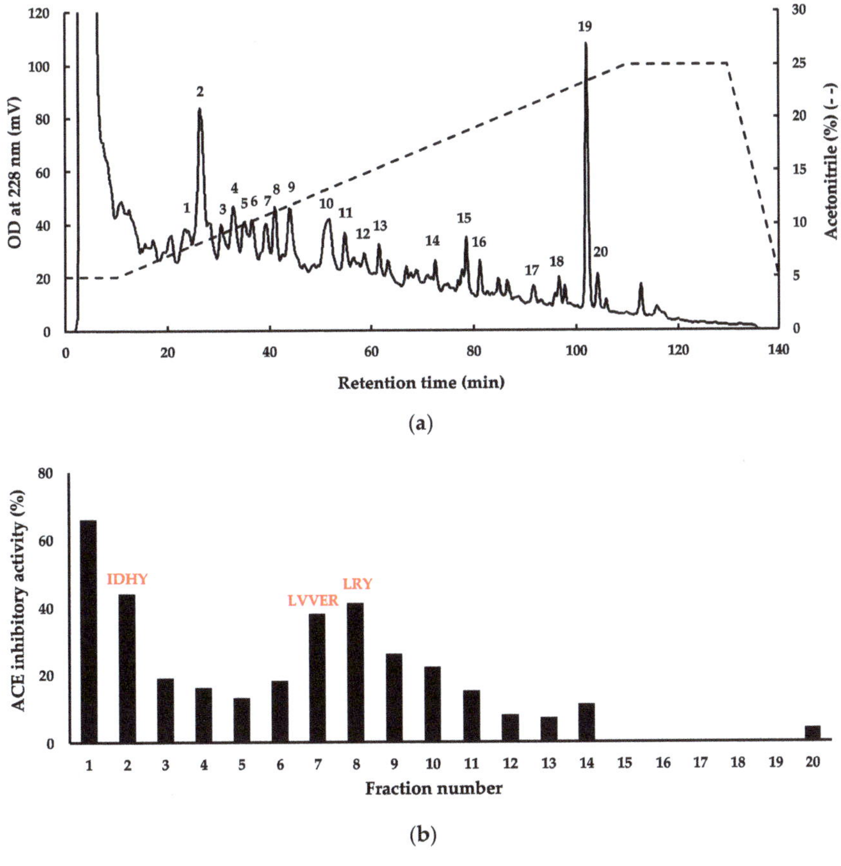

Figure 3. (**a**) Isolation of ACE inhibitory peptides from *G. chorda* WSP hydrolysate by RP-HPLC; (**b**) evaluation of ACE inhibitory activity of the pooled fractions 1–20.

Table 1. Bioactive peptides found in *G. chorda* soluble proteins following hydrolysis by thermolysin.

						Properties				Secondary Structure [a]
	Sequence	**Occurrence**	**Position**	**IC_{50} (μM)**	**Proteins**	**$[M+H]^+$**	**Solubility [b]**	**SAS in nm^2 [c]**	**Peptide Ranker Score [d]**	
Detected	IDHY	1	86–89	-	PE-α	547.25	Good	0.381	0.285	Helix
	LRY	1	90–92	5.1	PE-β	451.26	Good	0.486	0.512	Helix
	LVVER	1	159–163	-	RuBisCo-L	615.35	Good	0.316	0.044	Helix
Potential [e]	AR	1/1/1	36–37, 56–57, 15–16	96	PE-α/ PC-β/ APC-α	245.14	Good	0.125 0.700 0.865	0.394	Helix Helix -
	VR	1/1	164–165, 38–39	52.8	PE-γ/ APC-β	273.17	Good	0.579 1.091	0.115	Helix Helix
	LEE	1	115–117	100	PC-α	389.17	Good	0.809	0.0350	Helix
	FQ	1	59–60	51.23	APC-γ	293.13	Poor	0.843	0.916	Helix
	IW	1	285–286	4.7	RuBisCo-L	317.16	Poor	0.453	0.944	Helix
	VK	1	134–135	13.0	RuBisCo-L	245.16	Good	0.662	0.033	Beta strand

[a] PDBSUM was used to generate the secondary structure of peptides in the protein. [b] Solubility was predicted by INNOVAGEN peptide calculator (https://pepcalc.com/peptide-solubility-calculator.php, accessed on 10 November 2022). [c] Solvent accessible surface (SAS) for each residue was calculated by the SASA script in Gromacs. [d] Predicted score by PeptideRanker (http://distilldeep.ucd.ie/PeptideRanker/, accessed on 14 November 2022).[e] Potential bioactive peptides with IC_{50} < 100 μM were considered. -: Non defined.

2.3. Structural Characterization of G. chorda WSP and Structure-Function Relationship

To optimize the application of *G. chorda* WSP in the preparation of hydrolysate with high ACE inhibitory activity by in silico analysis, it is important to elucidate the structure of WSP. However, *G. chorda* contained relatively high amounts of polysaccharides. In addition, the phycobiliproteins are very hydrophobic and adsorb to the column resin, resulting in very low yields. For these reasons, it was very difficult to isolate and purify the major proteins of WSP. Therefore, we needed to approach the elucidation of their primary structure by genetic analysis. Since the genes of phycobiliproteins and RuBisCo, major proteins of WSP, are encoded in chloroplast DNA, as in previous studies [4,20], we determined the complete chloroplast genome and manually annotated it. The genes of the main WSP were found, and their amino acid sequences were deduced (Supplementary Material, Figure S1a–d, AP017366 in NCBI). It was noteworthy that PE possessed a gamma subunit (PE-γ) in addition to α and β subunits (PE-α, PE-β), i.e., we obtained 28,573 contigs by next generation sequencing of *G. chorda* DNA and we found the contig (LC713007 in NCBI) containing PE-γ gene encoded in nuclear DNA. The α and β subunits of PE construct $(\alpha\beta)_6$ as described above. On the other hand, PE-γ is placed in the central space of the $(\alpha\beta)_6$ hexamer complex as linker protein to form part of the rod of the phycobilisome. Compared to the α and β subunits, there have been fewer structural and functional studies of the γ subunits, because the gene is encoded in the nucleus [21]. APC also presented three subunits, namely α, β and γ (APC-α, APC-β, and APC-γ). PC α and β subunits (PC-α, PC-β) and RuBisCo-L and -S genes were also encoded in *G. chorda* chloroplast genome. From the deduced amino acid sequences, the amino acid compositions of these proteins were analysed. High percentages of total hydrophobic amino acids (31.0–46.5%) and total aromatic amino acids (5.1–10.1%) were observed in *G. chorda* phycobiliproteins and RuBisCo (Table 1). In addition, Pro was found at 1.7–4.1%, and Trp was particularly abundant in RuBisCo-L (1.6%). High hydrophobic amino acid content was also found in Japanese dulse chloroplast proteins [4]. The important role of bulky hydrophobic amino acids (Pro, Phe, Tyr, and Trp) at the C-terminal, and the N-terminal aliphatic amino acid for di- and tripeptides for high ACE inhibitory activity is well known [19]. Moreover, the calculated molecular weight of WSP on the basis of their amino acid composition was found in accordance with SDS-PAGE analysis, and the calculated pI confirmed their water solubility (Table S1, Supplementary Material).

The origin of detected ACE inhibitory peptides was determined by mapping their sequences in the primary sequence of WSP (Table S1). It was found that the sequences of IDHY, LRY and LVVER were, respectively, detected in the primary structure of PEα, PEβ and RuBisCo-L, in a single occurrence. Presence of other potential ACE inhibitory peptides after hydrolysis of *G. chorda* WSP by thermolysin was predicted using the BIOPEP tool. Five peptides with $IC_{50} \leq 100$ µM were detected and resulting from the primary structure of PE-α, PE-β, PC-α, PC-β, APC-α, APC-β, APC-γ, and RuBisCo-L (Table S1).

In addition, it was observed that the peptides IW and IK with lower IC_{50} were found in the primary structure of RuBisCo-L. Afterwards, the 3D structure of *G. chorda* WSP was predicted in silico to understand the structural factors that contributed to the release of ACE inhibitory peptides. The modeled structures are then presented in Figure 4a–d and their secondary structure was analysed by PDBsum (Table 2). It was observed that phycobiliproteins were rich in alpha helix (7 to 14) secondary structure, and also contained beta turns (2 to 13) and gamma turns. PE-γ was the more complex phycobiliprotein with 14 helices (62.1%), 13 beta turns and 1 gamma turn (Table 2). This secondary structure is common to phycobiliproteins in many red algae species and the high number of alpha helices is essential for the building of phycobilisomes rod-shape structure [12]. The secondary structure of RuBisCo was more complex. RuBisCo-L contained 25 alpha helices and 27 beta turns, but also 15 strands and 2 beta hairpins. RuBisCo-S also contained 4 strands and 2 beta hairpins, in addition to alpha helix (3) and beta turns (5). Generally, the sheet secondary structure is less susceptible to enzymatic hydrolysis than the helix one, and presence of beta hairpins conferred additional stability of the structure [11].

Table 2. Secondary structure in G. chorda WSP [a].

	PE			PC		APC			RuBisCo	
	α	β	γ	α	β	α	β	γ	L	S
Secondary structure descriptors [b]										
helices	10 (74.4%) [c]	10 (74.9%)	14 (62.1%)	9 (76.6%)	10 (71.2%)	9 (78.1%)	7 (78.3%)	9 (77.5%)	25 (42.2%)	3 (20.3%)
beta hairpins	-	-	-	-	-	-	-	-	2	2
beta sheets	-	-	-	-	-	-	-	-	3	2
beta strands	-	-	-	-	-	-	-	-	15 (14.8%)	4 (40.5%)
beta bulges	-	-	-	-	-	-	-	-	3	2
Helix–helix interactions	18	17	14	17	18	19	13	20	22	-
beta turns	5	4	13	2	4	6	7	6	27	5
gamma turns	1	-	1	-	-	-	-	-	3	-

[a] Secondary structure was generated by PDBsum (https://www.ebi.ac.uk/thornton-srv/databases/pdbsum/Generate.html, accessed on 5 December 2022). [b] Number of secondary structures. [c] Rate of amino acid residues involved in secondary structure formation among total amino acid residues. -: Non defined.

Peptides with ACE inhibitory activity were further mapped on the secondary structure of *G. chorda* WSP to analyze their structural environment in the protein (Figure 4 and Table 1). It was found that all the detected and potential peptides were located in the helix region of different proteins, except for the peptide VK which is located in sheet. Solvent accessible surface (SAS) is an additional tool to analyze the accessibility of peptides encrypted in the protein structure to proteases. Generally, the region with SAS < 0.3 is buried and those with SAS > 0.3 are exposed [22]. Then, as expected, all the detected peptides were located in exposed regions. Potential ACE inhibitory peptides were also exposed to the solvent, excepted for the peptide AR located in PE-α. Solubility of the peptides was finally predicted to evaluate recovery of the released peptides in water. It was found that all the detected peptides were soluble in water. In contrary, peptides IW and FQ were less soluble in water.

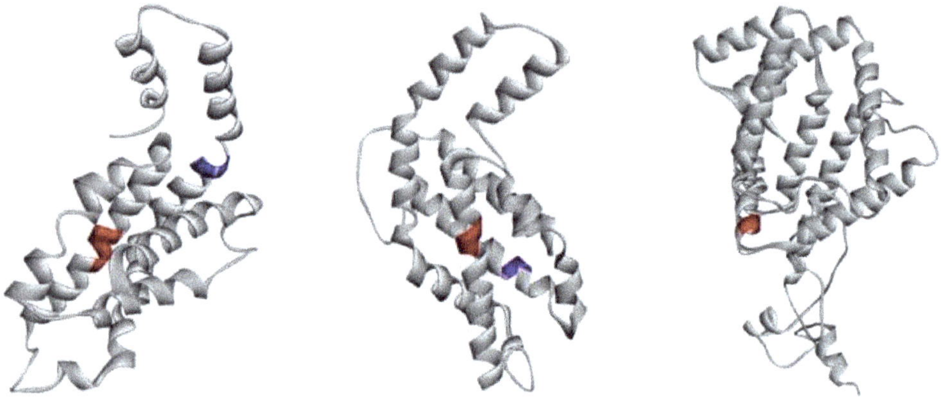

(1) (2) (3)
(a)

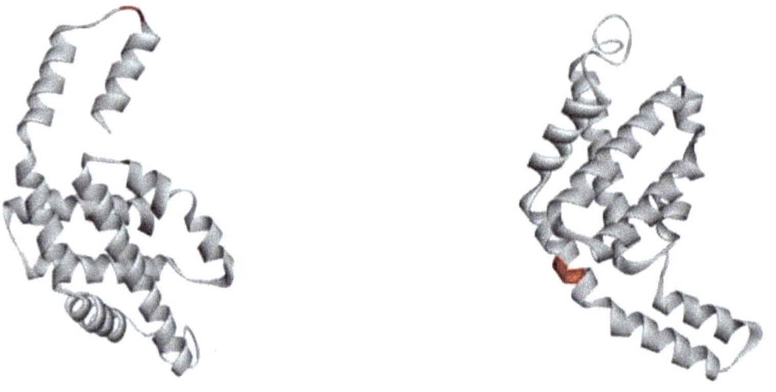

(1) (2)
(b)

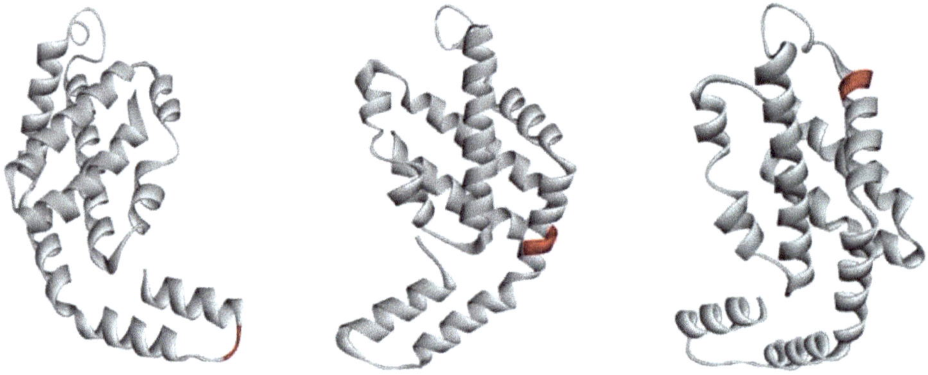

(1) (2) (3)
(c)

Figure 4. *Cont.*

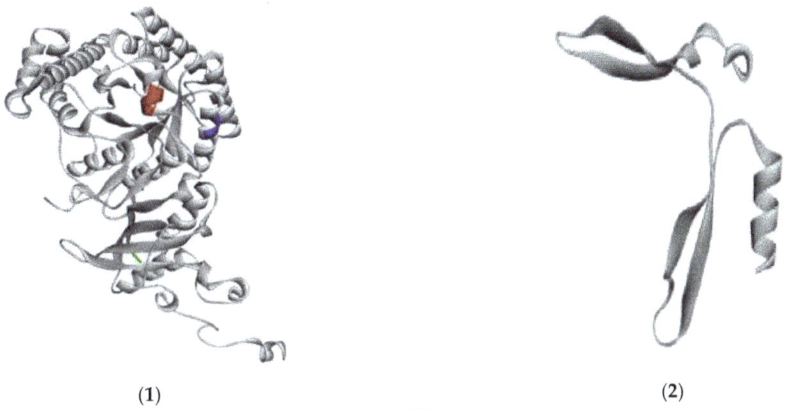

(d)

Figure 4. Predicted 3D structure of G. chorda phycobiliproteins and RuBisCo, and location of bioactive peptides. (**a**) (**1**)PE-α showing IDHY (red) and AR (blue); (**2**) PE-β showing LRH (red); (**3**) PE-γ showing VR (red); (**b**) (**1**) PC-α showing LEE (red); (**2**) PC-β showing AR (red); (**c**) (**1**) APC-α showing AR (red); (**2**) APC-β showing VR (red); (**3**) APC-γ showing FQ (red); (**d**) (**1**) RuBisCo-L showing LVVER (red); IW (blue); VK (green); (**2**) RuBisCo-S.

2.4. Prediction of the Interaction between New Bioactive Peptides and Human ACE

To confirm the potential of a new peptide to inhibit ACE, generally in vitro or in vivo experiments are required. However, recent simulation of the interaction between ACE and different peptides by using in silico methods gave good correlation with results obtained in vitro. In addition, the *in silico* methods produced an overview of the interaction at the atomic level [23]. This is convenient to make a decision. Therefore, inhibition of human ACE by IDHY and LVVER was evaluated by molecular docking, and results were compared to those of lisinopril and captopril (Table 3 and Figure 5). Docking methodology was valid because RMSD was less than 1 Å. The affinity energy between ACE and the peptides was lower for IDHY (−9.5 kcal/mol) compared to LVVER (−6.9 kcal/mol). As a result, IDHY interacted with ACE through 7 hydrogen bonds and 2 bonds with Zn^{2+} ion, while ACE interacted with LVVER through 6 hydrogen bonds. Zn^{2+} ion plays an important role in the activity of ACE because it facilitates the binding of the substrate to the Zn^{2+}-binding motif HEXXH at the active site which includes His383, His387 and Glu411. In addition, Zn^{2+} ion assists the nucleophilic attack from an activated water molecule, with the reaction being initiated by the carboxyl group of Glu384 [23]. Therefore, potent ACE inhibitors should bind to specific amino acid residues at the active site, together with coordinating Zn^{2+}, in order to prevent the fixation of the substrate to the active site. In this regard, IDHY coordinated with the Zn^{2+} ion and also interacted with Glu384 through a hydrogen bond of 2.926 Å. Moreover, IDHY was linked to His387 and Glu411 by salt bridges (Figure 5). No interaction was observed between the specific amino acid residues at the active site and LVVER. Furthermore, the number of non-bonded contact was also important, because interaction of inhibitor with a high number of amino acid residues near the active site could alter the conformation structure and then prevent the fixation of the substrate. On the other hand, Lisinopril interacted with ACE through coordination bonds with Zn^{2+} ions, hydrogen bonds and non-bonded interactions with specific residues at the active site, as well as those near the active site (Figure 5c).

Table 3. Molecular docking results of the interaction of IDHY and LVVER from G. chorda against crystal structure of ACE.

Ligand	Number Clusters	Affinity (kcal/mol) [a]	RMSDi in A	Number of Bonds with Zn^{2+}	Hydrogen Bonds [b]			Number of Non-Bonded Contacts
					Number	Residues	Length (Å)	
IDHY	10	−9.50	0.0	2	7	TYR523	3.323	102
						GLU403	3.189	
						GLU403	2.568	
						GLU384	2.926	
						ALA356	2.847	
						SER355	2.958	
						ALA354	3.067	
LVVER	10	−6.9	0.0	0	6	SER517	2.681	62
						SER516	2.994	
						GLU143	2.998	
						GLU143	2.941	
						ARG124	2.741	
						ASP121	2.619	
Lisinopril	-	-	-	2	8	TYR523	2.775	48
						TYR520	2.556	
						HIS513	3.109	
						LYS511	2.934	
						HIS387	3.327	
						ALA354	2.917	
						HIS353	2.760	
						HIS353	3.241	
Captopril	-	-	-	1	5	TYR520	2.657	36
						HIS513	2.694	
						LYS511	2.730	
						HIS353	2.542	
						GLN281	3.074	

[a] Affinity energy was calculated by AutoDockFR suite suite version 1.0 (The Scripps Research Institute, Centre For Computational Structural Biology, California, USA). The hit with the lower energy was considered. [b] Number of hydrogen bonds and non-bonded contact was calculated by LigPlotPlus software and Discovery Studio using default parameters. -: Non defined.

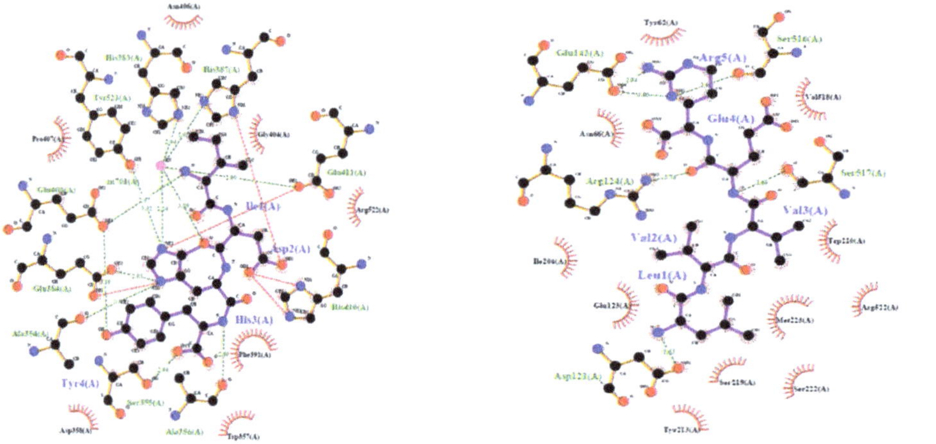

(a) (b)

Figure 5. *Cont.*

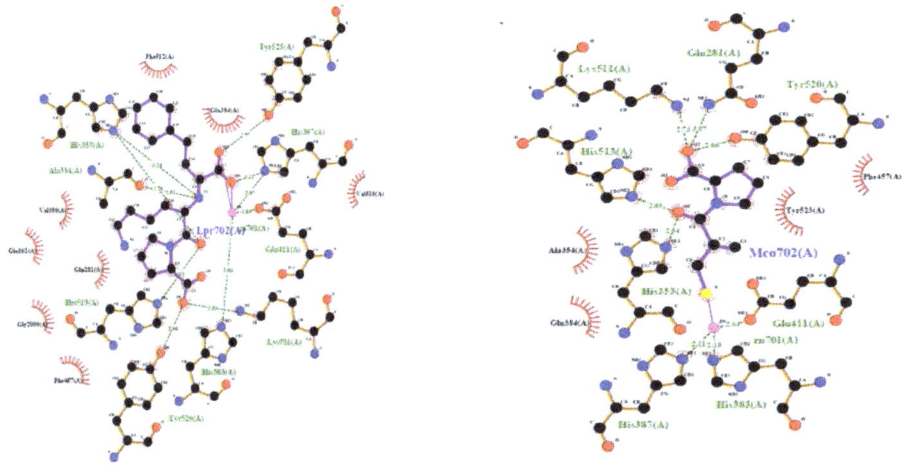

(**c**) (**d**)

Figure 5. 2D view of the interaction of human ACE with ACE inhibitory peptides: (**a**) IDHY; (**b**) LVVER; (**c**) Lisinopril; (**d**) Captopril.

3. Materials and Methodsw

3.1. Materials

Samples (*G. chorda*) were collected on the coast of Hakodate, Hokkaido Prefecture, Japan. Hexadecyltrimethylammonium Bromide (CTAB), tris-[hydroxymethyl]amino-methane (Tris), ethylenediamine-*N*,*N*,*N*′,*N*′-tetraacetic acid, disodium salt, dihydrate (EDTA), Proteinase K (EC 3.4.21.64, from *Tritirachium album*), RNase A (EC 3.1.27.5, from bovine pancreas), porcine stomach pepsin (EC 3.4.23.1) and bovine pancreatic trypsin (EC 3.1.21.4) were purchased from FUJIFILM Wako Pure Chemical (Osaka, Japan). Phenol-chloroform-isoamyl alcohol (25:24:1) was purchased from NACALAI TESQUE, INC (Kyoto, Japan). Ala-Pro-*p*-nitroanilide (Ala-Pro-*p*NA) were also obtained from Bachem AG (Bubendorf, Switzerland). All other regents were purchased from FUJIFILM Wako Pure Chemical (Osaka, Japan).

3.2. Preparation of G. chorda WSP Hydrolysate

The WSP from *G. chorda* were prepared according to the same method as in our previous paper [3]: i.e., frozen *G. chorda* was lyophilized and ground into a fine powder. To this powder, 20 v/w distilled water was added and proteins were extracted at 4 °C for 7 h. The extract was centrifuged at 4 °C, 15,000× *g* for 10 min, and then the supernatant was used as *G. chorda* WSP. The visible ray absorption spectrum of *G. chorda* WSP was analyzed by a spectrophotometer (UV-1800, Shimadzu, Kyoto, Japan). *G. chorda* WSP hydrolysate were prepared as previously reported [3,13]. The WSP were hydrolyzed by 1.0 wt% of thermolysin at 70 °C for 3 h, and the reaction was ended by heat treatment at 100 °C for 5 min. Subsequently, the solution was centrifuged at 4 °C, 15,000× *g* for 10 min. The supernatant was dried by lyophilisation into *G. chorda* peptides.

For analysis of protein composition, sodium dodecyl sulfate-polyacrylamide gel electrophoresis (SDS-PAGE) was carried out using a 0.1% SDS-13.75% polyacrylamide slab-gel by the method of Laemmli [24]. The gel was stained with 0.1% Coomassie Brilliant Blue R-250 in 50% methanol-7% acetic acid and the background of the gel was destained with 7% acetic acid. Fluorescence of phycobiliprotein on slab-gel was detected by gel documentation LED illuminator (VISIRAYS AE-6935GN: ATTO, Tokyo, Japan).

3.3. ACE Inhibitory Assay

ACE inhibitory assay was carried out according to the method of Cheng and Cushman [25], with some modifications. Fifteen microliters of sample solution (3.2 mg/mL) were added to 30 μL of ACE (0.2 units/mL), and the mixture was pre-incubated at 37 °C for 5 min. Thirty microliters of Hip-His-Leu solution (12.5 mM in 0.1 M sodium borate buffer containing 400 mM NaCl at pH 8.3) were added to the mixture. After incubation at 37 °C for 1 h, the reaction was stopped by adding 75 μL of 1.0 M HCl. The released hippuric acid was extracted with 450 μL of ethyl acetate. Four hundred microliters of the upper layer were evaporated, and then the hippuric acid was dissolved in 1.5 mL of distilled water. The absorbance at 228 nm of the solution was measured by a spectrophotometer. The inhibition was calculated from the following equation: $[1 - (As - Asb)/(Ac - Acb)] \times 100$, where Ac is the absorbance of the buffer, Acb is the absorbance when the stop solution was added to the buffer before the reaction, As is the absorbance of the sample, and Asb is the absorbance when the stop solution was added to the sample before the reaction.

3.4. DPP-IV Inhibitory Assay

Preparation of the recombinant dipeptidyl peptidase-IV (DPP-IV, EC 3.4.14.5) from human kidney was carried out according to the method of Hatanaka et al. [26]. DPP-IV inhibitory activities with *G. chorda* protein and peptides were analysed by a slight modification of the method of Hatanaka et al. [26]: dried samples were dissolved with 20 mM Tris-HCl (pH 7.5) (16.6 mg/mL). Thirty micro liters of each sample (0.5 mg, final concentration of 5 mg/mL) was added to 20 μL (0.029 U, final concentration of 0.29 U/mL) of DPP-IV in 20 mM Tris-HCl (pH 7.5), and then the mixture was pre-incubated at 37 °C for 3 min. The enzymatic reaction was initiated by adding 50 μL (final concentration of 0.5 mg/mL) of 1.0 mg/mL Ala-Pro-*p*NA in 20 mM Tris-HCl (pH 7.5). This mixture was incubated at 37 °C for 10 min and measured the increased absorbance at 405 nm using a UV-1800 spectrophotometer (Shimazu, Kyoto, Japan). One unit (U) of the enzyme activity was defined as the amount of enzyme that liberates 1 μmol *p*-nitroaniline per min under the assay conditions. The percentage of inhibition was determined relative to the enzyme activity without samples.

3.5. DPPH Radical Scavenging Assay

DPPH radical scavenging assay was carried out according to the method of Sharma and Bhat [27] with some modifications. Sample or distilled water were mixed with 1.0 mL of 500 μM DPPH solution (in 99.5% ethanol) and 800 μL of 100 mM Tris-HCl buffer (pH 8.0). The mixture was incubated at room temperature in dark condition for 20 min. After the incubation, the solution was centrifuged (3500, KUBOTA, Osaka, Japan) at 4 °C, 2000× *g* for 10 min, and the supernatant was measured absorbance at 517 nm. DPPH radical scavenging activity was calculated from the following equation: $[1 - (As - Asb)/Aw] \times 100$, where As is the absorbance of sample mixed with DPPH solution and Asb is the absorbance of sample mixed with ethanol, and Aw is the absorbance of distilled water mixed with DPPH solution. All the assays were performed in triplicate.

3.6. Separation of G. chorda WSP Hydrolysate

The *G. chorda* hydrolysate was dissolved in ultrapure water containing 0.1% trifluoroacetic acid (TFA) and applied to sequential filtration by Millex-GV (pore size: 0.22 μm) and Millex-LG (pore size: 0.20 μm). Peptides in the filtrate were isolated by reversed phase-HPLC (RP-HPLC) with a Mightysil RP-18GP column (4.6 × 150 mm) (Kanto Kagaku, Tokyo, Japan) using a linear gradient of acetonitrile (1–20%) containing 0.1% TFA at a flow rate of 1.0 mL/min.

The amino acid sequences of the ACE inhibitory peptides were analysed by MALDI-TOF/MS/MS using a 4700 Proteomics Analyser mass spectrometer with *DeNovo* Explorer ver. 3.6 (Applied Biosystems, CA, USA).

3.7. Statistical Analysis

All experiments were replicated at least three times. Mean values with standard deviations were reported. Means were compared by one way ANOVA and Tukey post hoc was applied to check the significant differences among means. The computer software used in this study was SPSS (version10.1, 2000, SPSS Inc., Chicago, IL, USA).

3.8. Isolation and Sequencing of *G. chorda* DNA

DNA was extracted from *G. chorda* according to the CTAB DNA extraction method with some modifications [28]. First, the fresh sample was thoroughly washed with ultrapure water and freeze-dried. Then, approximately 10 mg dried sample was well ground into a powder and added to a 2.0 mL tube. The sample was suspended in 1 mL Tris-EDTA (TE) buffer, vortexed, and then placed on ice for 10 min. After that, the sample was centrifuged at 4 °C, 15,000× *g* for 1 min. The supernatant was collected in a new 2.0 mL tube containing 1% SDS and 0.1 mg/mL proteinase K and then incubated at 37 °C for 1 h. After the incubation, the sample containing 0.7 M NaCl and 1% CTAB was incubated at 65 °C for 10 min. Then the sample was added to an equal volume of phenol-chloroform-isoamyl alcohol, vortexed and centrifuged at 4 °C, 15,000× *g* for 5 min. Afterward, the supernatant (water-layer) was moved to a new 2.0 mL tube containing an equal volume of chloroform, vortexed and centrifuged at 4 °C, 15,000× *g* for 5 min. The supernatant (water-layer) was moved to a new 1.5 mL tube containing 0.6 volume of 2-propanol, mixed gently, centrifuged at 4 °C, 15,000× *g* for 5 min, and then discard the supernatant. The pellet was rinsed with 70% ethanol, centrifuged at 4 °C, 12,000× *g* for 5 min, then discard the supernatant and air-dried on a clean bench for 10 min. The DNA sample was dissolved in TE buffer containing 20 ng/mL RNase A in the final concentration approximately 100 ng/µL DNA concentration and incubate at 37 °C for 30 min. Finally, the concentration and purity of *G. chorda* DNA were analysed by NanoDrop 2000 Spectrometer (Thermo Fisher Scientific, Waltham, MA, USA).

The nucleotide sequences of the DNA were analysed by using a next generation sequencer, Ion PGM System (Thermo Fisher Scientific, Waltham, MA, USA). The data were assembled with CLC Genomics Workbench 9.5.4 (QIAGEN, Hilden, Germany). The gap in PE-γ gene was filled by Sanger sequencing. Nucleotide and deduced amino acid sequences of the PE subunits from *G. chorda* were aligned using EMBL-EBI Clustal Omega [29]. Molecular weight and isoelectric point of *G. chorda* phycobiliproteins were calculated from deduced amino acid sequences by using the compute pI/Mw tool, ProtParam (https://web.expasy.org/protparam/, accessed on 5 December 2022).

3.9. In Silico Analysis

3.9.1. Building 3D Structure of *G. chorda* Phycobiliproteins and RuBisCo

The 3D structures of *G. chorda* phycobiliproteins and RuBisCo were predicted using SWISS-MODEL server (http://swissmodel.expasy.org/); the predicted structure was output by PyMOL version 2.5.2 (Schrödinger, LLC, NY, USA) [30], and the secondary structures were analysed by PDBsum webserver [31].

3.9.2. Ligand Preparation

The peptides IDHY and LVVER were found potential inhibitors of ACE and selected for *molecular docking* analysis. Their 3D structure was built in Biovia Discovery Studio Client v19.1.0.18287 (Dassault Systèmes, San Diego, CA, USA), and energy was minimized. The peptides were then prepared for the flexible docking software using AutoDock tools version 1.5.7.

3.9.3. Protein Preparation

The appropriate 3D structures of ACE (identity 1O86) in complex with Lisinopril were retrieved from Protein Data Bank (https://www.rcsb.org/), as well as the structure of ACE with Captopril (1UZF). All the ligands were removed using Biovia Discovery Studio v19.1

software and the protein was prepared for docking using AutoDock tools and Kollman charges were used.

3.9.4. Grid Generation and Molecular Docking

The grid was centered on the crystallized ligand in the crystal structure of ACE using AGFR 1.0 tool, dedicated software for flexible docking preparation. The dimensions of the box were: 32 Å × 32 Å × 32 Å, center-x = 40.915 Å, center-y = 39.340 Å, center-z = 42.338 Å. Docking was performed at 2×10^6 evaluations in 6 runs each using AutoDockFR software. Results were analysed using PyMOL version 2.5.2, Biovia Discovery Studio and LigPlot plus version 2.2.5 (Cambridgeshire, UK) for the 2D interaction diagram.

4. Conclusions

It has been demonstrated in this study that *G. chorda* WSP contained a high amount of PE, but also PC, APC and RuBisCo. Their hydrolysis by thermolysin produced bioactive peptides with DPP-IV inhibitory and DPPH scavenging activities, and particularly ACE inhibitory activity. Fractionation and identification of peptides in the thermolysin hydrolysate produced three peptides with high potential for ACE inhibition and among them two new peptides. Molecular docking analysis of the interaction between the new peptide IDHY and ACE revealed it was a promising inhibitor. In addition, the 3D structures of phycobiliproteins and RuBisCo were predicted, and the location of bioactive peptides with ACE inhibitory activity was mapped to the structure. The structural information surrounding bioactive peptides in the protein structure such as solvent accessible area, the type of secondary conformation and solubility was then determined, to understand the structure–function relationship of *G. chorda* WSP. From these results, it could be expected that *G. chorda* protein hydrolysates finds application as an ingredient in the prevention of hypertension, and bioactive peptides as a component in functional foods.

Supplementary Materials: The following supporting information can be downloaded at: https://www.mdpi.com/article/10.3390/md21010049/s1, Figure S1a–d: Amino acid sequences of the main WSP of *G. chorda*: (a) PE-α, -β, and -γ; (b) PC-α and -β; (c) APC-α, -β, and -γ (d) RuBisCo-L and -S. Table S1: Amino acid composition and distribution of *G. chorda* phycobiliproteins and RuBisCo.

Author Contributions: H.K. conceived and designed the research; Y.K. contributed to sample collection; Y.M., Y.K., M.A.M.M., W.M. and T.S. performed the experiments and analysed the data. H.K., M.A.M.M. and Y.K. contributed to writing and editing the manuscript. All authors have read and agreed to the published version of the manuscript.

Funding: This research received no external funding.

Institutional Review Board Statement: Not applicable.

Informed Consent Statement: Not applicable.

Conflicts of Interest: The authors declare no conflict of interest.

References

1. Sanjeewa, K.K.; Lee, W.; Jeon, Y.J. Nutrients and bioactive potentials of edible green and red seaweed in Korea. *Fish. Aquat. Sci.* **2018**, *21*, 19. [CrossRef]
2. Layse, C.; Almeida, F.; Falcão, H.D.S.; Lima, G.R.D.M.; Montenegro, C.D.A.; Lira, N.S.; de Athayde-Filho, P.F.; Rodrigues, L.C.; de Souza, M.F.V.; Barbosa-Filho, J.M.; et al. Bioactivities from marine algae of the genus Gracilaria. *Int. J. Mol. Sci.* **2011**, *12*, 4550–4573. [CrossRef]
3. Furuta, T.; Miyabe, Y.; Yasui, H.; Kinoshita, Y.; Kishimura, H. Angiotensin I converting enzyme inhibitory peptides derived from phycobiliproteins of dulse *Palmaria palmata*. *Mar. Drugs* **2016**, *14*, 32. [CrossRef]
4. Kumagai, Y.; Miyabe, Y.; Takeda, T.; Adachi, K.; Yasui, H.; Kishimura, H. *In silico* analysis of relationship between proteins from plastid genome of red alga *Palmaria* sp. (Japan) and angiotensin I converting enzyme inhibitory peptides. *Mar. Drugs* **2019**, *17*, 190. [CrossRef]
5. Fitzgerald, C.; Mora-Soler, L.; Gallagher, E.; O'Connor, P.; Prieto, J.; Soler-Vila, A.; Hayes, M. Isolation and characterization of bioactive pro-peptides with *in vitro* renin inhibitory activities from the macroalga *Palmaria palmata*. *J. Agric. Food Chem.* **2012**, *60*, 7421–7427. [CrossRef]

6. Sato, N.; Furuta, T.; Takeda, T.; Miyabe, Y.; Ura, K.; Takagi, Y.; Yasui, H.; Kumagai, Y.; Kishimura, H. Antioxidant activity of proteins extracted from red alga dulse harvested in Japan. *J. Food Biochem.* **2018**, *43*, e12709. [CrossRef]
7. Miyabe, Y.; Furuta, T.; Takeda, T.; Kanno, G.; Shimizu, T.; Tanaka, Y.; Gai, Z.; Yasui, H.; Kishimura, H. Structural properties of phycoerythrin from dulse *Palmaria palmata*. *J. Food Biochem.* **2017**, *41*, e12301. [CrossRef]
8. Morikawa, R.; Toji, K.; Kumagai, Y.; Kishimura, H. ACE inhibitory effect of the protein hydrolysates prepared from commercially available nori product by pepsin–trypsin digestion. *Eur. Food Res. Technol.* **2022**, *248*, 243–251. [CrossRef]
9. Windarto, S.; Lee, M.C.; Nursyam, H.; Hsu, J.L. First report of screening of novel angiotensin-I converting enzyme inhibitory peptides derived from the red alga *Acrochaetium* sp. *Mar. Biotechnol.* **2022**, *24*, 882–894. [CrossRef]
10. Joel, C.H.; Sutopo, C.C.; Prajitno, A.; Su, J.H.; Hsu, J.L. Screening of angiotensin-I converting enzyme inhibitory peptides derived from *Caulerpa lentillifera*. *Molecules* **2018**, *23*, 3005. [CrossRef]
11. Carbonaro, M.; Maselli, P.; Nucara, A. Structural aspects of legume proteins and nutraceutical properties. *Food Res. Int.* **2015**, *76*, 19–30. [CrossRef]
12. Zhang, J.; Ma, J.; Liu, D.; Qin, S.; Sun, S.; Zhao, J.; Sui, S.F. Structure of phycobilisome from the red alga *Griffithsia pacifica*. *Nature* **2017**, *551*, 57–63. [CrossRef] [PubMed]
13. Kumagai, Y.; Toji, K.; Katsukura, S.; Morikawa, R.; Uji, T.; Yasui, H.; Shimizu, T.; Kishimura, H. Characterization of ACE Inhibitory peptides prepared from *Pyropia pseudolinearis* protein. *Mar. Drugs* **2021**, *19*, 200. [CrossRef] [PubMed]
14. Bennett, A.; Bogorad, L. Complementary chromatic adaptation in a filamentous blue-green alga. *J. Cell Biol.* **1973**, *58*, 419–435. [CrossRef]
15. Cermeño, M.; Stack, J.; Tobin, P.R.; O'Keeffe, M.B.; Harnedy, P.A.; Stengel, D.B.; FitzGerald, R.J. Peptide identification from a *Porphyra dioica* protein hydrolysate with antioxidant, angiotensin converting enzyme and dipeptidyl peptidase IV inhibitory activities. *Food Funct.* **2019**, *10*, 3421–3429. [CrossRef] [PubMed]
16. Harnedy, P.A.; O'Keeffe, M.B.; FitzGerald, R.J. Purification and identification of dipeptidyl peptidase (DPP) IV inhibitory peptides from the macroalga *Palmaria palmata*. *Food Chem.* **2015**, *172*, 400–406. [CrossRef]
17. Mune Mune, M.A.; Minka, S.R.; Henle, T. Investigation on antioxidant, angiotensin converting enzyme and dipeptidyl peptidase IV inhibitory activity of Bambara bean protein hydrolysates. *Food Chem.* **2018**, *250*, 162–169. [CrossRef]
18. Rudolph, S.; Lunow, D.; Kaiser, S.; Henle, T. Identification and quantification of ACE-inhibiting peptides in enzymatic hydrolysates of plant proteins. *Food Chem.* **2017**, *224*, 19–25. [CrossRef]
19. Wu, J.; Aluko, R.E.; Nakai, S. Structural requirements of angiotensin I-converting enzyme inhibitory peptides: Quantitative structure−activity relationship study of di-and tripeptides. *J. Agri. Food Chem.* **2006**, *54*, 732–738. [CrossRef]
20. Sumikawa, K.; Takei, K.; Kumagai, Y.; Shimizu, T.; Yasui, H.; Kishimura, H. *In silico* analysis of ACE inhibitory peptides from chloroplast proteins of red alga *Grateloupia asiatica*. *Mar. Biotechnol.* **2020**, *22*, 391–402. [CrossRef]
21. Apt, K.E.; Metzner, S.; Grossman, A.R. The γ subunits of phycoerythrin from a red alga: Position in phycobilisomes and sequence characterization. *J. Phycol.* **2001**, *37*, 64–70. [CrossRef]
22. Vecchi, B.; Añon, M.C. ACE inhibitory tetrapeptides from *Amaranthus hypochondriacus* 11S globulin. *Phytochemistry* **2009**, *70*, 864–870. [CrossRef] [PubMed]
23. Fan, H.; Liao, W.; Wu, J. Molecular interactions, bioavailability, and cellular mechanisms of angiotensin-converting enzyme inhibitory peptides. *J. Food Biochem.* **2019**, *43*, e12572. [CrossRef] [PubMed]
24. Laemmli, U.K. Cleavage of structural proteins during the assembly of the head of bacteriophage e T4. *Nature* **1970**, *227*, 680–685. [CrossRef] [PubMed]
25. Cheung, H.S.; Cushman, D.W. Inhibition of homogeneous angiotensin-converting enzyme of rabbit lung by synthetic venom peptides of *Bothrops jararaca*. *Biochim. Biophys. Acta (BBA)-Enzymol.* **1973**, *293*, 451–463. [CrossRef]
26. Hatanaka, T.; Inoue, Y.; Arima, J.; Kumagai, Y.; Usuki, H.; Kawakami, K.; Kimura, M.; Mukaihara, T. Production of dipeptidyl peptidase IV inhibitory peptides from defatted rice bran. *Food Chem.* **2012**, *134*, 797–802. [CrossRef]
27. Sharma, O.P.; Bhat, T.K. DPPH antioxidant assay revisited. *Food Chem.* **2009**, *113*, 1202–1205. [CrossRef]
28. Wilson, P.J.; Grewal, S.; McFadden, T.; Chambers, R.C.; White, B.N. Mitochondrial DNA extracted from eastern North American wolves killed in the 1800s is not of gray wolf origin. *Canadian J. Zool.* **2003**, *81*, 936–940. [CrossRef]
29. Madeira, F.; Park, Y.M.; Lee, J.; Buso, N.; Gur, T.; Madhusoodanan, N.; Basutkar, P.; Tivey, A.R.N.; Potter, S.C.; Finn, R.D.; et al. The EMBL-EBI search and sequence analysis tools APIs in 2019. *Nucl. Acids Res.* **2019**, *47*, W636–W641. [CrossRef]
30. DeLano, W.L.; Bromberg, S. *PyMOL User's Guide*; DeLano Scientific LLC: South San Francisco, CA, USA, 2004.
31. Laskowski, R.A. PDBsum new things. *Nucl. Acids Res.* **2009**, *37*, D355–D359. [CrossRef]

marine drugs

Article

Immunoenhancing Effects of *Cyclina sinensis* Pentadecapeptide through Modulation of Signaling Pathways in Mice with Cyclophosphamide-Induced Immunosuppression

Rui Zhao [1], Xiao-Xia Jiang [1], Qiao-Ling Zhao [2], Han-Wei Ye [1], Yi Lin [1], Ju Huang [1,3,*] and Yun-Ping Tang [1,*]

1 Zhejiang Provincial Engineering Technology Research Center of Marine Biomedical Products, School of Food and Pharmacy, Zhejiang Ocean University, Zhoushan 316022, China
2 Zhoushan Institute for Food and Drug Control, Zhoushan 316000, China
3 Key Laboratory of Health Risk Factors for Seafood of Zhejiang Province, Zhejiang Ocean University, Zhoushan 316022, China
* Correspondence: qiuqiu20130621@163.com (J.H.); tangyunping1985@zjou.edu.cn (Y.-P.T.)

Abstract: Our study aimed to investigate the immune-enhancing mechanism of the pentadecapeptide (RVAPEEHPVEGRYLV) from *Cyclina sinensis* (SCSP) in a cyclophosphamide (CTX)-induced murine model of immunosuppression. Our results showed that SCSP treatment significantly increased mouse body weight, immune organ indices, and the production of serum IL-6, IL-1β, and tumor necrosis factor (TNF)-α in CTX-treated mice. In addition, SCSP treatment enhanced the proliferation of splenic lymphocytes and peritoneal macrophages, as well as phagocytosis of the latter in a dose-dependent manner. Moreover, SCSP elevated the phosphorylation levels of p38, ERK, JNK, PI3K and Akt, and up-regulated IKKα, IKKβ, p50 NF-κB and p65 NF-κB protein levels, while down-regulating IκBα protein levels. Our results indicate that SCSP has immune-enhancing activities, and that it can activate the MAPK/NF-κB and PI3K/Akt pathways to enhance immunity in CTX-induced immunosuppressed mice.

Keywords: *Cyclina sinensis*; pentadecapeptide; immunomodulatory; cyclophosphamide; mechanism

Citation: Zhao, R.; Jiang, X.-X.; Zhao, Q.-L.; Ye, H.-W.; Lin, Y.; Huang, J.; Tang, Y.-P. Immunoenhancing Effects of *Cyclina sinensis* Pentadecapeptide through Modulation of Signaling Pathways in Mice with Cyclophosphamide-Induced Immunosuppression. *Mar. Drugs* **2022**, *20*, 560. https://doi.org/10.3390/md20090560

Academic Editors: Chang-Feng Chi and Bin Wang

Received: 8 August 2022
Accepted: 28 August 2022
Published: 31 August 2022

1. Introduction

The immune system, composed of a complete set of immune organs, cells, and active substances, constantly monitors the body for foreign entities and maintains the continuous and healthy operation of the entire body [1]. However, factors such as obesity [2], stress [3], mood [4], and lifestyle [5] have been shown to affect its normal functioning. Immunotherapy can artificially enhance or suppress the body's immunological responses in cases of low or hyperactive conditions in order to return the immune system to its physiologic status [6]. Compared with the instability and adverse effects of chemically synthesized immunomodulators, natural products with immunomodulatory activity offer a way of effectively avoiding these risk factors [7,8]. Therefore, it is necessary to identify safe and effective natural immune modulators.

In the field of natural active product development, the marine environment offers a treasure trove of natural compounds with distinctive biological characteristics, due to its high biodiversity and complex ecological relationships [9]. Marine peptides have attracted much attention due to their unique biological properties, such as antihypertensive [10], antioxidant [11], antitumor [12], and antidiabetic activities [13]. Immunomodulatory peptides identified from different marine sources have shown significant immune-enhancing activities [14–16]. For example, Li et al. [17] purified two peptides (DNSIAMESMK and LLQLGSG) from oyster hydrolysate and showed that these two peptides markedly promoted the proliferation of murine lymphocytes and the phagocytic ability of macrophages. Cai et al. [18] isolated two peptides (HIAEEADRK and AEQAESDKK) from trypsin hydrolysates of tuna and showed that these two peptides could bind to the active sites of

TLR2 and TLR4 and stimulate macrophage activation. Xu et al. [19] purified a peptide (YVMRF) with immunoregulatory activity from *Stolephorus chinensis* and confirmed that YVMRF could stimulate RAW 264.7 differentiation and increase the concentrations of nitric oxide (NO), TNF-α, IL-6, and IL-1β. In previous studies, we purified an immunomodulatory peptide (RVAPEEHPVEGRYLV) from *Cyclina sinensis* (SCSP) and demonstrated that SCSP showed significant immune-enhancing activities in mice with CTX-induced immunosuppression [20]. However, the mechanisms underlying the immunomodulatory effects of SCSP have not been elucidated.

Several signaling pathways have been shown to play crucial roles in immune activation, including MAPK, PI3K/Akt, and downstream NF-κB pathways [21–23]. Yu et al. [24] demonstrated that sulfate-modified *Cyclocarya paliurus* polysaccharide could enhance the secretion of TNF-α, IL-10 and NO in immunosuppressed mice by modulating the MyD88-dependent MAPK/NF-κB/PI3K-Akt signaling pathway. He et al. [25] verified that low-molecular-weight peptides from *Mytilus coruscus* exerted immunomodulatory effects on macrophages by regulating the NF-κB/MAPK pathway. Yao et al. [26] reported that European eel (*Anguilla anguilla*)-derived peptides promoted the production of NO, inducible nitric oxide synthase (iNOS) and cytokines by modulating the NF-κB and MAPK pathways in macrophages. Moreover, the hexapeptide RNPFLP isolated from *Lepidium meyenii* protein hydrolysate activated RAW 264.7 cells via TLR2 and TLR4 receptor-mediated activation of the NF-κB and MAPK pathway [27]. In this study, we focused on the MAPK/NF-κB and PI3K/Akt pathways to investigate the potential mechanisms underlying the immune-enhancing effects of SCSP in mice with CTX-induced immunosuppression. Our results provide an explanation for the effects of SCSP and support its use as a novel immunomodulator candidate or immune adjuvant.

2. Results

2.1. Effect of SCSP on Immune Organ Indices

Body weight and organ indices are often utilized as the primary metrics to examine the physiological conditions of experimental animals and the therapeutic impact of medications in the early stages of research [28]. Our previous studies showed that the final murine body weight in the SCSP-treated groups was significantly higher than in the CTX group, suggesting that SCSP could improve CTX-induced murine body weight loss [29]. Moreover, SCSP treatment effectively increased the murine immune organ indices, showing that SCSP could alleviate immune organ damage by CTX (Figure 1).

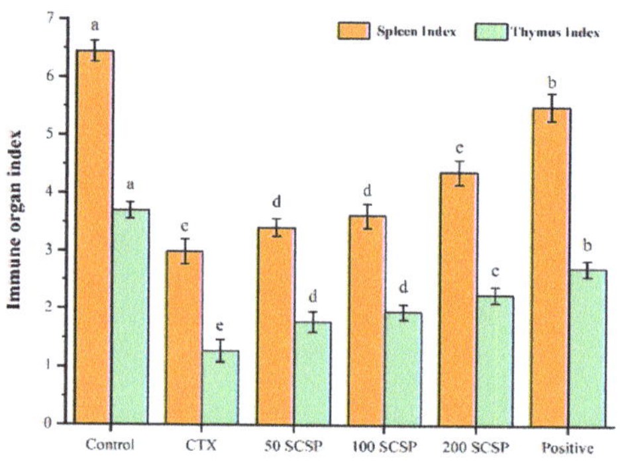

Figure 1. Effect of SCSP on immune organ indices in CTX-induced mice (n = 10). Different letters over bars indicate statistical significance between two groups ($p < 0.05$), the same as below.

2.2. Effect of SCSP on Cytokine Production

As shown in Figure 2, CTX significantly inhibited the secretion of IL-1β (9.38 ± 0.21 ng/L vs. 16.30 ± 0.19 ng/L), IL-6 (12.79 ± 0.39 ng/L vs. 33.16 ± 0.82 ng/L), and TNF-α

(61.61 ± 1.88 ng/L vs. 94.27 ± 1.75 ng/L) when compared with the control group. Remarkably, higher concentrations of the three cytokines were observed (12.44 ± 0.26 ng/L, IL-1β; 30.22 ± 0.50 ng/L, IL-6; and 78.20 ± 2.12 ng/L, TNF-α) after treatment with 200 mg/kg of SCSP, although it was still lower than in the positive control group. The above results suggest that SCSP has an antagonistic effect on CTX-induced suppression of cytokine secretion.

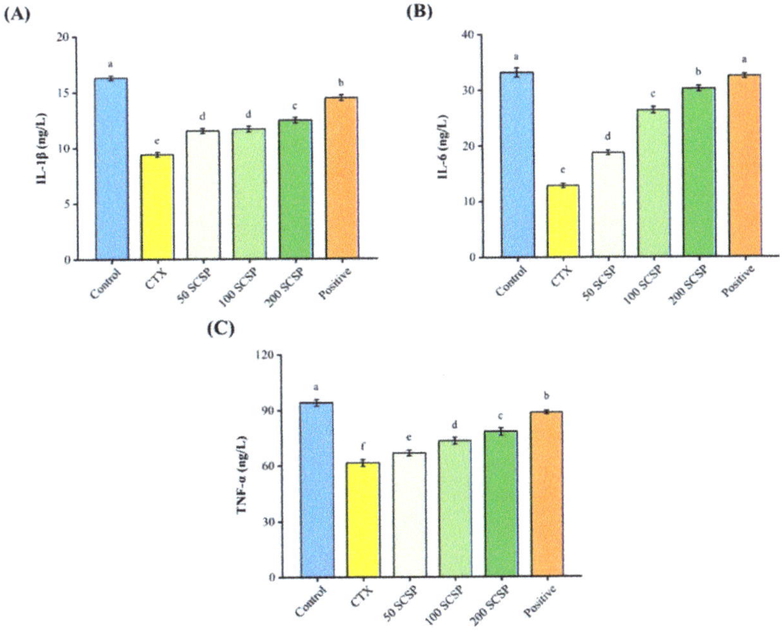

Figure 2. Effect of SCSP on serum levels of IL-1β (**A**), IL-6 (**B**), and TNF-α (**C**) in immunosuppressed mice (n = 10).

2.3. *Effects of SCSP on Cellular Immunity*

An experiment with splenic lymphocytes was carried out to determine the impact of SCSP on T and B cellular immune responses. As shown in Figure 3, CTX treatment significantly inhibited the proliferative activity of these two immune cell populations when compared with the control group (0.125 ± 0.009 vs. 0.226 ± 0.006, B cells; 0.116 ± 0.004 vs. 0.189 ± 0.007, T cells; $p < 0.05$). However, when animals were treated with different concentrations of SCSP, the proliferation of B and T cells improved substantially when compared with the CTX group ($p < 0.05$), indicating that SCSP enhanced cellular immune responses, increasing spleen lymphocyte proliferation. Otherwise, it was still lower than in the positive control group.

Proliferation (Figure 4A) and phagocytosis (Figure 4B) of mouse peritoneal macrophages were also analyzed to examine the regulatory effects of SCSP on immune cells. CTX significantly inhibited the proliferation and phagocytic activity of macrophages when compared with the control group. However, with increasing doses of SCSP, the proliferative rate of macrophages gradually increased, reaching its highest at 200 mg/kg of SCSP (0.324 ± 0.014), although it was still lower than in the positive control group (0.374 ± 0.019). On the other hand, SCSP considerably restored the phagocytic ability of macrophages when compared with the CTX-treated group, and this effect reached its highest at 200 mg/kg of SCSP. However, it was still lower than in the positive control group. These findings demonstrate that SCSP can enhance lymphocyte and macrophage activity to overcome CTX-induced immunosuppression.

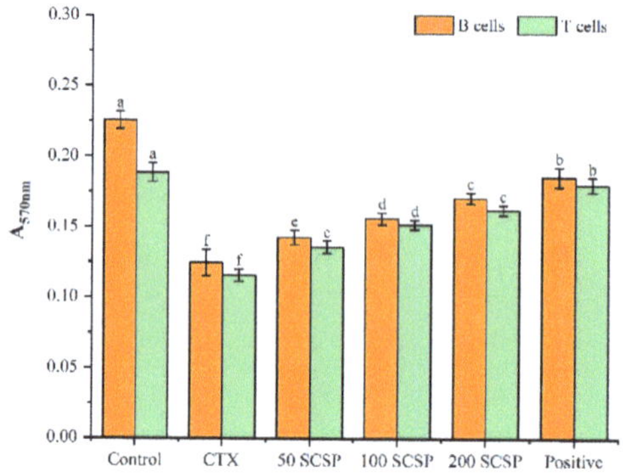

Figure 3. Effect of SCSP on the proliferative capacity of mouse spleen lymphocytes in vitro ($n = 10$).

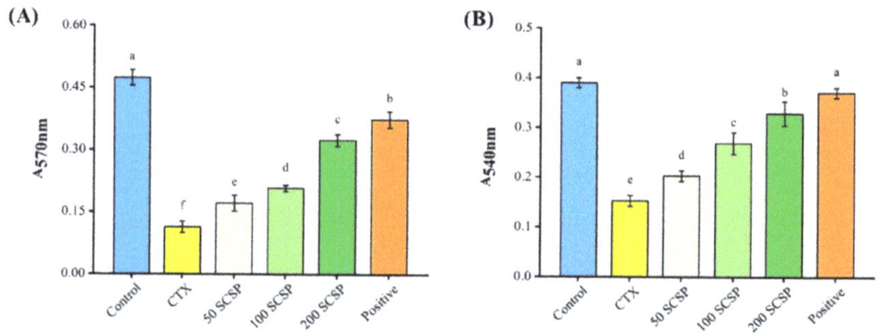

Figure 4. Effect of SCSP on the proliferative (**A**) and phagocytic (**B**) capacity of peritoneal macrophages in mice ($n = 10$).

2.4. Western Blot Analysis

To explore the mechanisms underlying the immunomodulatory effects of SCSP, the expression levels of proteins associated with the MAPK/NF-κB and PI3K/Akt pathways were analyzed in the spleen. In both pathways, CTX significantly inhibited the phosphorylation levels of the corresponding proteins ($p < 0.05$). After the administration of 200 mg/kg SCSP, the proportions of p-PI3K/PI3K and p-Akt/Akt were dramatically up-regulated in comparison with the CTX group (Figure 5B,C, $p < 0.05$), and the levels of up-regulation were higher than in the positive control group. Moreover, a notable enhancement in the phosphorylation levels of JNK, ERK and p38 was detected when SCSP (200 mg/kg) was administered (Figure 6B–D, $p < 0.05$).

As shown in Figure 7, NF-κB p50, NF-κB p65, IKKα, and IKKβ protein expression levels were markedly down-regulated after CTX treatment, while the expression level of IκBα increased, but not significantly. After treatment with 200 mg/kg of SCSP, the protein levels of NF-κB p50, NF-κB p65, IKKα, and IKKβ in the spleen of immunosuppressed mice increased considerably. Meanwhile, the expression of IκBα was clearly down-regulated ($p < 0.05$) when compared with the control. These results suggest that SCSP exerts its immunomodulatory effects in mice by activating the MAPK/NF-κB and PI3K/Akt pathways.

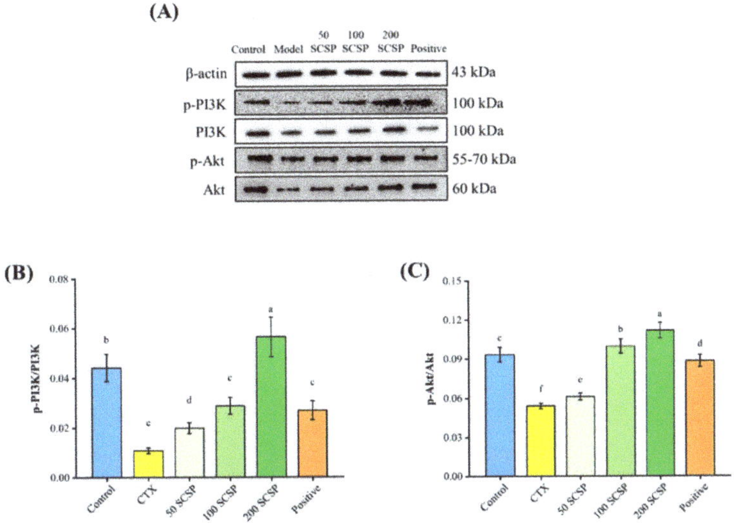

Figure 5. Effect of SCSP on the splenic PI3K/Akt pathway in mice (n = 10). (**A**) Western blotting of the related proteins in the PI3K/Akt pathway; (**B**) The expression of p-PI3K/PI3K; (**C**) The expression of p-Akt/Akt.

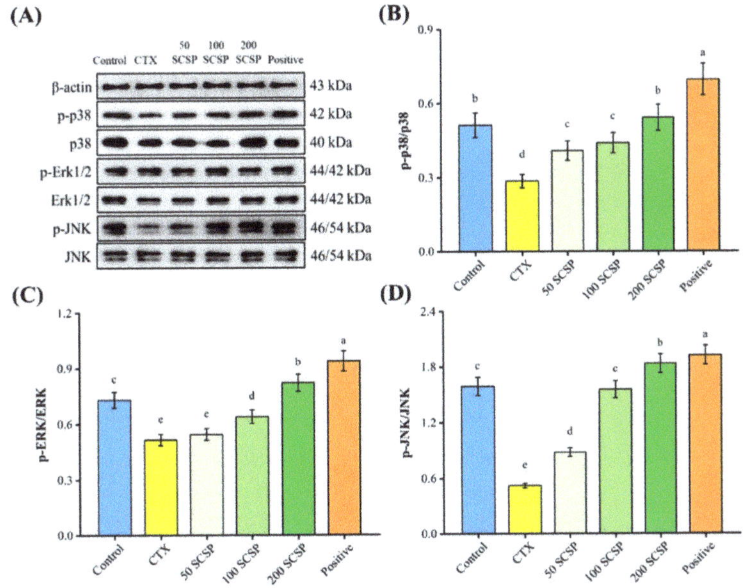

Figure 6. Effect of SCSP on the splenic MAPK pathway in mice (n = 10). (**A**) Western blotting of the related proteins in the MAPK pathway; (**B**) the expression of p-p38/p38; (**C**) the expression of p-ERk/ERk; (**D**) the expression of p-JNK/JNK.

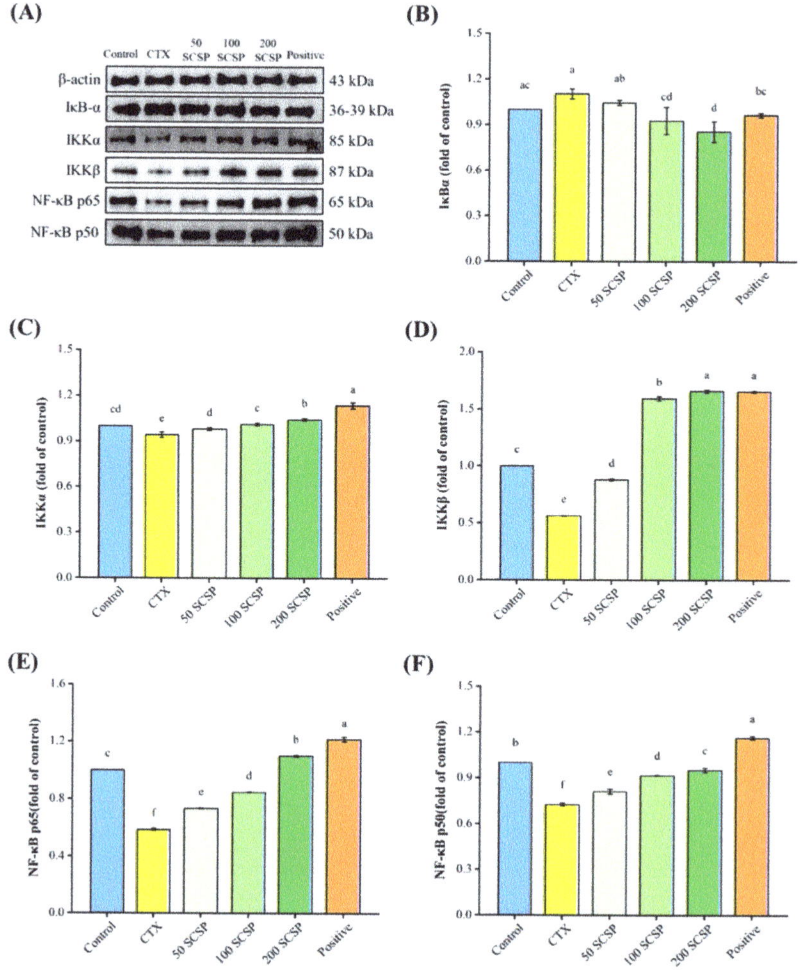

Figure 7. Effect of SCSP on the splenic NF-κB pathway in mice (n = 10). (**A**) Western blotting of the related proteins in the NF-κB pathway; (**B**) the expression of IκBα; (**C**) the expression of IKKα; (**D**) the expression of IKKβ; (**E**) the expression of NF-κB p65; (**F**) the expression of NF-κB p50.

2.5. Expression of NF-κB p65 in the Spleen

Immunohistochemical results showed that NF-κB p65 was highly expressed in the spleen of untreated mice, as evidenced by the brownish-yellow color in the cytoplasm and nucleus, whereas it was hardly observed in the CTX-immunosuppressed group. In contrast, the expression of NF-κB p65 increased gradually with higher SCSP doses (Figure 8). On the other hand, the expression level of NF-κB p65 in the positive control group was between that of the control and the SCSP-treated groups. These findings indicate that SCSP can increase NF-κB p65 expression in the spleen of CTX-immunosuppressed mice.

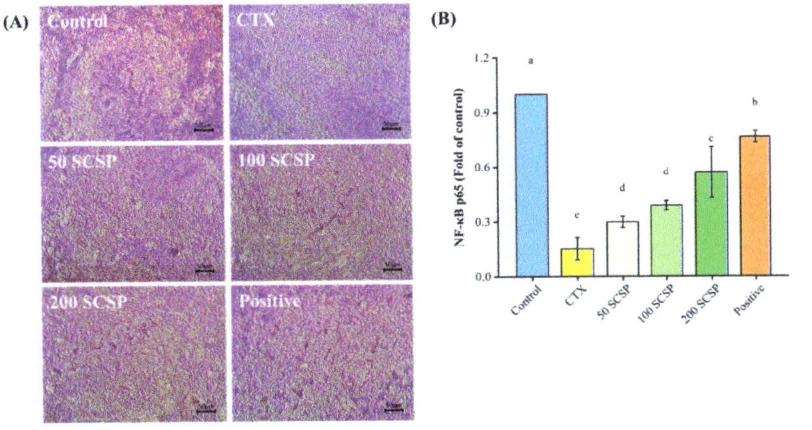

Figure 8. Effect of SCSP on NF-κB p65 expression in the spleen of mice (n = 10). (**A**) Immunohistochemistry of the spleen (×200); (**B**) semi-quantitative analysis of NF-κB p65.

2.6. Expression of p-PI3K in Spleen

The impact of SCSP on the expression of p-PI3K in the spleen of immunosuppressed mice is shown in Figure 9. The expression of p-PI3K in immunosuppressed mice was significantly lower than that in the untreated control group, as evidenced by the almost complete disappearance of brown granules in the cytoplasm. In contrast, some recovery of brown particles was observed following administration of SCSP (200 mg/kg), suggesting that SCSP can enhance the weak expression of p-PI3K caused by CTX treatment.

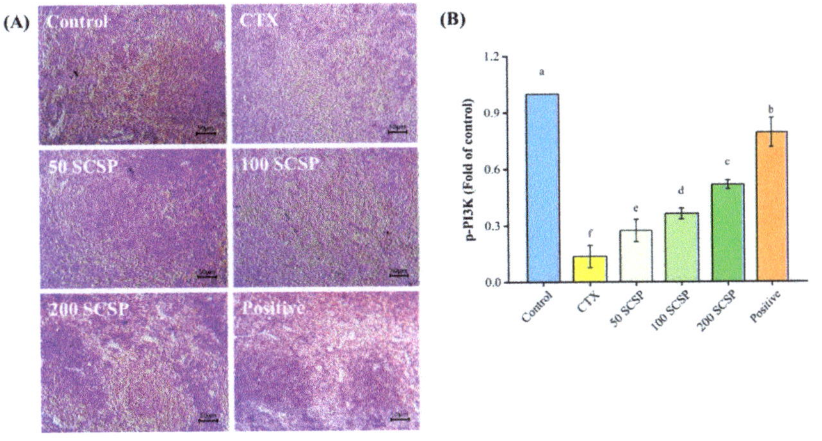

Figure 9. Effect of SCSP on p-PI3K expression in the spleen of mice (n = 10). (**A**) Immunohistochemistry of the spleen (×200); (**B**) semi-quantitative analysis of p-PI3K.

2.7. Expression of p-p38 in the Spleen

The expression of p-p38 in the spleen was also analyzed, and this was seen as a brownish-yellow region. Unlike the control group, the p-p38 protein was minimally expressed in the spleen of immunosuppressed mice (Figure 10A). However, it can be seen in the image that the brown particles in the SCSP and positive control groups clearly increased, and there was no noticeable difference between these two groups.

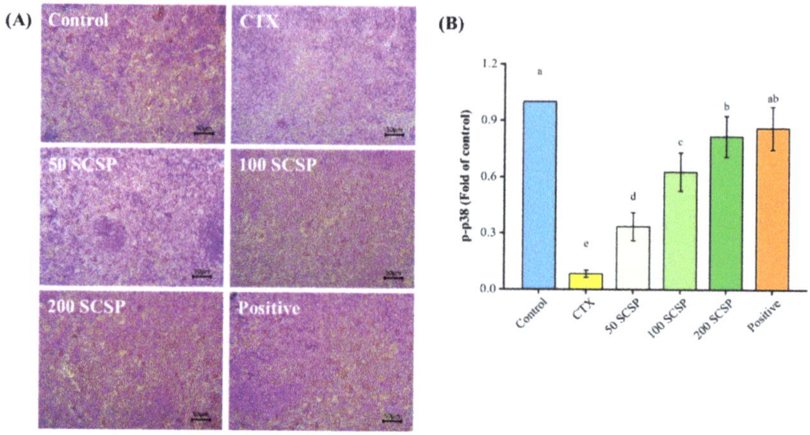

Figure 10. Effect of SCSP on p-p38 expression in the spleen of mice ($n = 10$). (**A**) Immunohistochemistry of the spleen (×200); (**B**) semi-quantitative analysis of p-p38.

3. Discussion

The immune system is an intricate network of immune organs, cells, and active substances that interact with each other to maintain the healthy operation of the body [1]. The rigorous regulation of the immune system is essential to ensure that the body mounts an appropriate response to pathogens while preventing excessive immune reactions. With the discovery of immunomodulators, immune regulation as a therapeutic approach against tumors, autoimmune diseases, and inflammatory diseases has become a reality [30]. CTX is the most commonly used chemotherapeutic drug against cancer in clinical practice, but it is associated with unwanted side effects such as immunosuppression [31]. To characterize an immunomodulator that can counteract this unwanted effect, we established a murine model of immunosuppression by intraperitoneally administering 80 mg/kg CTX for three continuous days. We used this model to explore the potential immunomodulatory mechanisms of SCSP.

Consistent with previous results [20], the suppression of immune function induced by CTX was reflected in the body weight and immune organ indices. The production of serum IL-1β, IL-6 and TNF-α, and the expression of NF-κB p65, p-PI3K and p-p38 in the spleen were all considerably lower than in the control group. Moreover, under the influence of CTX, the proliferative and phagocytic abilities of peritoneal macrophages and the proliferation of spleen lymphocytes were reduced, indicating that the CTX-induced immunosuppression model was successful.

As the largest immune organ in the body, the spleen is not only part of the lymphatic system, but also an important site for lymphocytes to migrate and receive antigenic stimulation to generate immune responses and immune effector molecules [32]. The thymus is the site for the differentiation, development and maturation of T lymphocytes. The development of all lymphoid organs and the generation of immunity in the body require the replenishment of T lymphocytes [28]. CTX can trigger immune organ atrophy and weight loss by reducing lymphocyte numbers in immune organs and inhibiting their proliferation and differentiation [31,33]. Our results showed that SCSP alleviated weight loss, splenic and thymic atrophy, and increased immune organ indices in immunosuppressed mice, suggesting that SCSP treatment has a significant immune-enhancing effect on immune organs.

Cytokines are small-molecular-weight proteins synthesized and secreted by immune cells. They perform critical functions, regulating cell interactions and the growth and differentiation of immune cells during immune responses [34]. It has been reported that polypeptides can stimulate several cellular immunological responses and regulate the secretion of different cytokines, thereby enhancing immune function in mice [35–37]. Our findings demonstrated that serum cytokines (IL-1β, IL-6, and TNF-α) in SCSP-treated mice increased in a dose-dependent manner. The lymphocyte is a major player in the immune response. T cells and B cells mediate cellular and humoral immunity, respectively, and their proliferation is directly correlated with the strength of specific immune responses [38]. Macrophages are involved in the recognition, phagocytosis and degradation of pathogens and trigger adaptive immune responses by presenting antigens to T cells [39]. Furthermore, in the initial stages of inflammation, macrophages play an indispensable role by releasing cytokines and chemokines [40]. Compared with the CTX-immunosuppressed group, SCSP significantly restored the proliferative rate of lymphocytes (T and B cells) and macrophages. Moreover, with increasing SCSP doses, the phagocytic capacity of peritoneal macrophages also increased. These results suggest that SCSP treatment reverses CTX-induced immune damage by enhancing immune cell function in mice.

NF-κB is a family of transcription factors involved in various biological processes such as inflammation, apoptosis, and proliferation [41,42]. The typical NF-κB pathway is considered to be a central regulator of inflammatory responses and has been extensively studied in human autoimmune diseases and cancer [43]. Akt serves as a key component of the PI3K/Akt signaling pathway, mediating multiple cellular functions, including metabolism, growth, and proliferation [44]. The activation of upstream PI3K enables Akt to regulate NF-κB signaling by phosphorylating IKK [45]. Our results showed that SCSP not only up-regulated the expression of important components of the NF-κB pathway in the spleen (including IKKα, IKKβ, NF-κB p50 and p65), but also enhanced the phosphorylation levels of PI3K and Akt proteins, and these results were consistent with the immunohistochemical results in splenic tissue. As one of the important pathways in the eukaryotic signal transmission network, the MAPK pathway modulates a number of crucial cellular physiological processes such as cell proliferation, differentiation, and inflammatory responses [46]. Western blotting results indicated that SCSP treatment of CTX-immunosuppressed animals increased the phosphorylation of JNK, ERK, and p38 proteins when compared with the CTX-immunosuppressed group. In addition, the immunohistochemical results also indicated that the SCSP group showed high expression of p-p38 protein. It has previously been reported that wild-simulated ginseng can activate mouse macrophages to produce immunomodulators (TNF-α, IL-1β, and IL-6) and intensify phagocytosis via the MAPK, NF-κB, and PI3K/Akt pathways [47]. Our overall results are consistent with the above reports, since the immune-enhancing effects of SCSP in CTX-immunosuppressed mice was achieved through activation of the MAPK/NF-κB and PI3K/Akt pathways.

4. Materials and Methods

4.1. Materials and Reagents

SCSP was provided by Wuxi MimoTopes Biotechnology (Wuxi, China) [20]. CTX was purchased from Hengrui Medicine (Lianyungang, China). The DAB immunohistochemistry kit was purchased from Boster (Wuhan, China). Neutral red staining solution and primary antibodies against β-actin, NF-κB p50, NF-κB p65, IKKα, IKKβ, and IκBα were supplied by Beyotime (Shanghai, China). The remaining primary antibodies were provided by Cell Signaling Technology Inc. (Beverly, MA, USA).

4.2. Animals and Treatment

A total of 60 male ICR mice (six-week-old, 20 ± 2 g) were purchased from the Zhejiang Academy of Medical Sciences (Hangzhou, China). All procedures in laboratory animals were authorized by the Animal Ethics Committee of Zhejiang Ocean University (SCXK ZHE 2019-0031). Mice were randomly assigned to six groups (n = 10) after the one-week adaptation period. With the exception of the control group, the remaining groups were treated with 80 mg/kg CTX continuously for three days [48]. Subsequently, the experimental groups were treated with different doses of SCSP (50, 100, and 200 mg/kg), while the positive control group received levamisole hydrochloride (25 mg/kg) at the same time for seven consecutive days (Figure 11). Twenty-four hours after the last feeding, blood samples were obtained using eyeball extirpation, and the mice were sacrificed by cervical dislocation.

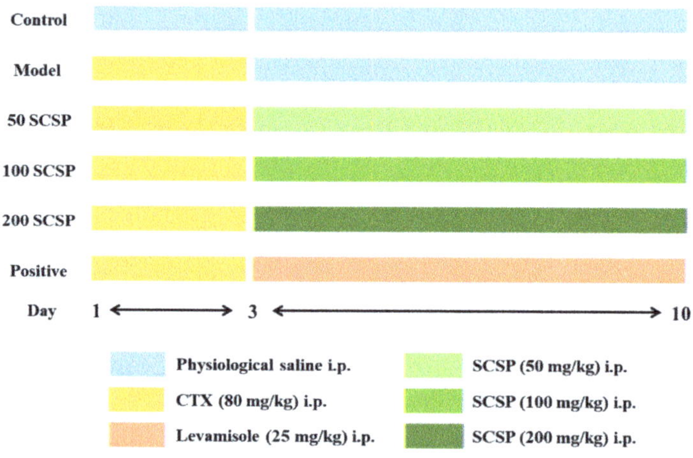

Figure 11. The experimental scheme and treatment of mice (n = 10). i.p., intraperitoneal injection.

4.3. Immune Organ Indices

The daily weight fluctuations of mice were monitored and recorded during the whole experiment. The collected spleens and thymuses were used to determine the organ indices using the following formula:

$$\text{Thymus or spleen index} = \text{thymus or spleen weight (mg)/body weight (g)} \qquad (1)$$

4.4. Cytokines Assays in Serum

Blood samples were collected in centrifuge tubes without anticoagulant treatment and placed in a refrigerator at 4 °C. After blood coagulation, serum was collected by centrifuging (6000× g, 5 min). The concentrations of IL-6, IL-1β, and TNF-α were determined following the guidelines by Solarbio (Beijing, China).

4.5. Splenic Lymphocyte Proliferation Assay

To evaluate the proliferative responses of T and B lymphocytes, splenic lymphocytes were stimulated with Con A and LPS, respectively [49,50]. The preparation of mouse spleen lymphocytes was carried out as described by Tang et al. [49,50]. The collected cells were seeded in a 96-well plate (1 × 10^6 cells/mL, 4 replicate wells in each group), Con A (5 μg/mL) or LPS (1 μg/mL) was added, and the plate was placed in an incubator (Forma 3111 CO_2 incubator, Thermo Forma, Waltham, MA, USA) at 37 °C with 5% CO_2 for 24 h. Then, 200 μL of MTT staining solution was added, and 150 μL of DMSO was added after incubating for 4 h. The absorbance at 570 nm was measured (SpectraMax M2 microplate reader, Molecular Devices, Silicon Valley, CA, USA).

4.6. Peritoneal Macrophage Proliferation Assay

The mice were intraperitoneally injected with sterile saline solution (5 mL), and the abdomen was gently pressed for 2 min, and the abdominal wall was cut open. Then, the abdominal fluid was sucked into a centrifuge tube, and the cell suspension was centrifuged (2000× g, 10 min) and resuspended with DMEM medium. After incubation at 37 °C with 5% CO_2 for 4 h, the supernatant was discarded to obtain purified macrophages [49,50]. The cell density was then adjusted (1 × 10^4 cells/mL), seeded in 96-well plates (200 μL per well), and incubated for 24 h. After discarding the supernatant from each well, 200 μL of PBS containing 10% MTT was added, and the plates were incubated for another 4 h. Then, 150 μL DMSO was added, and the optical density (OD) at 570 nm was measured to calculate the proliferation rate of macrophages.

4.7. Macrophage Phagocytic Capacity

Macrophage phagocytosis was examined by measuring neutral red uptake [50]. The collected peritoneal macrophages were seeded on a 96-well plate (5×10^5 cells/mL) and incubated for 24 h. Then, 200 μL of nutrient solution (excluding $NaHCO_3$), and 20 μL of neutral red staining solution was added. The supernatant was discarded after incubating for 2 h, lysis buffer was added, and the cells were incubated for another 10 min. The absorbance at 540 nm was measured, and the phagocytic index was calculated.

4.8. Western Blotting

The experimental procedures were conducted as previously described [31]. Briefly, the BCA protein assay kit was used to measure the amount of protein in each spleen homogenate supernatant, and 30 μg of proteins were loaded per lane. The proteins were separated using a 12% SDS-PAGE gel and then transferred to the PVDF membrane. Enhanced chemiluminescence (ECL) was utilized to detect the bands, and data processing was carried out using the Alphaview SA gel image analysis software (Fluor Chem FC3, ProteinSimple, San Jose, CA, USA).

4.9. Immunohistochemical Analysis

Paraffin sections of the mouse spleen were deparaffinized and rehydrated. Then, endogenous peroxidase was blocked with H_2O_2 and treated with antigen retrieval solution. After incubating with the primary antibody at 4 °C overnight, the secondary antibody was added, and the samples were incubated for 1 h. Finally, the DAB immunohistochemical staining kit was used for color development, and the staining characteristics of each group were analyzed with a CX31 biological microscope (Olympus, Tokyo, Japan).

4.10. Statistical Analysis

One-way analysis of variance (ANOVA) was performed on the experimental data using SPSS 22.0 software. All results are expressed as the mean ± standard deviation ($x \pm SD$) and differences between means were considered significant at $p < 0.05$.

5. Conclusions

In conclusion, SCSP enhanced immune responses by attenuating CTX-induced splenic and thymic damage in mice, enhancing the cellular functions of splenic lymphocytes and peritoneal macrophages, and promoting cytokine secretion. Moreover, SCSP activated the MAPK/NF-κB and PI3K/Akt pathways to enhance murine immunity (Figure 12). Our findings suggest that SCSP can effectively reverse CTX-induced murine immunosuppression, indicating that SCSP could be developed as a new immunomodulator or immune adjuvant in the future.

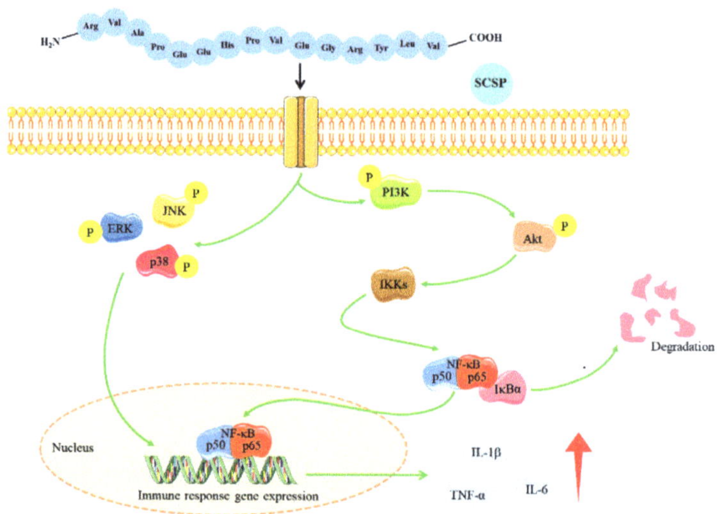

Figure 12. SCSP ameliorates CTX-induced immunosuppression possibly by regulating the MAPK/NF-κB and PI3K/Akt pathways.

Author Contributions: J.H. and Y.-P.T. conceived the study and designed the project. R.Z., X.-X.J., Q.-L.Z., H.-W.Y. and Y.L. experimented and analyzed the data. J.H. and Y.-P.T. revised the manuscript and supervised the whole study. All authors have read and agreed to the published version of the manuscript.

Funding: This work was financially supported by the National Natural Science Foundation of China (No. 41806153), the Zhejiang Province "Triple Agriculture Nine Aspects Cooperation" Science and Technology Cooperation Program (No. 2022SNJF064).

International Review Board Statement: All animal procedures were performed under the Animal Ethics Committee of Zhejiang Ocean University (No. SCXK ZHE 2019-0031).

Data Availability Statement: Data supporting our findings can be sent upon request.

Conflicts of Interest: The authors declare that the research was conducted in the absence of any commercial or financial relationships that could be construed as potential conflicts of interest.

References

1. Ploegh, H.L. Logic of the immune system. *Cancer Immunol. Res.* **2013**, *1*, 5–10. [CrossRef] [PubMed]
2. Barakat, B.; Almeida, M.E.F. Biochemical and immunological changes in obesity. *Arch. Biochem. Biophys.* **2021**, *708*, 108951. [CrossRef] [PubMed]
3. Ambrée, O.; Ruland, C.; Scheu, S.; Arolt, V.; Alferink, J. Alterations of the innate immune system in susceptibility and resilience after social defeat stress. *Front. Behav. Neurosci.* **2018**, *12*, 141. [CrossRef] [PubMed]
4. Herkenham, M.; Kigar, S.L. Contributions of the adaptive immune system to mood regulation: Mechanisms and pathways of neuroimmune interactions. *Prog. Neuro-Psychopharmacol. Biol. Psychiatry* **2017**, *79*, 49–57. [CrossRef]
5. Filgueira, T.O.; Castoldi, A.; Santos, L.E.R.; de Amorim, G.J.; de Sousa Fernandes, M.S.; Anastácio, W.d.L.d.N.; Campos, E.Z.; Santos, T.M.; Souto, F.O. The relevance of a physical active lifestyle and physical fitness on immune defense: Mitigating disease burden, with focus on COVID-19 consequences. *Front. Immunol.* **2021**, *12*, 587146. [CrossRef]
6. Zhou, B.; Liu, J.; Lin, M.; Zhu, J.; Chen, W.R. Recent advances in immunotherapy, immunoadjuvant, and nanomaterial-based combination immunotherapy. *Coord. Chem. Rev.* **2021**, *442*, 214009. [CrossRef]
7. Zhang, M.; Zhong, J.; Xiong, Y.; Song, X.; Li, C.; He, Z. Development of broad-spectrum antiviral agents—Inspiration from immunomodulatory natural products. *Viruses* **2021**, *13*, 1257. [CrossRef]
8. Nuzzo, G.; Senese, G.; Gallo, C.; Albiani, F.; Romano, L.; d'Ippolito, G.; Manzo, E.; Fontana, A. Antitumor potential of immunomodulatory natural products. *Mar. Drugs* **2022**, *20*, 386. [CrossRef]
9. Hamed, I.; Özogul, F.; Özogul, Y.; Regenstein, J.M. Marine bioactive compounds and their health benefits: A review. *Compr. Rev. Food Sci. Food Saf.* **2015**, *14*, 446–465. [CrossRef]

10. Pujiastuti, D.Y.; Ghoyatul Amin, M.N.; Alamsjah, M.A.; Hsu, J.-L. Marine organisms as potential sources of bioactive peptides that inhibit the activity of angiotensin I-converting enzyme: A review. *Molecules* **2019**, *24*, 2541. [CrossRef]
11. Chai, T.-T.; Law, Y.-C.; Wong, F.-C.; Kim, S.-K. Enzyme-assisted discovery of antioxidant peptides from edible marine invertebrates: A review. *Mar. Drugs* **2017**, *15*, 42. [CrossRef]
12. Xing, H.; Tong, M.; Jiang, N.; Zhang, X.; Hu, H.; Pan, H.; Li, D. Antitumour bioactive peptides isolated from marine organisms. *Clin. Exp. Pharmacol. Physiol.* **2017**, *44*, 1077–1082. [CrossRef]
13. Ngo, D.-H.; Vo, T.-S.; Ngo, D.-N.; Wijesekara, I.; Kim, S.-K. Biological activities and potential health benefits of bioactive peptides derived from marine organisms. *Int. J. Biol. Macromol.* **2012**, *51*, 378–383. [CrossRef]
14. Yu, F.; He, K.; Dong, X.; Zhang, Z.; Wang, F.; Tang, Y.; Chen, Y.; Ding, G. Immunomodulatory activity of low molecular-weight peptides from *Nibea japonica* skin in cyclophosphamide-induced immunosuppressed mice. *J. Funct. Foods* **2020**, *68*, 103888. [CrossRef]
15. Kang, H.K.; Lee, H.H.; Seo, C.H.; Park, Y. Antimicrobial and immunomodulatory properties and applications of marine-derived proteins and peptides. *Mar. Drugs* **2019**, *17*, 350. [CrossRef]
16. Ren, D.; Wang, M.; Shen, M.; Liu, C.; Liu, W.; Min, W.; Liu, J. In vivo assessment of immunomodulatory activity of hydrolysed peptides from *Corylus heterophylla* Fisch. *J. Sci. Food Agric.* **2016**, *96*, 3508–3514. [CrossRef]
17. Li, W.; Xu, C.; Zhang, C.; Cao, W.; Qin, X.; Gao, J.; Zheng, H. The purification and identification of immunoregulatory peptides from oyster (*Crassostrea hongkongensis*) enzymatic hydrolysate. *RSC Adv.* **2019**, *9*, 32854–32863. [CrossRef]
18. Cai, B.; Chen, H.; Wan, P.; Luo, L.; Ye, Z.; Huang, J.; Chen, D.; Pan, J. Isolation and identification of immunomodulatory peptides from the protein hydrolysate of tuna trimmings (*Thunnas albacares*). *LWT* **2022**, *164*, 113614. [CrossRef]
19. Xu, B.; Ye, L.; Tang, Y.; Zheng, J.; Tian, X.; Yang, Y.; Yang, Z. Preparation and purification of an immunoregulatory peptide from *Stolephorus chinensis* of the East Sea of China. *Process Biochem.* **2020**, *98*, 151–159. [CrossRef]
20. Yu, F.; Zhang, Z.; Ye, S.; Hong, X.; Jin, H.; Huang, F.; Yang, Z.; Tang, Y.; Chen, Y.; Ding, G. Immunoenhancement effects of pentadecapeptide derived from *Cyclina sinensis* on immune-deficient mice induced by Cyclophosphamide. *J. Funct. Foods* **2019**, *60*, 103408. [CrossRef]
21. Xu, Z.; Chu, M. Advances in immunosuppressive agents based on signal pathway. *Front. Pharmacol.* **2022**, *13*, 917162. [CrossRef]
22. Arakelyan, A.; Nersisyan, L.; Poghosyan, D.; Khondkaryan, L.; Hakobyan, A.; Löffler-Wirth, H.; Melanitou, E.; Binder, H. Autoimmunity and autoinflammation: A systems view on signaling pathway dysregulation profiles. *PLoS ONE* **2017**, *12*, e0187572. [CrossRef]
23. Mohseni, A.H.; Casolaro, V.; Bermúdez-Humarán, L.G.; Keyvani, H.; Taghinezhad-S, S. Modulation of the PI3K/Akt/mTOR signaling pathway by probiotics as a fruitful target for orchestrating the immune response. *Gut Microbes* **2021**, *13*, 1886844. [CrossRef]
24. Yu, Y.; Mo, S.; Shen, M.; Chen, Y.; Yu, Q.; Li, Z.; Xie, J. Sulfated modification enhances the immunomodulatory effect of *Cyclocarya paliurus* polysaccharide on cyclophosphamide-induced immunosuppressed mice through MyD88-dependent MAPK/NF-κB and PI3K-Akt signaling pathways. *Food Res. Int.* **2021**, *150*, 110756. [CrossRef] [PubMed]
25. He, K.; Zeng, Y.; Tian, H.; Zhang, Z.; Zhang, H.; Huang, F.; Yu, F. Macrophage immunomodulatory effects of low molecular weight peptides from *Mytilus coruscus via* NF-κB/MAPK signaling pathways. *J. Funct. Foods* **2021**, *83*, 104562. [CrossRef]
26. Yao, L.; Yang, P.; Luo, W.; Li, S.; Wu, Y.; Cai, N.; Bi, D.; Li, H.; Han, Q.; Xu, X. Macrophage-stimulating activity of European eel (*Anguilla anguilla*) peptides in RAW264.7 cells mediated *via* NF-κB and MAPK signaling pathways. *Food Funct.* **2020**, *11*, 10968–10978. [CrossRef] [PubMed]
27. He, P.; Pan, L.; Wu, H.; Zhang, L.; Zhang, Y.; Zhang, Y.; Yang, J.; Lin, Z.; Zhang, M. Isolation, identification, and immunomodulatory mechanism of peptides from *Lepidium meyenii* (maca) protein hydrolysate. *J. Agric. Food Chem.* **2022**, *70*, 4328–4341. [CrossRef] [PubMed]
28. Liu, Y.; Wu, X.; Wang, Y.; Jin, W.; Guo, Y. The immunoenhancement effects of starfish *Asterias rollestoni* polysaccharides in macrophages and cyclophosphamide-induced immunosuppression mouse models. *Food Funct.* **2020**, *11*, 10700–10708. [CrossRef]
29. Jiang, X.; Yang, F.; Zhao, Q.; Tian, D.; Tang, Y. Protective effects of pentadecapeptide derived from *Cyclaina sinensis* against cyclophosphamide-induced hepatotoxicity. *Biochem. Biophys. Res. Commun.* **2019**, *520*, 392–398. [CrossRef]
30. Talmadge, J.E. Natural product derived immune-regulatory agents. *Int. Immunopharmacol.* **2016**, *37*, 5–15. [CrossRef]
31. Zhang, J.; Zhou, H.-C.; He, S.-B.; Zhang, X.-F.; Ling, Y.-H.; Li, X.-Y.; Zhang, H.; Hou, D.-D. The immunoenhancement effects of sea buckthorn pulp oil in cyclophosphamide-induced immunosuppressed mice. *Food Funct.* **2021**, *12*, 7954–7963. [CrossRef]
32. Liu, N.; Dong, Z.; Zhu, X.; Xu, H.; Zhao, Z. Characterization and protective effect of *Polygonatum sibiricum* polysaccharide against cyclophosphamide-induced immunosuppression in Balb/c mice. *Int. J. Biol. Macromol.* **2018**, *107*, 796–802. [CrossRef]
33. Zhang, J.; Gao, S.; Li, H.; Cao, M.; Li, W.; Liu, X. Immunomodulatory effects of selenium-enriched peptides from soybean in cyclophosphamide-induced immunosuppressed mice. *Food Sci. Nutr.* **2021**, *9*, 6322–6334. [CrossRef]
34. Liu, F.; Zhang, L.; Feng, X.; Ibrahim, S.A.; Huang, W.; Liu, Y. Immunomodulatory activity of carboxymethyl pachymaran on immunosuppressed mice induced by cyclophosphamide. *Molecules* **2021**, *26*, 5733. [CrossRef]
35. Wang, S.; Huang, S.; Ye, Q.; Zeng, X.; Yu, H.; Qi, D.; Qiao, S. Prevention of cyclophosphamide-induced immunosuppression in mice with the antimicrobial peptide sublancin. *J. Immunol. Res.* **2018**, *2018*, 4353580. [CrossRef]

36. Khan, A.I.; Rehman, A.U.; Farooqui, N.A.; Siddiqui, N.Z.; Ayub, Q.; Ramzan, M.N.; Zexu, W.; Zhang, X.; Yu, Y.; Xin, Y.; et al. Shrimp peptide hydrolysate modulates the immune response in cyclophosphamide immunosuppressed mice model. *J. Food Biochem.* **2022**, e14251. [CrossRef]
37. Zeng, Y.; Hu, X.; Yu, Z.; Wang, F.; Zhang, Z.; He, K.; Tian, H.; Yu, F. Immune enhancement and antioxidant effects of low molecular-weight peptides derived from *Nibea japonica muscles* on immune-deficient mice induced by cyclophosphamide. *Process Biochem.* **2021**, *102*, 42–50. [CrossRef]
38. Li, M.-Z.; Huang, X.-J.; Hu, J.-L.; Cui, S.W.; Xie, M.-Y.; Nie, S.-P. The protective effects against cyclophosphamide (CTX)-induced immunosuppression of three glucomannans. *Food Hydrocoll.* **2020**, *100*, 105445. [CrossRef]
39. Niu, Y.; Dong, J.; Jiang, H.; Wang, J.; Liu, Z.; Ma, C.; Kang, W. Effects of polysaccharide from *Malus halliana* Koehne flowers in cyclophosphamide-induced immunosuppression and oxidative stress on mice. *Oxidative Med. Cell. Longev.* **2020**, *2020*, 1603735. [CrossRef]
40. Yang, Q.; Huang, M.; Cai, X.; Jia, L.; Wang, S. Investigation on activation in RAW264.7 macrophage cells and protection in cyclophosphamide-treated mice of *Pseudostellaria heterophylla* protein hydrolysate. *Food Chem. Toxicol.* **2019**, *134*, 110816. [CrossRef]
41. Xu, Q.; Yu, J.; Jia, G.; Li, Z.; Xiong, H. Crocin attenuates NF-κB-mediated inflammation and proliferation in breast cancer cells by down-regulating PRKCQ. *Cytokine* **2022**, *154*, 155888. [CrossRef]
42. Luo, X.; Zhang, H.; Wei, X.; Shi, M.; Fan, P.; Xie, W.; Zhang, Y.; Xu, N. Aloin suppresses lipopolysaccharide-induced inflammatory response and apoptosis by inhibiting the activation of NF-κB. *Molecules* **2018**, *23*, 517. [CrossRef]
43. Barnabei, L.; Laplantine, E.; Mbongo, W.; Rieux-Laucat, F.; Weil, R. NF-κB: At the borders of autoimmunity and inflammation. *Front. Immunol.* **2021**, *12*, 3169. [CrossRef]
44. Caforio, M.; de Billy, E.; De Angelis, B.; Iacovelli, S.; Quintarelli, C.; Paganelli, V.; Folgiero, V. PI3K/Akt pathway: The indestructible role of a vintage target as a support to the most recent immunotherapeutic approaches. *Cancers* **2021**, *13*, 4040. [CrossRef]
45. Yang, D.; Yang, L.; Cai, J.; Li, H.; Xing, Z.; Hou, Y. Phosphoinositide 3-kinase/Akt and its related signaling pathways in the regulation of tumor-associated macrophages polarization. *Mol. Cell. Biochem.* **2022**. [CrossRef]
46. Wei, J.; Wang, B.; Chen, Y.; Wang, Q.; Ahmed, A.F.; Zhang, Y.; Kang, W. The immunomodulatory effects of active ingredients from *Nigella sativa* in RAW264.7 cells through NF-κB/MAPK signaling pathways. *Front. Nutr.* **2022**, *9*, 899797. [CrossRef]
47. Um, Y.; Eo, H.J.; Kim, H.J.; Kim, K.; Jeon, K.S.; Jeong, J.B. Wild simulated ginseng activates mouse macrophage, RAW264.7 cells through TRL2/4-dependent activation of MAPK, NF-κB and PI3K/AKT pathways. *J. Ethnopharmacol.* **2020**, *263*, 113218. [CrossRef]
48. Xu, D.; Lin, F.; Zhu, X.Y.; Liu, W.Y.; Chen, X.W.; Feng, J.Q.; Fan, A.Q.; Cai, M.Y.; Xu, Y.J. Immunomodulatory effect of oyster peptide on immunosuppressed mice. *J. Peking Univ. (Health Sci.)* **2016**, *48*, 392–397.
49. Tang, Y.P.; Pu, Q.Y.; Zhao, Q.L.; Zhou, Y.F.; Jiang, X.X.; Han, T. Effects of fucoidan isolated from *Laminaria japonica* on immune response and gut microbiota in cyclophosphamide-treated mice. *Front. Immunol.* **2022**, *13*, 916618. [CrossRef]
50. Han, L.R.; Lei, H.N.; Tian, Z.W.; Wang, X.; Cheng, D.; Wang, C.L. The immunomodulatory activity and mechanism of docosahexenoic acid (DHA) on immunosuppressive mice models. *Food Funct.* **2018**, *9*, 3254. [CrossRef]

marine drugs

Article

Investigation of the In Vivo, In Vitro, and In Silico Wound Healing Potential of *Pinctada martensii* Purified Peptides

Ting Zhang [1,†], Faming Yang [1,2,†], Xiaoming Qin [1,3,4,5,6,7,*], Xianmei Yang [1], Chaohua Zhang [1,3,4,5,6,7], Zhaoyi Wan [1] and Haisheng Lin [1,3,4,5,6,7]

1 College of Food Science and Technology, Guangdong Ocean University, Zhanjiang 524088, China; zhting95@163.com (T.Z.); yangfm0123@163.com (F.Y.); 13414884976@163.com (X.Y.); zhangch2@139.com (C.Z.); spring5water@163.com (Z.W.); haishenglin@163.com (H.L.)
2 Marine College, Shandong University, Weihai 264209, China
3 Guangdong Provincial Key Laboratory of Aquatic Product Processing and Safety, Guangdong Ocean University, Zhanjiang 524088, China
4 National Research and Development Branch Center for Shellfish Processing (Zhanjiang), Zhanjiang 524088, China
5 Guangdong Province Engineering Laboratory for Marine Biological Products, Guangdong Ocean University, Zhanjiang 524088, China
6 Guangdong Provincial Engineering Technology Research Center of Marine Food, Guangdong Ocean University, Zhanjiang 524088, China
7 Collaborative Innovation Center of Seafood Deep Processing, Dalian Polytechnic University, Dalian 116034, China
* Correspondence: qinxm@gdou.edu.cn; Tel.: +86-0759-2396027
† These authors contributed equally to this work.

Abstract: Previous studies found that both oral and topical administration of enzymatic digestion products < 3 K Da ultrafiltration fractions of *Pinctada martensii* mantle (PMPs) had pro-healing effects. Thus, we further purified them by Sephadex-G25 and screened them by cellular assays to obtain *Pinctada martensii* purified peptides (PMPPs). In this study, we explored the mechanism of PMPPs on wound healing by in vivo, in vitro, and in silico experiments. LC-MS/MS results showed that PMPPs consisted of 33 peptides with molecular weights ranging from 758.43 to 2014.04 Da, and the characteristic peptide was Leu-Asp. The results of cellular assays showed that PMPPs promoted the proliferation of human skin fibroblasts (HSF) (135%) and human immortalized keratinocyte (HaCaT) cells (125%) very significantly at 12.5 μg/mL. The in vivo results showed that PMPPs could achieve scarless healing by inhibiting the inflammatory response, accelerating the epithelialization process, and regulating collagen I/III ratio. The optimal peptide sequence FAFQAEIAQLMS of PMPPs was screened for key protein receptors in wound healing (EGFR1, FGFR1, and MMP-1) with the help of molecular docking technique, which also showed to be the key pro-healing active peptide sequence. Therefore, it may provide a therapeutic strategy with great potential for wound healing.

Keywords: *Pinctada martensii* purified peptides; molecular docking; traceless healing

Citation: Zhang, T.; Yang, F.; Qin, X.; Yang, X.; Zhang, C.; Wan, Z.; Lin, H. Investigation of the In Vivo, In Vitro, and In Silico Wound Healing Potential of *Pinctada martensii* Purified Peptides. *Mar. Drugs* **2022**, *20*, 417. https://doi.org/10.3390/md20070417

Academic Editors: Chang-Feng Chi and Bin Wang

Received: 3 May 2022
Accepted: 24 June 2022
Published: 26 June 2022

1. Introduction

Wound repair involves three cross-linking phases: inflammatory response, cell proliferation, and tissue reconstruction [1]. After the skin is traumatized, an inflammatory reaction period begins, which lasts 3–5 days. Neutrophils accumulate at the wound site, cleaning up tissue debris and bacteria [2], which can lead to cell migration, proliferation and differentiation, and form granulation tissue, as well as promote the regeneration of collagen products and endothelial cells [3]. Finally, in the post-traumatic tissue remodeling period, a large amount of extracellular matrix (ECM) and type III collagen is gradually degraded, and type I collagen is meanwhile generated [4]. However, if wounds are not treated in time, it can cause wound infection, pain, the formation of thickened scars, and slow wound healing to affect esthetics and quality of life [5]. Therefore, accelerating skin wound closure and suppressing scarring are essential for patients with tissue defects.

Marine active substances have unique functions due to marine biodiversity and extremely complicated living environments [6]. Hence, these substances have great potential of use in the fields of food, medicine, health care, and cosmetics [7–9]. Presently, marine active substances are extracted from marine organisms such as fish, shrimp, sponges, seaweed, fungi, and so on [10] to develop marine drugs [11]. For example, oral salmon collagen peptides promote skin wound healing and angiogenesis in mice [12,13]. Oral low-molecular-weight peptides from *Theragra chalcogramma* can promote skin wound healing [14]. In addition, our previous study showed that oral and topical active peptides of *Pinctada martensii* could accelerate skin wound healing [15,16]. However, there is still a lack of reports of natural peptide drugs and products with clear structures that promote healing, which is hampered by the complex process of drug discovery. Excitingly, application of molecular docking technology can efficiently screen drug candidates, and save time and cost [17].

Noteworthy, purified peptides derived from *Pinctada martensii* or even marine shellfish to promote healing had received less reports and attention. In this study, we further separated and purified the obtained ultrafiltration fractions through gel chromatography and verified the activity using cellular experiments. The peptides fractions were identified by LC-MS/MS, and animal experiments were selected to investigate their healing-promoting mechanisms. Finally, the optimal peptide sequences were screened by molecular docking and their molecular mechanisms were analyzed. The aim is to provide new drugs and new ideas for wound healing treatment.

2. Results

2.1. Screening and Purification of Peptides Fractions

In vitro cellular experiments are an effective means of activity verification and fraction screening [15,16]. Firstly, effect of the obtained PMPs on HSF and HaCaT cells proliferation were explored (Figure 1A,B). Figure 1A showed that the positive control group (Human FGF-basic) and each concentration of PMPs significantly promoted the proliferation of HSF cells ($p < 0.01$). At the concentration of 100 $\mu g \cdot mL^{-1}$, the proliferation rate of HSF cells (165.31%) was the highest and significantly higher than that of the positive control group ($p < 0.01$). Simultaneously, at the concentration of 25 $\mu g \cdot mL^{-1}$, the proliferation rate of HaCaT cells (142%) was significantly different ($p < 0.05$) and significantly higher than that of the positive control group (rhEGF) compared with the blank control group ($p < 0.01$) (Figure 1B).

Therefore, Sephadex G-25 gel chromatography was selected for separation and purification of PMPs (Figure 1C). Four components were respectively collected and named as PMPs-1, PMPs-2, PMPs-3, and PMPs-4 (protein contents were 3.087 $mg \cdot mL^{-1}$, 3.395 $mg \cdot mL^{-1}$, 3.494 $mg \cdot mL^{-1}$, and 3.912 $mg \cdot mL^{-1}$). Samples were lyophilized and reserved for cell experiments.

Figure 1D showed that the positive control group (Human FGF-basic) significantly promoted the proliferation of HSF cells ($p < 0.01$), and the proliferation rate was higher than in other groups. In addition, all groups of PMPs also significantly promoted the proliferation of HSF cells, with the PMPs-4 component being the most effective in promoting the proliferation of HSF cells.

Figure 1E showed the positive control group (rhEGF) (administration concentration of 10 $\mu g \cdot mL^{-1}$, the proliferation rate of 130%) significantly promoted the proliferation of HaCaT cells ($p < 0.01$). The proliferation rate of PMPs-1, PMPs-2, and PMPs-3 components were the highest at the concentration of 50 $\mu g \cdot mL^{-1}$. However, when the concentration of PMPs-4 was 12.5 $\mu g \cdot mL^{-1}$, the increment rate was 125%, which was higher than that of F1, F2, and F3. So, the PMPs-4 component has the best effect in promoting the proliferation of HaCaT cells. Accordingly, PMPs-4 component as *Pinctada martensii* purified peptides (PMPPs) was selected for subsequent studies in this study.

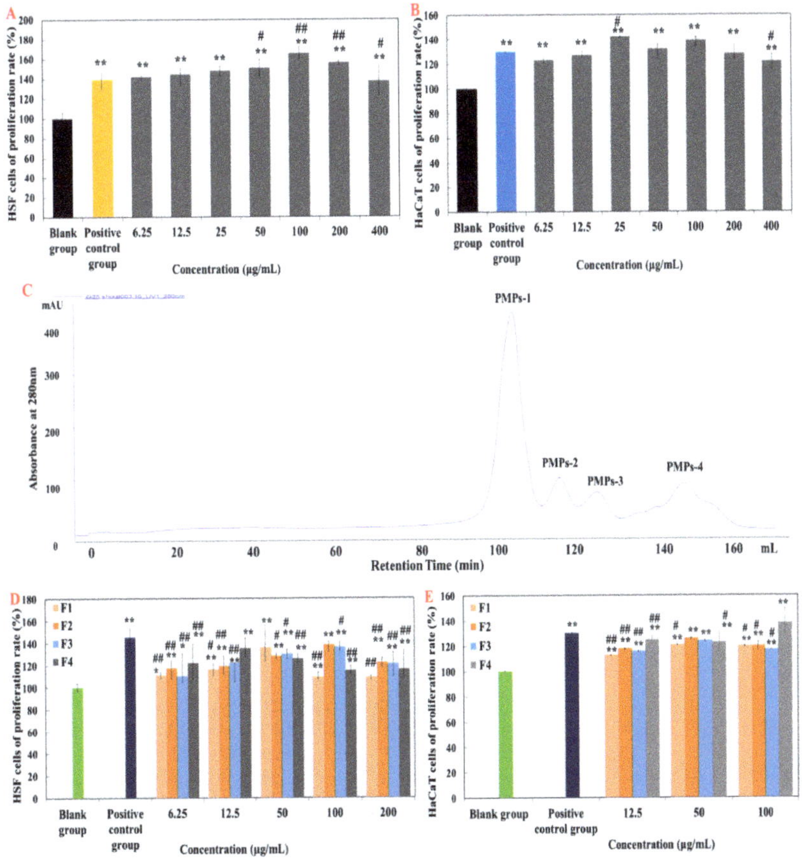

Figure 1. Effects of purified peptides on cells proliferation. (**A**,**B**) Effects of PMPs on cells proliferation. (**C**) Gel permeation chromatogram of PMPs on a Sephadex G-25 column. (**D**,**E**) Effects of PMPPs on cells proliferation. Note: "*" means significantly different compared with control group ($p < 0.05$), "**" means highly significant difference compared with control group ($p < 0.01$), "#" means significantly different compared with positive control group ($p < 0.05$), "##" means highly significant difference compared with positive control group ($p < 0.01$). The concentration of the positive control group is 10 ng·mL^{-1}.

2.2. Identification of PMPPs Peptide Sequences by LC-MS/MS

By primary mass spectrometry, it was found that PMPPs of 33 peptides had molecular weight ranging from 758.43 to 2014.04 Da (Figure 2).

Peptide fingerprinting of 20 characteristic peptides in the PMPPs was analyzed using an LC-MS/MS. The molecular weight of PMPPs was in the range 947.43–1992.06 Da (amino acid residue 7–17) (Table 1). One peptide fragment of Leu-Asp recurred in the 20 characteristic peptide sequences of PMPPs; Phe, Lys, and Arg recurred at the beginning of the characteristic peptide; and Glu reappeared at the tail of the characteristic peptide. Additionally, Leu, Ser, and Lys were found in the middle of PMPPs characteristic peptides.

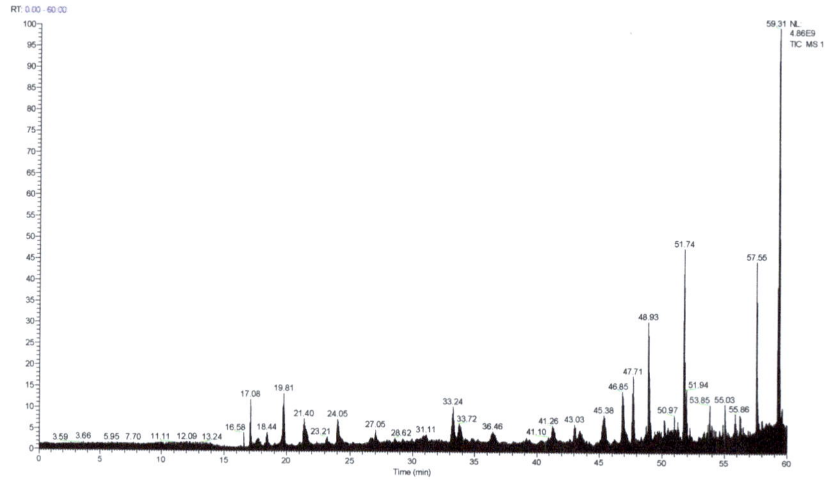

Figure 2. Total ion chromatogram of PMPPs.

Table 1. Main peptide sequences analysis of PMPPs.

Sequence	Peptide Sequence of PMPPs	Molecular Mass (Da)	Score
1	RGVVDSEDLPLNISRE	1512.78	58.46
2	KEAFSLFDKDGDGTITTKE	1843.89	56.77
3	FIMDNCEELIPEYLN	1653.73	47.74
4	RYESLTDPSKLDSGKD	1538.75	46.45
5	RELISNSSDALDKIRY	1559.82	45.27
6	FAFQAEIAQLMS	1136.56	42.91
7	RELISNSSDALDKI	1290.63	41.91
8	FAFQAEIAQLMS	1120.56	41.40
9	KFYEQFSKN	947.43	39.76
10	KHFSVEGQLEFRA	1347.66	39.38
11	LISNSSDALDKIRYE	1480.75	38.97
12	KLTDEEVDEMIRE	1348.62	38.78
13	FIMDNCEELIPEYLN	1637.73	36.49
14	KYRHPDGSYSA	1080.46	36.41
15	FLRELISNSSDALDKIRYE	1992.06	33.79
16	YSNKEIFLRELI	1247.69	33.05
17	KLTDEEVDEMIRE	1364.62	32.39
18	YESLTDPSKLD	988.51	31.40
19	RHVMTNLGEKL	1043.51	30.61
20	WEDHLAVKHFS	1094.55	30.55

Note: Scores obtained by scoring a known protein database to measure the similarity between theoretical mass spectra and experimental mass spectra. Peptide sequences scoring ≥30 or more were considered to be present with higher confidence.

2.3. *Effect of PMPPs on Wound Healing in Mice*

2.3.1. Macroscopic Effects of PMPPs on Wound Healing

Figure 3A,B visualized the healing process of each group of wounds, in which the topical administration of PMPPs significantly accelerated the wound healing. Figure 3C showed that there was no significant difference in the wound healing rate among the groups 4–6 days after modeling ($p > 0.05$). On days 8–14, topical administration of PMPPs significantly promoted the epithelialization process of the wounds compared with the control group and completed wound healing on day 14 ($p < 0.05$). However, wound healing was achieved in the control group on day 18, also demonstrating the advantages of topically administered PMPPs.

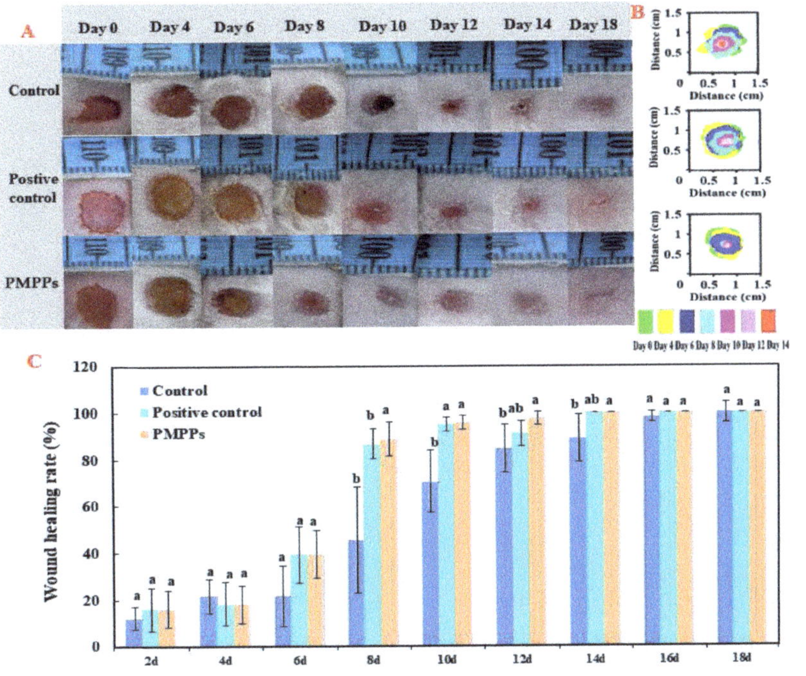

Figure 3. Effect of PMPPs on skin wound healing in mice. (**A**) Photographs of representative wounds on mice on days 0, 4, 6, 8, 10, 12, 14, and 18. (**B**) The area traces of wound healing in each group on days 0, 4, 6, 8, 10, 12, 14, and 18. (**C**) Wound healing rate of each group (calculated every two days). Values are expressed as mean ± SD, $n = 6$. Note: The same superscript letters indicate no significant difference ($p > 0.05$), and different superscript letters indicate significant differences ($p < 0.05$). The drug of positive control group was Jing Wanhong ointment.

2.3.2. Effects of the PMPPs on Wound Cytokines in Mice

The results of the inflammatory factor assay in Figure 4A,B showed that the topical administration of PMPPs at day 3 achieved an anti-inflammatory effect by inhibiting the secretion of the pro-inflammatory factor IL-1β ($p > 0.05$) and significantly promoting the secretion of the anti-inflammatory factor IL-10 ($p < 0.05$), while matching and decreasing the trend at day 5.

Moreover, the results of growth factors assay showed that topical administration of PMPPs significantly promoted the secretion of CCND1 and FGF-2 compared with the two control groups ($p < 0.05$) (Figure 4C,D).

2.3.3. Effects of PMPPs on Wound Tissue Regeneration

Figures 5 and S1 demonstrate the effect of topical administration of PMPPs on skin wound healing in mice by H&E staining microscopy results. On day 3, inflammatory cells from the two control groups infiltrated the wounds. However, the inflammatory response was weaker in the PMPPs group, which is consistent with the results in Figure 4A,B. At 7th days, the epidermal layer of the wounds in the negative control group was not completely healed, and collagen fibers in the dermis were sparse and few. In the positive control and PMPPs groups, the wounds formed a coherent epidermis and more granulation tissue in the dermis. Eighteen days after mock-up, the epidermis and dermis of the positive control and PMPPs groups were repaired similarly to normal skin compared to the negative control group, which is consistent with the results in Figure 3A.

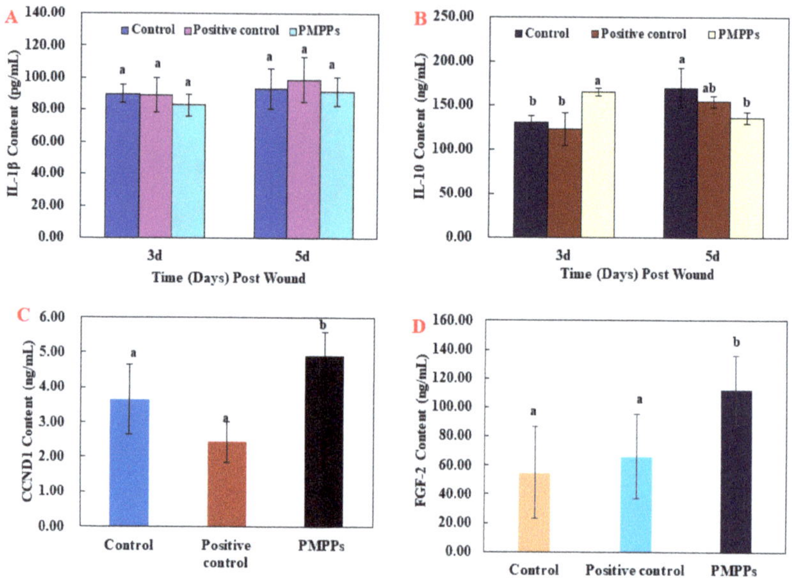

Figure 4. The effect of the PMPPs on wound cytokines in mice. (**A**) IL-1β content of mice in each experimental group on the 3rd and 5th day after animal model establishment. (**B**) IL-10 content of mice in each experimental group on the 3rd and 5th day after animal model establishment. (**C**) CCND1 content of mice in each experimental group on the 7th day after animal model establishment. (**D**) FGF-2 content of mice in each experimental group on the 7th day after animal model establishment. Note: the same superscript letters indicate no significant difference ($p > 0.05$).

As shown in Figure 6, immunohistochemistry was chosen to evaluate fibroblasts (FGF), epidermopoietic cells (EGF), and vascular regeneration (CD31) during trauma repair. Topical administration of PMPPs significantly promoted the expression of FGF and CD31 at day 7 compared with the control and positive control groups ($p < 0.05$), which is consistent with the results in Figure 4C,D. However, at day 18, the groups gradually converged, which is consistent with the results in Figures 3 and 5. However, there was no significant difference in the expression of EGF in the PMPPs group at day 7 compared to the other groups ($p > 0.05$). This suggests that topical administration of PMPPs accelerates the process of wound epithelialization by promoting fibroblast proliferation and vascular regeneration.

2.4. *Effects of PMPPs on Wound Collagen and Scar Formation*

The scar reduction rate, the image of Sirius red staining, and the ratio of type I/III collagen were analyzed as the important basis for the degree of scar reduction in each experimental group. Under a polarized light microscope, type I fibers are tightly packed, show strong birefringence, and appear as yellow or red fibers. Type III fibers show weak birefringence and appear green.

Firstly, Figure 7A,B visualize the effect of each group on the scar residue on the wounds; compared with the control group, all the administered groups effectively inhibited the scar residue, which is consistent with the results in Figure 7C. Then, Figure 7D showed the microscopic results denoting that compared with the two control groups, the I/III collagen in the PMPPs group was uniform in composition, and the collagen was knitted orderly and densely on day 18. Figure 7E showed that the I/III collagen ratio in the PMPPs group was significantly lower than that in the negative control group on the 18th day ($p < 0.05$).

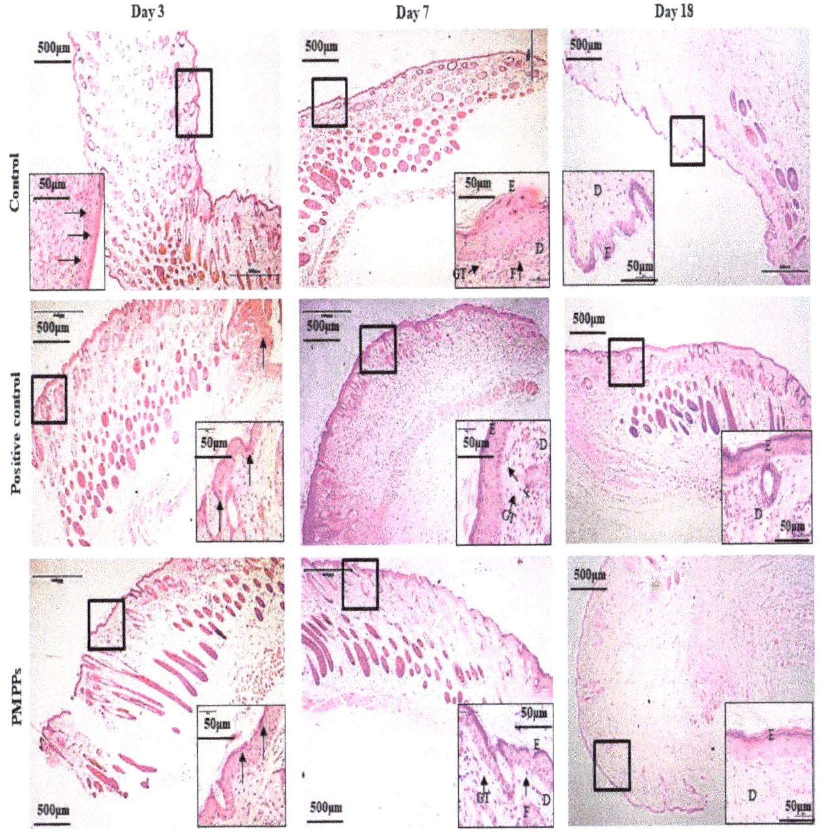

Figure 5. H&E stain histological analysis (4×). Note: Black thick arrows indicate inflammatory cell infiltration. Letters D, E, F, and GT represent the dermis layer, the epidermal layer, fibroblasts, and granulation tissue, respectively.

By measuring the content of TGF-β1, TβRII, and Smad 7 (It was an important inhibitory regulatory protein), the effect of PMPPs on the TGF-β/Smad signaling pathway was studied. ELISA results revealed that the protein expression levels of TGF-β and TβRII in the PMPPs group were significantly higher than those in the negative control group ($p < 0.05$) (Figure S2). Figure S2C showed that the Smad 7 content of the PMPPs group was significantly lower than that of the positive control group ($p < 0.05$). Although there was no significant difference in the content of Smad 7 among the groups, the PMPPs group had the lowest content of Smad 7 ($p > 0.05$). This indicated that topical administration of PMPPs could promote collagen secretion through the TGF-β/Smad signaling pathway.

2.5. Molecular Docking

Based on the results in Table 1, we selected a total of eight peptide sequences with scores ≥ 40 (the higher the peptide sequence score in the mass spectrometry results, the higher the reliability) in PMPPs and docked them with wound healing-related protein receptors EGFR1, FGFR1, and MMP-1 for the purpose of screening key peptide sequences and further elucidating the healing-promoting mechanism of PMPPs.

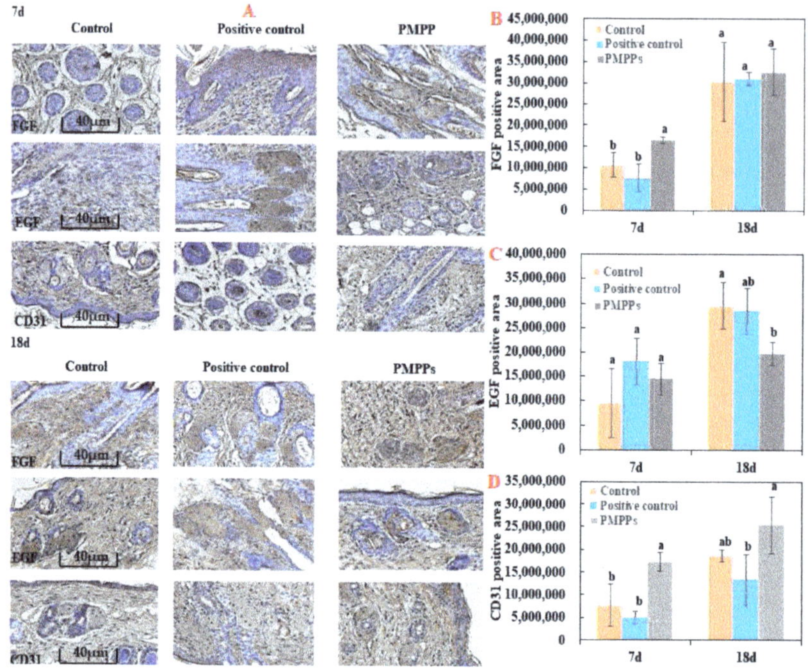

Figure 6. Immunohistochemical analysis of the marine bioactive peptide PMPPs on skin wounds in mice. (**A**) Representative images of FGF, EGF, and CD31 immunostaining of wounds in each group on days 7 and 18. (**B**) On the 7th and 18th day, the expression of FGF in wounds of each group after trauma. (**C**) EGF expression in wounds of each group after 7 days and 18 days of trauma. (**D**) CD31 expression in wounds of each group after 7 days and 18 days of trauma. Note: the same superscript letters indicate no significant difference ($p > 0.05$).

The optimal binding model of PMPPs (FAFQAEIAQLMS)—MMP-1 is shown in Figure 8A, with a minimum binding energy of 5.12 kcal/mol, indicating that a stable complex was formed between PMPPs (FAFQAEIAQLMS) and MMP-1, as lower energy indicates that ligands and proteins form a complex with a higher binding affinity and greater stability. The docking interaction diagram of the optimal active site of the enzyme is shown in Figure 8A1,A2, and in 2D and 3D docking views, the interaction of MMP-1 amino acid residues with PMPPs is revealed (Figure 8).

Figure 8A3 show the interactions between PMPPs and the conventional hydrogen bonds, pi-alky and pi-sulfur bonds formed by PMPPs with amino acid residues His 228 were found. Van der Waals forces were also observed between AAPs and amino acid residues: Gln 186, Thr 230, Ser 229, Ser 227, Asn 160, Ser 172, Asn 171, Pro 173, and His 183. In addition, the alky was also observed between Pro 238 and PMPPs.

The optimal binding model of PMPPs (FAFQAAEIAQLMS)-EGFR1/FGFR1 is shown in Figure S3 with minimum binding energies of 8.76 kcal/mol and 7.93 kcal/mol, respectively (the lower the energy, the easier the pep-tide binds to the receptor protein). Therefore, it can be concluded that hydrogen bonding, Van der Waals forces, and covalent bond interactions are the primary interaction forces involved in the binding of PMPPs and MMP-1. These findings support and further confirm the results of tests conducted in vivo and in vitro.

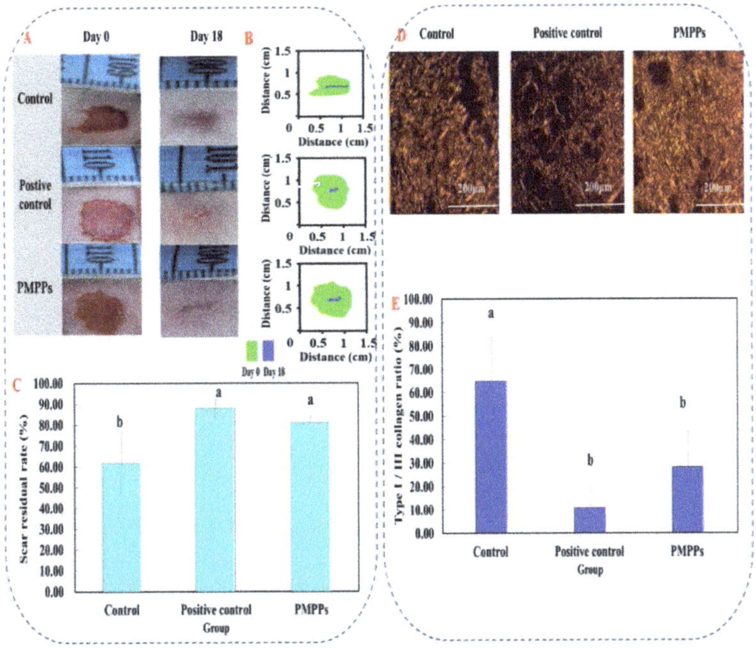

Figure 7. Effects of topical administration of PMPPs on wound collagen and scar formation. (**A**) Photographs of representative wounds in mice on days 0 and 18. (**B**) The area traces of scar reduction in each group on days 0, 4, 6, 8, 10, 12, 14, and 18. (**C**) The rate of scar reduction in each group. (**D**) Representative Sirius red-stained photos in collagen synthesis (magnification: ×200). Collagen III was green and collagen I was yellowish red. (**E**) The expression of collagen I/III after 18 days of modeling. Note: Different superscript letters on the same day indicate significant ($p < 0.05$) and non-significant ($p > 0.05$) differences between groups, respectively.

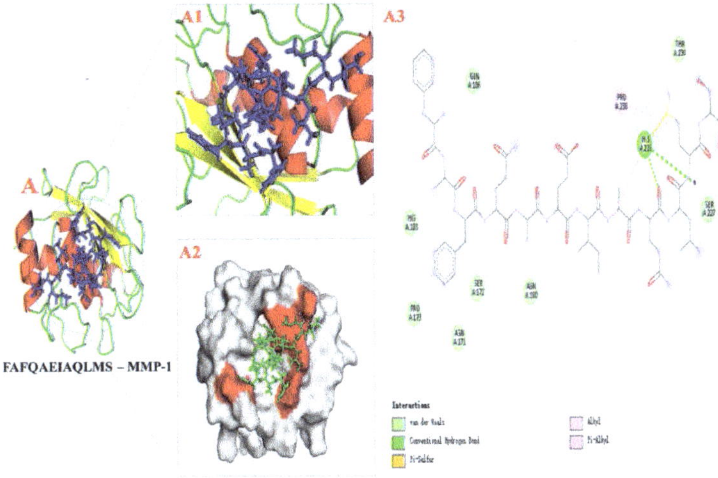

Figure 8. The docking results of PMPPs (FAFQAEIAQLMS) with protein receptors MPP-1. (**A1,A2**) 3D structure of PMPPs—MMP-1 and the process of binding interaction between them. (**A3**) 2D interaction diagram of PMPPs—MMP-1.

3. Discussion

Wound repair is a complex and distinct process involving multiple cells and cytokines. The skin as a human body barrier is damaged for a series of complications such as ulcers, infections, scars, and even chronic wounds [18]. Clearly, this has prompted the need to develop drugs or products that meet the functional requirements of each stage of the healing process. At the same time, our results showed that topical and oral PMPs could both promote wound healing and inhibit scar formation, which was closely related to shortening the time of hemostasis and epithelialization, promoting angiogenesis, regulating cytokines, depositing collagen, and remodeling collagen fiber [15,16]. Hence, we purified the PMPs by gel chromatography, their biological activities were demonstrated by in vitro cellular assays, and the best fraction PMPs-4 (PMPPs) was screened by this method (Figure 1). This is closely related to the peptide sequence composition of PMPPs (Table 1), which is beneficial for promoting cell proliferation and laying a solid foundation for subsequent studies.

Molecular docking is an effective and reliable computational technique for predicting possible binding modes and studying the ligand binding mechanism between small molecules and proteins. Molecular docking is widely used in structural molecular biology and drug discovery [19], which is a useful technology to identify the binding mode or force of ligand protein complexes. Binding energy is also an important criterion for considering the interaction between proteins and ligands, and the lowest binding energy is considered to be more stable. Epidermal growth factor receptor (EGFR1), fibroblast growth factor (FGFR1), and matrix metalloproteinase (MMP-1) play important roles in cell proliferation, tissue remodeling, and wound healing [20]. Thus, it not only helped us to screen for the best peptide sequence FAFQAEIAQLMS, but also further elucidated the mechanism of the significant cell proliferation promotion by PMPPs.

Wound healing includes three phases that are intertwined in space and time, namely the inflammatory phase, the proliferative phase, and the tissue remodeling phase [21,22]. During the inflammatory period, macrophages secrete pro-inflammatory factors (IL-1β, TNF-α, IL-6, etc.) and anti-inflammatory factors (IL-10) to clear the necrotic tissue and prevent infection at the wound site [23,24]. On the third day after the trauma, macrophages in the skin tissue entered the injured area. Besides phagocytosing pathogens, they also secreted various growth factors and cytokines, as well as neutrophils [25]. Furthermore, the H&E microscopy showed that compared with the two control groups, the PMPPs group significantly inhibited the inflammatory response (Figure 5), which was closely related to the significant promotion of IL-10 secretion in the PMPPs group (Figure 4A,B).

The greatest feature of the proliferative period is the granulation tissue formed by fibroblasts, endothelial cells, and keratinocytes [26]. Meanwhile, at this stage, macrophages induce fibroblast proliferation by secreting TGF-β, and then some skin tissues produce collagen under the stimulation of TGF-β and regulate tissue repair by depositing the type III collagen [27,28]. The TGF-β/Smad signaling pathway plays an important role in cell growth, differentiation, migration, apoptosis, and repair after injury [29]. In addition, fibroblast growth factor-2 (FGF-2) and cyclin 1 (CCND1) play important roles in cell proliferation and tissue regeneration [30]. In this study, coated administration of PMPPs was effective in accelerating the process of wound epithelialization (Figure 5), and this was closely related to its significant promotion of the secretion of growth factors TGF-β, FGF-2, and CCND1, thereby favoring fibroblasts, epidermopoietic cells, and angiogenesis (Figures 4 and 6). Importantly, the topical administration of PMPPs showed great potential to meet the functional requirements of all phases of wound healing, which are verified with the results of tissue remodeling (Figures 8 and S3).

During the tissue remodeling period, macrophages secrete metalloproteinases, degrade excess fibers in the wound, induce apoptosis, and clear fibroblasts [31]. Meanwhile, collagen III levels increased significantly after the inflammatory phase, which can reduce scar formation. Type III collagen in the connective tissue is replaced by type I collagen in the remodeling period [32,33]. This was closely related to the fact that the PMPPs group significantly promoted the proliferation of CD31 and FGF (Figure 6), and enhanced collagen synthesis through the TGF-β/Smad signaling pathway (Figure S2). In addition, by shortening the inflammatory period, the PMPPs significantly promoted the secretion of TGF-β and cleverly coordinated the proportion of collagen in the wound, thereby inhibiting scar formation in PMPPs-treated mice, as evidenced through the results summarized in Figures 3 and 7 [34]. Although positive drugs could promote skin wound healing and inhibit scar residue, the mechanism of action was different from PMPPs, which is consistent with the main efficacy reported: it was suitable for mild wound healing, and had the functions of promoting blood circulation, detoxification, pain relief, etc.

4. Materials and Methods

4.1. Materials

Pinctada martensii mantle were purchased from Dongfeng Market, Zhanjiang City, China. Neutral protease (3×10^4 U/g) was purchased from Pangbo Biological Engineering Co., Ltd. (Nanning, China). Jing Wanhong ointment (Chinese medicine certificate Z20023137) was provided by Tianjin Da Rentang Jing Wanhong Pharmaceutical Co., Ltd. ELISA kits (Nanjing Jiancheng Biotechnology Research Institute); HaCaT and HSF cells were purchased from Beijing Beina Chuanglian Biotechnology Research Institute. IL-1β (interleukin-1β), TGF-β (transforming growth factor β1), TβRII (transforming growth factor beta 1 type II receptor), and Smad 7 (signal transduction molecule 7) were purchased from Mlbio, Shanghai, China. IL-10 (interleukin-10) was purchased from Nanjing Institute of Bioengineering, Nanjing, China. Human FGF-basic, purchased from Pepro Teck Company, USA. rhEGF was purchased from Meilun Biotechnology Co., Ltd., Dalian, China. Iodoacetamide, dithiothreitol, ammonium bicarbonate, and formic acid were purchased from Sigma Company, USA. Acetonitrile (>99.9%) was purchased from Fisher Chemical Company, USA. Fetal bovine serum, DMEM medium, PBS, 2.5%. Trypsin-EDTA, and penicillin-streptomycin double antibody were purchased from Thermo Fisher Scientific, USA. Sephadex G-25 was purchased from GE, USA. RPMI 1640 medium was purchased from Gibco, USA. BCA protein concentration determination kit (enhanced) was purchased from Shanghai Biyuntian Biotechnology Co., Ltd., China. The other chemicals used in this experiment were of analytical grade and are commercially available.

4.2. Preparation of PMPs

The preparation methods of PMPs were as reported by Yang et al. [16]: the *Pinctada martensii* mantle were washed, drained, and ground before being dissolved in water with a ratio of 1:3 (mantle: water). The hydrolysis reaction was carried out using neutral protease at 1000 U/g (raw material) at 53 °C, pH 7 for 3–5 h while stirring was carried out. Next, the mixture was incubated in boiled water for 10 min and cooled immediately to inactivate the enzymes. Following inactivation, the hydrolysate was fractioned into <3 K Da group using ultrafiltration system (XX42PMINI, Millipore, Burlington, MA, USA) and the ultrafiltration membranes (Mili Pellicon, Millipore, Burlington, MA, USA) and CNPs were obtained by rotary evaporation (N-1300V, EYELA, Tokyo, Japan) and freeze-drying (FDU-2110, EYELA, Tokyo, Japan) in sequence.

4.3. Gel Permeation or Ultrafiltration Purification of PMPPs

A suitable amount of Sephadex G-25 dry gum (GE, Boston, MA, USA) was soaked in 20% ethanol for 24 h to activate it. A 65 cm × 2.6 cm (long × inner diameter) gel column was filled it by the AKTA Purifier protein purification instrument (AKTA Purifier, Thermo, Waltham, MA, USA). Ultrapure water as the eluent was used to balance the pressure of gel column for 24 h when the gel column pressure was stable. After the ultrafiltration component of PMPs was passed through 0.22 μm membrane, the elution was 5 mL at a fixed flow rate of 1.0 mg·mL^{-1}, and detected at 280 nm to obtain the small molecular purified peptides (PMPPs). The collected components were lyophilized for cell proliferation test.

4.4. Cell Proliferation Assay In Vitro

HaCaT (Human immortalized keratinocytes) and HSF (Human Skin fibroblast) cells were cultured in 25 cm^2 cell culture flasks. Complete medium consisted of 90% DMEM, 10% fetal bovine serum, and 1% double antibody. The cultured HaCaT and HSF cells were diluted into 2×10^5 cells·mL^{-1} and 100 μL per well was added into 96-well microplates and cultured at 5% CO_2 and 37 °C saturated humidity for 4 h. After the cells were completely adherent, the PBS was used to gradient formulation of SMPs and purified components of different concentrations. After passing the samples through 0.22 μm filter membrane, 10 μL of each was added to the adherent cells. WST-8 (tetrazolium salt 2-(2-methoxy-4-nitrophenyl)-3-(4-nitrophenyl)-5-(2,4-disulfophenyl) -2H-tetrazolium, monosodium salt (CCK-8)) diluted with 100 μL of culture medium was added after 24 h of culture for reaction for 1 h and then OD value was measured at 450 nm.

4.5. Peptide Sequence Analysis of PMPPs

The major peptide sequence analysis of PMPPs was as reported by Yang et al. [16]: The PMPPs lyophilized powder were reduced by 10 mM DTT for 1 h at 56 °C, then alkylated by 50 mM IAA in dark for 40 min at room temperature. Following the addition of the enzyme, the solution was incubated overnight at 37 °C. Salt from the peptide solution was removed using a C18 tip, and peptides were then lyophilized to near dryness. Finally, Peptide sequences were identified by electrospray ionization mass spectrometry and tandem mass spectrometry (ESI-MS/MS) in positive ion mode. After chromatography, ESI-MS/MS was carried out using a Q Exactive™ triple quadrupole instrument (Thermo Fisher Scientific, Waltham, MA, USA) equipped with an ESI source. Sequences of characteristic peptides were determined by analysis and comparison with secondary fragments of peptides from the collision-induced dissociation spectrum of the protonated molecule [M + H] + in the Uniprot database.

4.6. Animal Grouping and Establishment of Trauma Model

The study was approved by the Guangdong Ocean University (Zhanjiang, China), Experimental Animal Care Ethics Committee (Approval No.: 20190001, Approval Date: 17 June 2019). SPF male mice (4-weeks-old) were purchased from Pengyue Experimental Animal Breeding Co., Ltd. (Jinan, China) and the production license number was SCXK 20190003, Shandong, China. The laboratory license number was SYXK 2019-0204, Guangdong, China. All experiments were in accordance with the ARRIVE guidelines and were conducted in accordance with the National Institutes of Health guidelines for the care and use of laboratory animals (NIH Publication 8023, revised 1978).

The dorsal hair was shaved and sterilized before the experiment, and 1% pentobarbital was administered as sodium (50 mg/kg) to anesthetize the mice. A full skin defect model of 8 mm in diameter was made on the back of each SPF grade KM male mice (20.0 ± 2.0 g, 4 weeks old). Fifty-seven model mice were randomly divided into three groups: negative control group, positive control group (Jing Wanhong ointment was selected as the positive control drug, which has the effects of activating blood circulation, detoxifying, detumescence and pain relieving, and removing saprophytic muscles. The active ingredients are mainly Ampelopsis radix, Angelica dahurica and other traditional Chinese medicines; dose: 2–3 mg/day, administration method: Topical use), and PMPPs group (Topical use, peptides dose: 0.5–1 mg/day), and 19 rats were in each group. The negative control group was not administered after modeling, and the positive control group and the PMPPs group were administered on the day of modeling, and were applied once a day for 18 days.

4.7. Percentage of Wound Closure and Residual Scar Rate

Photographs were taken at a fixed height every two days, and the image processing software Image J (National Institutes of Health, Bethesda, MD, USA) was used to analyze and calculate the wound healing rate and observe the scab removal time and wound scar formation [15].

4.8. Tissue Preparation for Histological Assessment

Tissues were removed around each mouse wound, immersed in neutral formalin, and then dehydrated with a series of increasing concentrations of alcohol. Dehydrated tissue was embedded in paraffin to prepare sample sections for histopathological and histomorphological observation [16].

4.9. ELISA Analysis

After centrifugation at 10,000 rpm for 15 min at 4 °C, the supernatant of the homogenized tissue was collected as protein extract. Before the index detection, the protein content of each sample (Beyotime Biotechnology Co., Ltd., Shanghai, China) was measured and diluted to the same level. Quantification of IL-1β, TGF-β1, TβRII, Smad7, and IL-10 in 10% (*v*/*v*) dorsal skin homogenate supernatant was performed using ELISA kits (Nanjing Jiancheng, Nanjing, China) [15].

4.10. Hematoxylin and Eosin Staining for Microscopic Analysis

The tissue was taken from the injured part of the back of the mouse, and the tissue was immediately fixed in formalin. After dehydration with ethanol solution, the sections were stained with hematoxylin and eosin. In order to observe the histopathological changes, the sections were examined at a magnification of 40 times using Olympus microscope (Olympus IX51, Tokyo, Japan).

4.11. Immunohistochemistry

After dehydration, hydration, and hydrothermal antigen repair, the antigen was extracted with citrate buffer (pH 6.0). Goat serum was added to block the non-specific binding site and incubated at room temperature for 20 min. Next, 50–100 microliters of primary antibody (diluted 1:200, provided by Nanjing Institute of bioengineering, China) were added to the tissue sections drop by drop, and the slides were placed in a humidification chamber at 37 °C for 2 h. Then, 50 μL universal second-class IgG antibody Fab fragment HRP polymer (provided by Nanjing Institute of bioengineering, China), was added, followed by incubation at 37 °C for 30 min, washing with PBS for 3 times. After adding diaminobiphenylamine (DAB) to make it colored, CD31, EGF, and FGF were observed under optical microscope (Olympus IX51, Tokyo, Japan).

4.12. Sirius Red Picric Acid Dyeing

The steps of the Sirius red staining method were as follows [15]: Firstly, the sample was fixed in 10% formalin fixative and routinely dehydrated. Second, sample sections were stained with Sirius Red staining solution for 8–10 min. Subsequently, the running water was quickly rinsed to remove the stained surface of the section. Finally, the anhydrous ethanol was quickly dehydrated to transparency and sealed with a neutral gum.

4.13. Molecular Docking

The crystal structure of protein receptors linked to skin wound healing of EGFR1 (PDB code: 3POZ, resolution: 1.50 Å), FGFR1 (PDB code: 1AGW, resolution: 2.40 Å) [35] and MMP-1 (PDB code: 966C, resolution: 1.90 Å) [36] was obtained from RCSB Protein Data Bank (https://www.rcsb.org/, access on 13 September 2021). The initially crystal structure of EGFR1 was processed with AutoDock Tools 1.5.6 by removing non-polar water molecules, adding polar hydrogen, and saving the original charge of EGFR1/ FGFR1/ MMP-1 before exporting as a .pdbqt file, which was processed with AutoDock Tools 1.5.6 to form the .pdbqt file for the docking study. In the docking process, the receptor was kept rigid while making the ligands more flexibly during simulation.

The probable interaction between SMPPs (FAFQAEIAQLMS) and EGFR1/ FGFR1/ MMP-1 were explored through Autodock 4.2 with the grid box centered at the coordinates of x = 126, y = 126, and z = 126. The grid sizes along the X, Y, and Z axes were set to $60 \times 60 \times 60$ at a grid space of 0.375 Å (since the specific binding site of the peptide to the protein receptor was unknown, to avoid measures of optimal binding sites, a full domain boxing of the receptor was chosen for semi-flexible docking with the peptide). The docking calculations were performed 100 times by Lamarckian genetic algorithm, and the output was sorted by Lamarckian GA module. The protein–ligand complexation possesses the minimum energy scoring was selected for further visualization of the docked conformation with PyMOL and Discovery Studio.

4.14. Data Analysis

The wound area was calculated with Image J software (National Institutes of Health, Bethesda, Maryland, USA), and the experimental data were expressed as means ± standard deviation (mean ± S.D.). SPSS20 software (IBM, Armonk, NY, USA) was used for statistical analysis, and the LSD method was used for multiple comparisons between groups; *p*-values of less than 0.05 were considered to be statistically significant.

5. Conclusions

Studies showed that the PMPPs screened by gel chromatography purification and cellular assays were composed of 33 peptides that could achieve effective scarless healing though promoting the inhibition of inflammatory response and cytokine secretion, accelerating the epithelialization process, and activating the TGF-β/Smad pathway to coordinate the trauma type I/III collagen ratio. The molecular docking technique not only helped us to screen for the most promising peptide sequence FAFQAEIAQLMS, but also elucidated that FAFQAEIAQLMS played a role in promoting wound healing by docking easily with the protein receptor EGFR1/FGFR1/MPP-1, which enriches the pro-healing mechanism of PMPPs. This research aimed to provide new materials and new methods for the development of wound healing drugs.

Supplementary Materials: The following supporting information can be downloaded at: https://www.mdpi.com/article/10.3390/md20070417/s1, Figure S1: H&E stain histological analysis (40×); Figure S2: Effects of topical administration of PMPPs on TGF-β/Smad signaling pathway. Figure S3: Docking results of PMPPs (FAFQAEIAQLMS) with protein receptors EGFR1/FGFR1.

Author Contributions: Conceptualization, X.Q.; data curation, T.Z., X.Y. and Z.W.; formal analysis, F.Y.; funding acquisition, X.Q. and C.Z.; investigation, X.Y.; methodology, T.Z., F.Y. and Z.W.; project administration, X.Q.; resources, C.Z. and H.L.; software, F.Y.; supervision, X.Q. and C.Z.; validation, H.L.; visualization, Z.W.; writing—original draft, T.Z. and F.Y.; writing—review and editing, F.Y. All authors have read and agreed to the published version of the manuscript.

Funding: This research was financially supported by the China Agricultural Research System of MOF and MARA (CARS-49), Guangdong Ocean University "Haizhifan" starting plan for university students' scientific and technological innovation cultivating project (230419038), Guangdong Ocean University Graduate Education Innovation Program Excellent Dissertation Cultivation Project (521005036), High Value of Aquatic Products in Guangdong's Ordinary Higher Education Institutions Processing and Utilization Innovation Team Project (GDOU2016030503).

Institutional Review Board Statement: The animal study protocol was approved by the Guangdong Ocean University (Zhanjiang, China), Experimental Animal Care Ethics Committee (Approval No.: 20190001, Approval Date: 17 June 2019).

Informed Consent Statement: Not applicable.

Data Availability Statement: Not applicable.

Conflicts of Interest: The authors declare no conflict of interest.

References

1. Zhang, M.Z.; Zhai, X.Y.; Ma, T.F.; Huang, Y.K.; Yan, C.H.; Du, Y.P. Multifunctional cerium doped carbon dots nanoplatform and its applications for wound healing. *Chem. Eng. J.* **2021**, *423*, 130301. [CrossRef]
2. Boniakowski, A.E.; Kimball, A.S.; Jacobs, B.N.; Kunkel, S.L.; Gallagher, K.A. Macrophage-mediated inflammation in normal and diabetic wound healing. *J. Immunol.* **2017**, *199*, 17. [CrossRef]

3. Yang, F.M.; Zhao, D.; Zhang, K.; Wang, Z.C.; Wang, Y.X.; Wu, C.C.; Cui, S.H.; Guo, T.T.; Chen, L.Q.; Chen, J.D. Oral delivery of marine shellfish supramolecule peptides for skin wound healing. *Colloids Surf. B Biointerfaces* **2022**, *216*, 112592. [CrossRef]
4. Costa, A.M.A.; Peyrol, S.; Pôrto, L.C.; Comparin, J.-P.; Foyatier, J.-L.; Desmoulière, A. Mechanical forces induce scar remodeling: Study in Non-pressure-treated versus pressure-treated hypertrophic scars. *Am. J. Pathol.* **1999**, *155*, 1671–1679. [CrossRef]
5. Wu, K.K.; Fu, M.M.; Zhao, Y.T.; Gerhard, E.; Li, Y.; Yang, J.; Guo, J.S. Anti-oxidant anti-inflammatory and antibacterial tannin-crosslinked citrate-based mussel-inspired bioadhesives facilitate scarless wound healing. *Bioact. Mater.* **2023**, *20*, 93–110. [CrossRef]
6. Cheung, R.C.F.; Ng, T.B.; Wong, J.H. Marine Peptides: Bioactivities and Applications. *Mar. Drugs* **2015**, *13*, 4006–4043. [CrossRef]
7. Sridhar, K.; Inbaraj, B.S.; Chen, B.H. Recent developments on production, purification and biological activity of marine peptides. *Food Res. Int.* **2021**, *147*, 110468. [CrossRef]
8. Berthon, J.-Y.; Nachat-Kappes, R.; Bey, M.; Cadoret, J.-P.; Renimel, I.; Filaire, E. Marine algae as attractive source to skin care. *Free Radical Res.* **2017**, *51*, 555–567. [CrossRef]
9. Khotimchenko, Y. Pharmacological potential of sea cucumbers. *Int. J. Mol. Sci.* **2018**, *19*, 1342. [CrossRef]
10. Lazcano-Perez, F.; Roman-Gonzalez, S.A.; Sanchez-Puig, N.; Arreguin- Espinosa, R. Bioactive peptides from marine organisms: A short overview. *Protein Pept. Lett.* **2012**, *19*, 700–707. [CrossRef]
11. Anjum, K.; Abbas, S.Q.; Akhter, N.; Shagufta, B.I.; Shah, S.A.A.; Hassan, S.S.u. Emerging biopharmaceuticals from bioactive peptides derived from marine organisms. *Chem. Biol. Drug Des.* **2017**, *90*, 12–30. [CrossRef]
12. Zhang, Z.; Wang, J.; Ding, Y.; Dai, X.; Li, Y. Oral administration of marine collagen peptides from chum salmon skin enhances cutaneous wound healing and angiogenesis in rats. *J. Sci. Food Agric.* **2011**, *91*, 2173–2179. [CrossRef]
13. Sellimi, S.; Maalej, H.; Rekik, D.M.; Benslima, A.; Ksouda, G.; Hamdi, M.; Sahnoun, Z.; Li, S.; Nasri, M.; Hajji, M. Antioxidant, antibacterial and in vivo wound healing properties of laminaran purified from cystoseira barbata seaweed. *Int. J. Biol. Macromol.* **2018**, *119*, 633–644. [CrossRef]
14. Yang, T.; Zhang, K.; Li, B.; Hou, H. Effects of oral administration of peptides with low molecular weight from alaska pollock (theragra chalcogramma) on cutaneous wound healing. *J. Funct. Foods* **2018**, *48*, 682–691. [CrossRef]
15. Yang, F.; Qin, X.; Zhang, T.; Zhang, C.; Lin, H. Effect of oral administration of active peptides of pinctada martensii on the repair of skin wounds. *Mar. Drugs* **2019**, *17*, 697. [CrossRef]
16. Yang, F.; Qin, X.; Zhang, T.; Lin, H.; Zhang, C. Evaluation of small molecular polypeptides from the mantle of pinctada martensii on promoting skin wound healing in mice. *Molecules* **2019**, *24*, 4231. [CrossRef]
17. Crampon, K.; Giorkallos, A.; Deldossi, M.; Baud, S.; Steffenel, L.A. Machine-learning methods for ligand–protein molecular docking. *Drug Discov. Today* **2022**, *27*, 151–164. [CrossRef]
18. Chouhan, D.; Dey, N.; Bhardwaj, N.; Mandal, B.B. Emerging and innovative approaches for wound healing and skin regeneration: Current status and advances. *Biomaterials* **2019**, *216*, 119267. [CrossRef]
19. St-Cyr, D.; Ceccarelli, D.F.; Orlicky, S.; van der Sloot, A.M.; Tang, X.; Kelso, S.; Moore, S.; James, C.; Posternak, G.; Coulombe-Huntington, J.; et al. Identification and optimization of molecular glue compounds that inhibit a noncovalent E2 enzyme-ubiquitin complex. *Sci. Adv.* **2021**, *7*, eabi5797. [CrossRef]
20. Xu, J.; Zhang, S.; Wu, T.; Fang, X.; Zhao, L. Discovery of TGFBR1 (ALK5) as a potential drug target of quercetin glycoside derivatives (QGDs) by reverse molecular docking and molecular dynamics simulation. *Biophys. Chem.* **2022**, *281*, 106731. [CrossRef]
21. Qiu, H.; Liu, S.; Wu, K.; Zhao, R.; Cao, L.; Wang, H. Prospective application of exosomes derived from adipose-derived stem cells in skin wound healing: A review. *J. Cosmet. Dermatol.* **2020**, *19*, 574–581. [CrossRef] [PubMed]
22. Sorg, H.; Tilkorn, D.J.; Hager, S.; Hauser, J.; Mirastschijski, U. Skin wound healing: An update on the current knowledge and concepts. *Eur. Surg. Res.* **2017**, *58*, 81–94. [CrossRef] [PubMed]
23. Bhar, B.; Chakraborty, B.; Nandi, S.K.; Mandal, B.B. Silk-based phyto-hydrogel formulation expedites key events of wound healing in full-thickness skin defect model. *Int. J. Biol. Macromol.* **2022**, *203*, 623–637. [CrossRef]
24. Luo, M.; Wang, M.; Niu, W.; Chen, M.; Cheng, W.; Zhang, L.; Xie, C.; Wang, Y.; Guo, Y.; Leng, T.; et al. Injectable self-healing anti-inflammatory europium oxide-based dressing with high angiogenesis for improving wound healing and skin regeneration. *Chem. Eng. J.* **2021**, *412*, 128471. [CrossRef]
25. Zheng, G.; Zhang, D.; Tang, Q.; Ma, H.-W.; Dong, X.-Y.; Chen, Y.-L.; Ni, W.-F.; Wang, B.-L.; Xu, H.-Z.; Shen, L.-Y. Charge-switchable, anti-oxidative molecule tuned polyelectrolyte multilayered films: Amplified polyelectrolyte diffusivity and accelerated diabetes wound healing. *Chem. Eng. J.* **2021**, *416*, 129521. [CrossRef]
26. El Ayadi, A.; Jay, J.W.; Prasai, A. Current approaches targeting the wound healing phases to attenuate fibrosis and scarring. *Int. J. Mol. Sci.* **2020**, *21*, 1105. [CrossRef]
27. Kiritsi, D.; Nyström, A. The role of TGFβ in wound healing pathologies. *Mech. Ageing Dev.* **2018**, *172*, 51–58. [CrossRef]
28. Penn, J.W.; Grobbelaar, A.O.; Rolfe, K.J. The role of the TGF-β family in wound healing, burns and scarring: A review. *Int. J. Burns Trauma* **2012**, *2*, 18–28.
29. Wang, Y.; Feng, Z.; Yang, M.; Zeng, L.; Qi, B.e.; Yin, S.; Li, B.; Li, Y.; Fu, Z.; Shu, L.; et al. Discovery of a novel short peptide with efficacy in accelerating the healing of skin wounds. *Pharmacol. Res.* **2021**, *163*, 105296. [CrossRef]
30. Lavoie, H.; Gagnon, J.; Therrien, M. ERK signalling: A master regulator of cell behaviour, life and fate. *Nat. Reviews. Mol. Cell Biol.* **2020**, *21*, 607–632. [CrossRef]

31. Nosrati, H.; Khodaei, M.; Alizadeh, Z.; Banitalebi-Dehkordi, M. Cationic, anionic and neutral polysaccharides for skin tissue engineering and wound healing applications. *Int. J. Biol. Macromol.* **2021**, *192*, 298–322. [CrossRef] [PubMed]
32. Ling, Z.; Deng, J.; Zhang, Z.; Sui, H.; Shi, W.; Yuan, B.; Lin, H.; Yang, X.; Cao, J.; Zhu, X.; et al. Spatiotemporal manipulation of L-arginine release from bioactive hydrogels initiates rapid skin wound healing accompanied with repressed scar formation. *Appl. Mater. Today* **2021**, *24*, 101116. [CrossRef]
33. Li, D.; Sun, W.Q.; Wang, T.; Gao, Y.; Wu, J.; Xie, Z.; Zhao, J.; He, C.; Zhu, M.; Zhang, S.; et al. Evaluation of a novel tilapia-skin acellular dermis matrix rationally processed for enhanced wound healing. *Mater. Sci. Eng. Mater. Biol. Appl.* **2021**, *127*, 112202. [CrossRef] [PubMed]
34. Kisling, A.; Lust, R.M.; Katwa, L.C. What is the role of peptide fragments of collagen I and IV in health and disease? *Life Sci.* **2019**, *228*, 30–34. [CrossRef] [PubMed]
35. Martínez-Morales, P.L.; del Corral, R.D.; Olivera-Martínez, I.; Quiroga, A.C.; Das, R.M.; Barbas, J.A.; Storey, K.G.; Morales, A.V. FGF and retinoic acid activity gradients control the timing of neural crest cell emigration in the trunk. *J. Cell Biol.* **2011**, *194*, 489–503. [CrossRef]
36. Wongrattanakamon, P.; Nimmanpipug, P.; Sirithunyalug, B.; Chaiyana, W.; Jiranusornkul, S. Investigation of the Skin Anti-photoaging Potential of Swertia chirayita Secoiridoids Through the AP-1/Matrix Metalloproteinase Pathway by Molecular Modeling. *Int. J. Pept. Res. Ther.* **2018**, *25*, 517–533. [CrossRef]

marine drugs

MDPI

Article

Antioxidative Effect of *Chlorella Pyrenoidosa* Protein Hydrolysates and Their Application in Krill Oil-in-Water Emulsions

Yujia Liu [1,†], Yuli Qi [1,†], Qi Wang [1], Fawen Yin [2,3], Honglei Zhan [1], Han Wang [1], Bingnan Liu [1], Yoshimasa Nakamura [4] and Jihui Wang [1,5,*]

1 School of Biological Engineering, Dalian Polytechnic University, Dalian 116034, China; liuyuj@dlpu.edu.cn (Y.L.); qyl1123004@163.com (Y.Q.); wq2020ydsan@163.com (Q.W.); zhanhonglei121@163.com (H.Z.); hwang@dlpu.edu.cn (H.W.); lbnno158@foxmail.com (B.L.)
2 School of Food Science and Technology, Dalian Polytechnic University, Dalian 116034, China; yinfawen198@126.com
3 National Engineering Research Center of Seafood, Dalian 116034, China
4 Graduate School of Environmental and Life Science, Okayama University, Okayama 700-8530, Japan; yossan@cc.okayama-u.ac.jp
5 School of Chemical Engineering and Energy Technology, Dongguan University of Technology, Dongguan 523808, China
* Correspondence: lyj32731@126.com
† These authors contributed equally to this work.

Citation: Liu, Y.; Qi, Y.; Wang, Q.; Yin, F.; Zhan, H.; Wang, H.; Liu, B.; Nakamura, Y.; Wang, J. Antioxidative Effect of *Chlorella Pyrenoidosa* Protein Hydrolysates and Their Application in Krill Oil-in-Water Emulsions. *Mar. Drugs* **2022**, *20*, 345. https://doi.org/10.3390/md20060345

Academic Editors: Chang-Feng Chi and Bin Wang

Received: 22 March 2022
Accepted: 23 May 2022
Published: 25 May 2022

Abstract: *Chlorella pyrenoidosa* is an excellent source of protein, and in this research, we assessed the antioxidant and emulsifying effects of Chlorella protein hydrolysate (CPH) using neutral proteases and alkaline proteases, as well as the properties of CPH-derived krill oil-in-water (O/W) emulsions. The CPHs exhibited the ability to scavenge several kinds of free radicals, including 1,1-diphenyl-2-picrylhydrazyl (DPPH), O_2^-, hydroxyl, and ABTS. Additionally, the CPHs (5 mg/mL) scavenged approximately 100% of the DPPH and ABTS. The CPHs showed similar emulsifying activities to Tween 20 and excellent foaming activities (max FS 74%), which helped to stabilize the krill oil-in-water emulsion. Less than 10 mg/mL CPHs was able to form fresh krill oil-in-water emulsions; moreover, the CPHs (5 mg/mL) in a krill O/W emulsion were homogenous, opaque, and stable for at least 30 days. Based on their inhibitory effects on the peroxide value (POV) and thiobarbituric acid reactive substances (TRABS), the CPHs were found to be able to inhibit lipid oxidation in both emulsifying systems and krill O/W emulsions. Thus, the CPHs could improve superoxide dismutase (SOD) activities by 5- or 10-fold and decrease the high reactive oxygen species (ROS) level caused by the addition of H_2O_2 in vitro. In conclusion, health-promoting CPHs could be applied in krill oil-in-water emulsions as both emulsifiers and antioxidants, which could help to improve the oxidative and physical stability of emulsions.

Keywords: *Chlorella pyrenoidosa* protein hydrolysate; antioxidant activity; krill oil-in-water emulsion; lipid oxidation

1. Introduction

Antarctic krill (*Euphausia superba*), a well-known species, famous for its nutritional value, is considered one of the richest biomasses in the world, and the functional lipid content in krill has been proven to be approximately 12–50%. Therefore, Antarctic krill oil has an abundance of phospholipids, eicosapentaenoic acid (EPA), docosahexaenoic acid (DHA), and astaxanthin [1]. To date, Antarctic krill oil has been confirmed to have anti-inflammatory, anticancer, brain function-promoting, and cardiovascular disease-preventing functions [2]. DHA and EPA in krill oil are incorporated into phospholipids, and the bioavailability of krill oil improves as a result [3]. Developing different types of krill oil can provide more opportunities for Antarctic krill oil consumption.

An O/W emulsion is a classic oil form that is commonly used in food products. An O/W emulsion from oil can help change the water solubility and enrich the functional components of emulsions. In the food industry, O/W emulsions are usually stabilized by commercial emulsifiers such as Tween 20, Tween 80, and Span. However, O/W emulsions are easily oxidized because there are many components promoting lipid oxidation in the aqueous phase that require interfacial antioxidants for stable oxidation of emulsions. Additionally, some antioxidant proteins and protein hydrolysates can also be used as both emulsifiers and antioxidants for different kinds of oil and add to the nutritional value of emulsions. Shen et al. indicated that fish gelatin and milk protein Maillard reaction products can both stabilize and raise krill O/W emulsions' stability [4]. Additionally, whey protein and its hydrolysates were shown to be able to stabilize medium-chain triglyceride oil emulsions [5]. Various other protein hydrolysates, such as porcine bone protein hydrolysates [6], soy protein hydrolysate [7], and rice dreg protein hydrolysate [8], have demonstrated their inhibition effects on lipid oxidation and different emulsifying properties. Finding additional stabilized emulsifiers and antioxidants from protein hydrolysates will help in the process of developing more stable and functional O/W emulsions; stable krill O/W emulsions, in particular, require further investigation.

Chlorella pyrenoidosa (*C. pyrenoidosa*) is a green alga with a long history that is widely used as a food supplement worldwide. Most *C. pyrenoidosa* is found growing in fresh water environments; however, some marine types of *C. pyrenoidosa* can also be cultured in seawater [9–11]. The marine species of *C. pyrenoidosa* could possibly decrease the large inputs needed to a greater extent than freshwater species, because of the requirement of fresh water. More than 50% of the *C. pyrenoidosa* cell content is protein, which includes all essential amino acids [12]. Protein hydrolysates originating from the *C. pyrenoidosa* protein have been reported to have antioxidant effects and ameliorate the development of atherosclerosis [13]. A small number of studies have targeted the emulsifier behavior of these hydrolysates. It remains unknown whether these hydrolysates are suitable emulsifiers for deriving krill O/W emulsions and whether they could contribute to inhibiting lipid oxidation. In this study, we evaluated the emulsifying, antioxidant, and lipid peroxidation inhibitory properties and the cytoprotective effects of CPHs that were hydrolyzed by alkaline proteases and neutral proteases. These two protein hydrolysates were used to emulsify krill O/W emulsions, and their physical and oxidative stabilities were investigated. The purpose of this study was to apply CPHs in a krill oil emulsion as emulsifiers, which further increased their oxidative stabilities and added to the health-adding value of the emulsion.

2. Results and Discussion

2.1. Antioxidant Activities of CPHs

The DPPH and O_2^- radical scavenging activities are usually used to estimate the antioxidant activity of antioxidant components from food in vitro, since these free radicals are always found in biological systems. The effects of antioxidants on the scavenging of DPPH and O_2^- probably contribute to the weakening and termination of the chain reaction of lipid oxidation. The free radicals of the DPPH scavenging activities of the neutral protease Chlorella protein hydrolysate (NCPH), the alkaline protease Chlorella protein hydrolysate (ACPH), and ascorbic acid are shown in Figure 1A. A total of 1.25 mg/mL and 2.5 mg/mL NCPH exhibited a free radical scavenging ability of about 65% for DPPH, whereas 5, 10, and 20 mg/mL NCPH scavenged nearly 100% of DPPH radicals. Additionally, 1.25, 2.5, and 5 mg/mL ACPHs scavenged DPPH radicals in a dose-dependent manner. All of the 5, 10, and 20 mg/mL ACPHs showed 100% scavenging ability. DPPH, a steady hydrophobic free radical, was shown to be reduced and eliminated by a hydrogen atom-donating compound; while hydroxyl radicals are considered to have an important role in both hydrophilic systems and the early stages of lipid peroxidation [14]. In addition, the scavenging activity of other antioxidant emulsifiers in O/W emulsions, such as whey protein isolates, lotus seedpod proanthocyanin conjugate, and Cod (*Gadus morhua*) for the protein hydrolysates of different free radicals have been examined with DPPH [15].

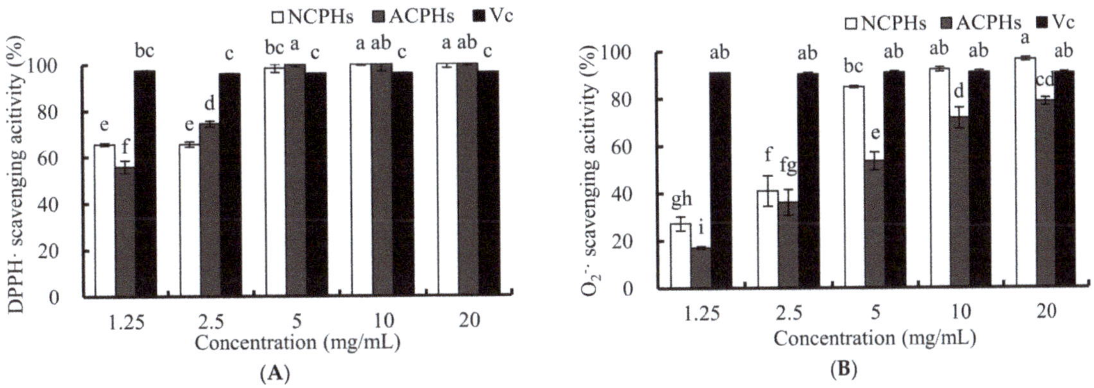

Figure 1. DPPH (**A**) and O_2^- (**B**) free radical scavenging activities of 0, 1.25, 2.5, 5, 10, and 20 mg/mL CPHs and VC. CPHs were obtained by neutral proteases (20,000 U) and alkaline proteases (20,000 U) for 5 h, separately. Different letters above values indicate different significances ($p < 0.05$).

The O_2^- free radical is an oxidant that can generate hydroxyl radicals that can abstract a hydrogen atom from other fatty acids from emulsions and forms a hydroperoxide (primary oxidation product) [16]. The scavenging activities of different concentration of CPHs on O_2^- are shown in Figure 1B. NCPHs and ACPHs similarly exhibited a dose-dependent O^{2-} free radical scavenging activity. We also found that in the O_2^- free radical scavenging experiment, NCPHs had a significantly higher antioxidant capacity than ACPHs for most concentrations of each sample. Moreover, a lower concentration (1.25 mg/mL) of NCPHs and ACPHs only showed approximately 20–30% O_2^- free radical scavenging activity, whereas the value reached 70–80% at concentrations of 10 and 20 mg/mL for NCPHs and ACPHs, respectively; suggesting that the increase in dosage had a strong influence on the O^{2-} free radical scavenging activity. Consequently, such proteins and hydrolysates can act as O_2^- free radical scavengers, including squid protein hydrolysates, in which the increase in the O_2^- free radical scavenging activity agreed with our results [17].

Therefore, based on the results of the O^{2-} and DPPH free radical scavenging activities, CPHs does not only act as a significant free radical scavenger for O_2^- and DPPH free radical-containing food or biological systems, such as in vitro and in vivo systems, but also exhibits a good potential antioxidant capability in solvent-containing systems, such as emulsion systems.

In addition, NCPHs and ACPHs have shown OH and ABTS radical scavenging activities (Supplementary Material Figure S1A,B), which proved that NCPHs and ACPHs are excellent antioxidants via multiple pathways.

2.2. Emulsifying and Foaming Activities of CPHs

To test the antioxidant activity of CPHs in emulsion, the emulsifying and foaming properties of CPHs should be preferentially determined. The EAI and ESI results of CPHs at 1.25, 2.5, 5, 10, and 20 mg/mL are shown in Figure 2A,B. In general, EAI decreased significantly and dose dependently, as did Tween 20 (positive control), whereas ESI showed no significant change. When comparing the NCPHs and ACPHs, the NCPHs seemed to have higher EAI values than those of the ACPHs at lower concentrations (1.25, 2.5, and 5 mg/mL), but they had no significant differences at higher concentrations, suggesting that neutral proteases might be more suitable for manufacturing emulsifying system-based hydrolysates. Several other hydrolysates have also been proven to have the same tendency of a decline in their emulsifying capability at higher concentrations [18,19]. Generally, there are two processes involved in the progression of emulsification, and these processes include the disruption and deformation of lipid droplets that determine the emulsion's distinct surface area; and the emulsifier helps to stabilize this interface. Based on these two points, the protein adsorption at the oil–water interface is a diffusion method that is more easily controlled at low protein concentrations; whereas a higher protein concentration attenuates migration by the activation of an energy barrier in diffusion-dependent situations [20], which points to a decrease in emulsifying activity. This would also explain why, at high concentrations, NCPHs and ACPHs resulted in no significant differences in EAIs (Figure 2A), because extra proteins were blocked and there was no additional emulsifying activity. Moreover, the ESI results also suggested that concentration had no influence on the emulsion stability and that the NCPHs and ACPHs retained a higher emulsion stability, without exhibiting any differences from each other.

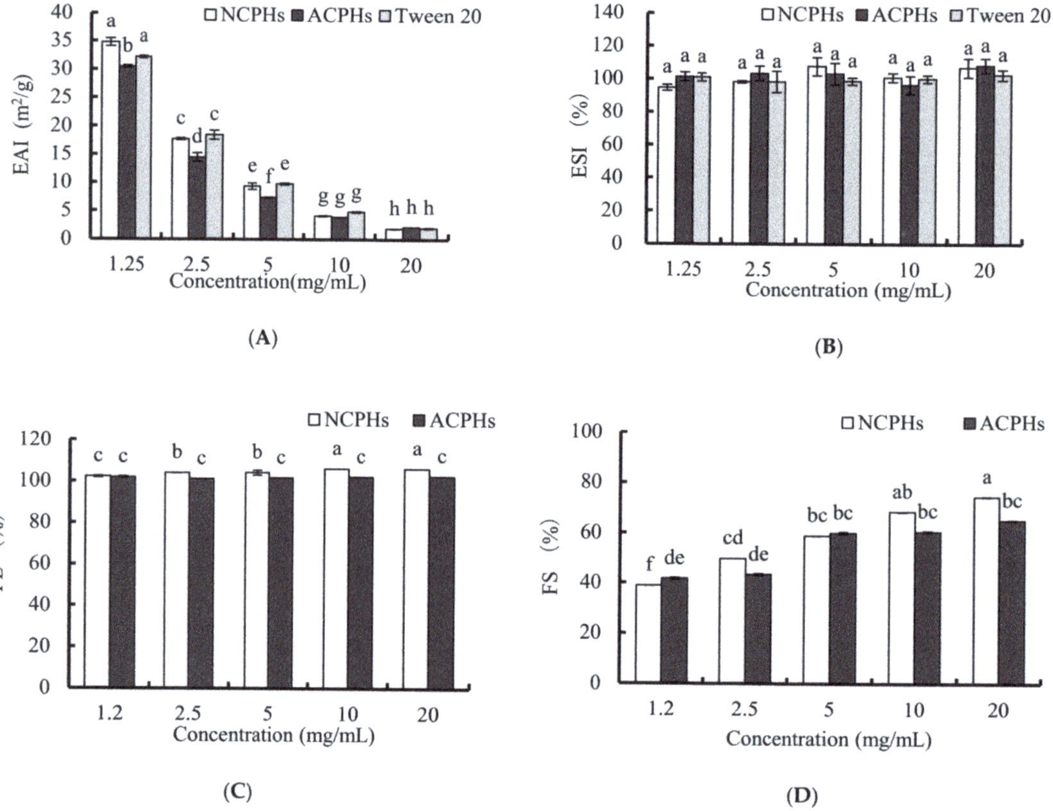

Figure 2. EAI (**A**) and ESI (**B**) of NCPHs, ACHPs, and Tween 20 at 0, 1.25, 2.5, 5, 10, and 20 mg/mL. FE (**C**) and FS (**D**) of NCPHs and ACHPs at 0, 1.25, 2.5, 5, 10, and 20 mg/mL. Different letters (a–h) above values indicate different significances ($p < 0.05$).

The results of the FE and FS tests of the samples with CPHs at 1.25, 2.5, 5, 10, and 20 mg/mL are shown in Figure 2C,D. In the NCPHs, the values of FE and FS increased slightly and dose-dependently and reached their maximum values at 20 mg/mL, whereas the FE value of the ACPHs did not significantly change with increasing concentration, and the FS value of the ACPHs only significantly increased at concentrations of 2.5 and 5 mg/mL. Furthermore, the FS and FE values of the NCPHs were dramatically higher than those of the ACPHs at higher concentrations (10 and 20 mg/mL), and the tendencies were similar and comparable between these two groups in the results of EAI (Figure 2A). Both FS and FE are critical foam properties that can be mediated by small-molecular-weight surfactants, such as peptides or hydrolysates. Generally, molecules' penetration, transportation, and reorganization are involved in foam formation, which can be enhanced by the adsorption of proteins or peptides and can trigger a rapid reduction in surface tension. In some ways, the enzymatic hydrolysis of proteins, not only strongly increases their solubility, but also enhances their foaming properties, which consequently modify three major structures, as follows: a lower molecular mass, a higher amount of the ionizable group, and the essential involvement of hydrophobic structures [21]. Our results revealed that higher amounts of hydrolysates led to a better foaming ability, which was probably due to the higher speed of adsorption of the hydrolysates at the surface, which was consistent with previous reports on the foaming capability of other protein hydrolysates [18]. In addition, the emulsifying ability of the NCPHs was better than that of the ACPHs overall, indicating that neutral proteases might be more suitable for producing *Chlorella pyrenoidosa*-derived hydrolysates with a better emulsifying ability.

2.3. Intracellular Antioxidant Activity of CPHs In Vitro

Intracellular ROS are generated by various cell metabolite pathways in the human body. Antioxidants can regulate antioxidant enzymes in cells or directly mitigate ROS-induced damage. SOD is one of the most important antioxidant enzymes; it is ubiquitously expressed in human cells and plays a detoxifying role against superoxide radicals [22]. SODs convert superoxide radicals into O_2 and hydrogen peroxide, and then the hydrogen peroxide catalases to oxygen and water. Therefore, we used the MDA-MB-231 cell line to assess the effect of CPHs on cellular SOD activities and H_2O_2-induced oxidative stress. As shown in Figure 3A, both the NCPHs and ACPHs increased SOD activity in a dose-dependent manner. Treatment with 0.25 and 0.5 mg/mL NCPHs significantly increased SOD activity in comparison to the control group (without the hydrolysate treatment), whereas treatment with 0.125, 0.25, and 0.5 mg/mL ACPHs significantly induced SOD activity. The SOD activity induced by the ACPHs was significantly higher than that induced by the NCPHs. These results indicate that NCPHs and ACPHs show antioxidant effects through intracellular detoxification. Furthermore, the antioxidant effects of the NCPHs and ACPHs against H_2O_2-induced cellular damage were also investigated using a DCFH-DA kit (Figure 3B,C). The cell-permeant reagent DCFH-DA is a fluorogenic dye that can reflect the peroxyl, hydroxyl, and other ROS activity in cells. After cellular uptake, internal esterase can deacetylate DCFH-DA to a non-fluorescent compound, which is later oxidized by ROS into the fluorescent compound 2′-7′dichlorofluorescein (DCF). The results indicated that the accumulation of green fluorescence was significantly enhanced by H_2O_2 treatment, whereas without the CPHs or H_2O_2 treatment, green fluorescence was hardly detected. In comparison, pretreatment with NCPHs and ACPHs dramatically attenuated H_2O_2-induced green fluorescence in MDA-MB-231 cells, suggesting that H_2O_2-induced oxidative stress was dramatically decreased. In addition, when comparing the NCPHs and ACPHs, the NCPHs were found to have better antioxidant effects against cellular oxidative damage in the MDA-MB-231 cell line, since the intensity of green fluorescence of the NCPHs was lighter than that of the ACPHs at each concentration and seemed to vanish at 0.5 mg/mL. Additionally, the peptides from protein hydrolysates in Monkfish [23] and salmon collagen hydrolysate [24] had similar effects on SOD activity or ROS mitigation effects. In this figure, we show the SOD activities induced by NCPHs and ACPHs, which could convert harmful superoxide to hydrogen peroxide, while hydrogen peroxide could also be cleaved by NCPHs and ACPHs. These data demonstrate that the NCPHs and ACPHs exerted protective effects by inducing antioxidant defenses and reducing oxidative stress. Other peptides derived from *Chlorella* sp., such as the peptide (Leu-Asn-Gly-Asp-Val-Trp) from *Chlorella ellipsiodea*, have peroxyl radical and DPPH radical scavenging antioxidant activities in vitro, and intracellular radical scavenging activity in monkey kidney cells [25]. Another peptide (Val-Glu-Cys-Tyr-Gly-Pro-Asn-Arg-Pro-Gln-Phe) from *Chlorella vulgaris* demonstrated its antioxidant activity in vitro or and in cell-based assays [26]. Antioxidant peptides NIPP-1 (Pro-GlyTrp-Asn-Gln-Trp-Phe-Leu) and NIPP-2 (Val-Glu-Val-Leu-Pro-Pro-Ala-Glu-Leu) from microalgae *Navicula incerta* have shown their cytoprotective activities in HepG2/CYP2E1 cells [27]. In addition, the abundance of aromatic amino acids (Tyr, Trp, Met, Lys, Cys, His), hydrophobic amino acids (Leu, Val), and a particular functional group (sulfhydryl group of Cys) is thought to facilitate a higher antioxidant capacity of peptides [28]. In our study, the most abundant amino acids of NCPH and ACPH were Leu, Pro, Ala, Glu, and Asp (data not shown); of which, Leu and Pro are also found in peptides of *Chlorella ellipsiodea* and *Chlorella vulgaris* and majorly facilitate higher antioxidant activities.

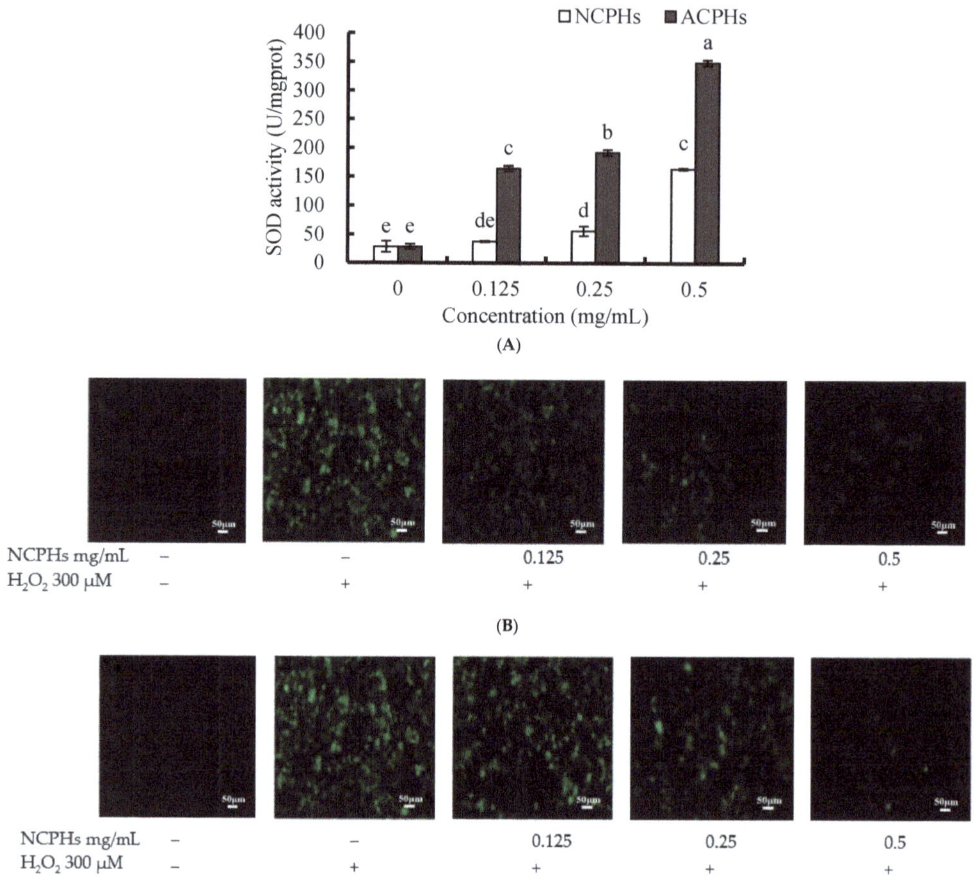

Figure 3. A total of 1×10^6 MDA-MB-231 cells were treated with 0, 0.125, 0.25, and 0.5 mg/mL NCPHs and ACPHs for 3 h. They were then pretreated with 0 or 300 μM H_2O_2 for another 3 h. (**A**) SOD activities of MDA-MB-231 cells after NCPH and ACPH treatments. (**B**) ROS level of MDA-MB-231 cells after treatment with H_2O_2 or NCPHs. (**C**) ROS level of MDA-MB-231 cells after treatment with H_2O_2 or ACPHs. Different letters (a–e) above values indicate different significances ($p < 0.05$).

2.4. Lipid Peroxidation Inhibition Assay

The enzymatic hydrolysates of proteins in oil-dispersion products have been confirmed to have antioxidant effects on lipid oxidation, because of their radical scavenging activity and their capability for sequestering pro-oxidative metal ions. To assess the antioxidant activity of each sample in hydrophobic systems, the effects of the NCPHs and ACPHs on lipid peroxidation were evaluated by determining the levels of POV and TRABS, and the results are shown in Figure 4. The results showed that the NCPHs and ACPHs exhibited a dose-dependent POV inhibitory effect on linoleic acid oxidation, as well as a similar tendency in the TBARS inhibition experiments; which was consistent with previous reports [29]. When comparing every two days, out of six days of incubation, the inhibitory effects of the NCPHs and ACPHs against oxidation gradually increased and reached a level approximately the same as that of ascorbic acid (the positive control); whereas the antioxidant effect of ascorbic acid started to decrease from the beginning, suggesting that these two hydrolysates might have more advantages in oil–water emulsion systems with long-term inhibition activity against lipid peroxidation. When comparing these two samples, it is worth noting that the ACPHs exhibited comparatively higher inhibitory effects than those of the NCPHs based on the level of POV, even though the free radical scavenging activities of the NCPHs were higher than those of the ACPHs; this means that the antioxidant abilities of the hydrolysates in aqueous environments and emulsifying systems were equivalent but not completely the same. Therefore, determining the antioxidant capability of NCPHs and ACPHs in an oil-in-water emulsifying system is necessary.

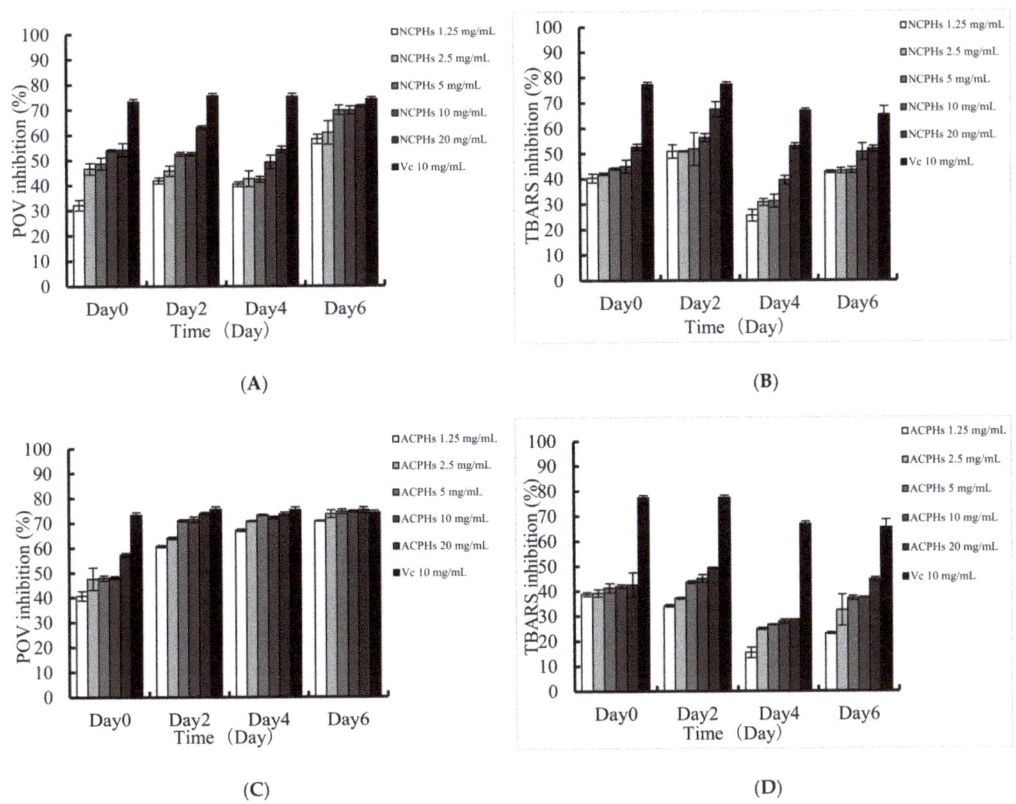

Figure 4. Effect of different concentrations of NCPHs and ACPHs on linoleic acid oxidation were measured at 40 °C for 6 days. Lipid peroxidation inhibition assay of CPHs: POV inhibition of NCPHs (**A**) and ACPHs (**C**) in concentrations of 1.25, 2.5, 5, 10, and 20 mg/mL for 0, 2, 4, and 6 days. TRABS inhibition of NCPHs (**B**) and ACPHs (**D**) in concentrations of 1.25, 2.5, 5, 10, and 20 mg/mL for 0, 2, 4, and 6 days.

2.5. CPH-Loaded Antarctic Krill Oil Emulsion

2.5.1. Particle Size and Zeta Potential of CPH-Loaded Antarctic Krill Oil Emulsions

Here, we chose CPHs (1.25, 2.5, 5, and 10 mg/mL) as the emulsifiers for the Antarctic krill oil emulsions, based on their emulsifier properties. The choice of emulsifier affects the physicochemical, sensorial, and functional properties of the emulsion produced. Particle size, polymerization, and zeta potential were used to identify the emulsion's stability. The particle sizes of the CPH-loaded Antarctic krill oil emulsions with different concentrations are shown in Figure 5A. The 1.25, 2.5, 5, and 10 mg/mL CPHs increased the particle size of the KO emulsion in a dose-dependent manner. The 1.25 and 2.5 mg/mL NCPHs-KO emulsion and the ACPHs-KO emulsion showed similar particle sizes, close to 120 nm. The NCPHs and ACPHs (10 mg/mL) clearly increased the particle size of the KO emulsions, which were approximately 257 nm and 201 nm, respectively. The zeta potentials of the different concentrations of CPH-loaded KO emulsions were all negative, and between −30 mV and −45 mV. There were no significant differences between the different concentration groups or different protease-loaded groups.

These particle sizes of the emulsion indicated that less than 5 mg/mL CPH could form small droplets, which helped in allowing active delivery, thereby boosting the rapid absorption and release of hydrophobic bioactive ingredients such as phospholipids and omega 3 fatty acids [5]. There were significant differences between the particle sizes of the NCPH-KO emulsion and the ACPH-KO emulsion, probably due to these peptides having different numbers of hydrophobic regions produced by different enzymes. The adsorption of peptides onto droplet interfaces depends on their hydrophobic properties, mainly their surface hydrophobicity [30].

The progress of the enzymatic hydrolysis of soy proteins and whey protein can produce smaller peptides that contain a partially exposed hydrophobic core and fewer secondary and tertiary structures, making them excellent emulsifiers [31]. These properties account for their increased dispersion in the oil–water interface and the maintenance of the physical and chemical stability of emulsions [31]. However, sometimes, a protein hydrolysate alone, such as porcine bone protein hydrolysates, cannot obtain the stabilities achieved in O/W emulsions [6].

2.5.2. Morphology of CPH-Loaded KO Emulsions

The different concentrations of the CPH-loaded KO emulsions showed that both the NCP- and ACP-loaded KO emulsions were homogenous, opaque, and stable on day 0. With the addition of CPHs, the initial reddish colloids turned brownish, which possibly occurred because the color of the CPHs changed the color of the emulsions (Figure 5C). During the 30-day storage time, the 1.25, 2.5, and 10 mg/mL NCPH- and ACPH-loaded KO emulsions had different degrees of creaming or separation from the first three days. The 10 mg/mL NCP- and ACP-loaded KO emulsions had the most obvious signs of separation (data not shown). However, the 5 mg/mL NCPH- and ACPH-loaded KO emulsions remained stable at room temperature for 30 days (Figure 5D). These results may be because an adequate surface hydrophobicity of CPHs is needed for strong and cohesive films to form around droplets, and 1.25 mg/mL and 2.5 mg/mL were not sufficient for the CPHs to function as good emulsifiers. The exceeded protein load at the interface led to extra protein escaping from the interface, to form flocculation via a hydrophobic interaction, making the 10 mg/mL CPH-loaded emulsion easy to cream and separate.

The microstructure of the CPH-loaded KO emulsions with different concentrations was observed using CSLM. Using the CSLM image, the protein (which exhibited green fluorescence) and oil droplet (which exhibited red fluorescence) distributions were obtained. As shown in Figure 5E, the 1.25, 2.5, and 5 mg/mL NCPH-loaded KO emulsions and ACPH-loaded KO emulsions had a relatively uniform distribution of oil droplets, with small particles and good dispersions. The 10 mg/mL NCPH-loaded KO emulsions and ACPH-loaded KO emulsions had larger particles and more protein in the oil droplets.

These results were consistent with the particle results in Figure 5A and indicate that NCPHs and ACPHs can be applied in KO emulsions as emulsifiers.

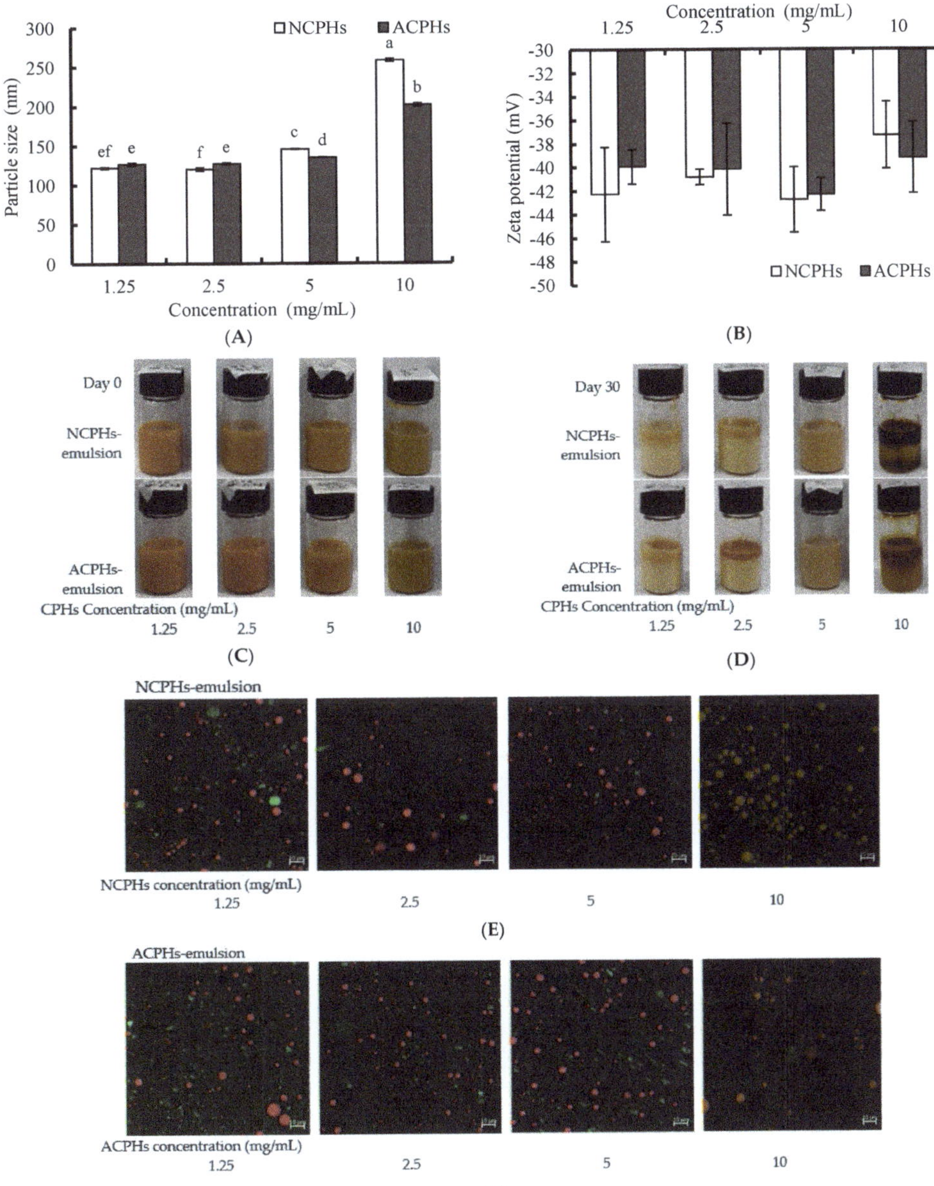

Figure 5. NCPHs and ACPHs in concentrations of 1.25, 2.5, 5, 10, and 20 mg/mL in water were used to form a KO emulsion containing 10% krill oil. (**A**) Particle size of CPH-derived KO emulsions. (**B**) Zeta potential of CPH-derived KO emulsions. (**C**) Photograph of CPH-derived KO emulsions at day 0. (**D**) Photograph of CPH-derived KO emulsions at day 30. (**E**) CLSM micrographs of NCPH-derived KO emulsions. (**F**) CLSM micrographs of ACPH-derived KO emulsions. Different letters (a–f) above values indicate different significances ($p < 0.05$).

2.6. Oxidative Stability of the Emulsion

The enzymatic hydrolysate of protein in oil-dispersion products has been reported to suppress lipid oxidation, due to their peptide radical scavenging and pro-oxidative metal ion sequestering capability. The NCPHs and ACPHs showed antioxidant activities against KO oxidation (Figures 1 and 4). However, the oxidative stability of the NCPH- and ACPH-loaded emulsions remains unknown. Here, we used the levels of POV and TBARS to represent the oxidative stability. The KO emulsion and Tween 20 emulsion were used as controls. After different the KO emulsions were stored at 40 °C for six days, the POV value of the KO emulsion and Tween 20 emulsion increased from 3.43 meq/kg to 3.77 meq/kg, and 2.56 meq/kg to 3.62 meq/kg, respectively. However, the POV value of the NCPH-loaded emulsion increased from 1.21 meq/kg to 1.59 meq/kg, and the POV value of the ACPH-loaded emulsion increased from 1.01 meq/kg to 1.19 meq/kg. These results indicate that the POVs of the NCPH- and ACPH-loaded emulsions were both significantly lower than those of the KO emulsions, which was probably due to the lipid oxidation inhibitory effect. After six days of storage at 40 °C, the TRABS values of the KO emulsion and the Tween 20-, NCPH-, and ACPH-loaded KO emulsions were significantly increased and finally reached 25.65 mg/kg, 19.04 mg/kg, 12.76 mg/kg, and 9.58 mg/kg, respectively (Figure 6B). These results indicate that Tween 20, NCPHs, and ACPHs significantly inhibited the TRABS formation in the KO emulsions.

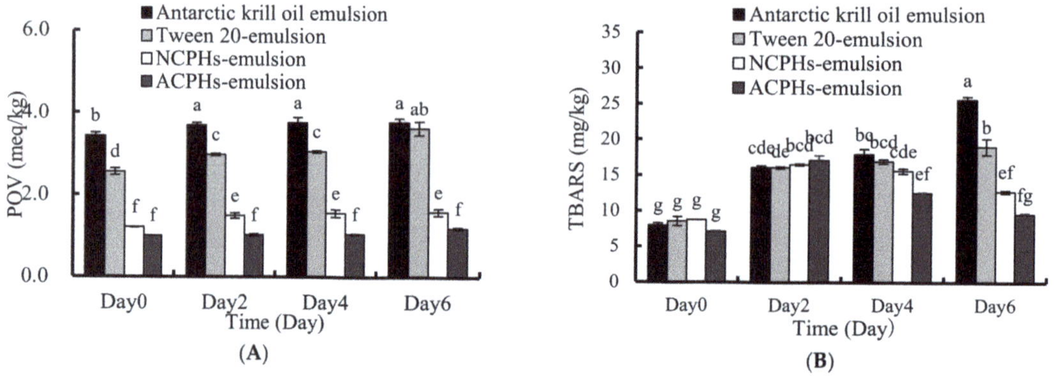

Figure 6. Accelerated oxidation of CPH-derived emulsion, KO emulsions, and Tween 20 KO emulsions at 40 °C for 6 days. Lipid peroxidation value: (**A**) POV value of KO emulsion, Tween 20 emulsion, and CPH-derived emulsion over 6 days. (**B**) TRABS value of KO emulsion, Tween 20 emulsion, and CPHs derived emulsion over 6 days. The significance was analyzed by one-way ANOVA followed by Tukey's HSD using SPSS 16.0. The different letters (a–g) above the bars indicate significant differences among the treatments for each condition ($p < 0.05$).

We hypothesize that the Tween 20-loaded KO emulsions decreased the POV and TRABS values, probably through physical effects, because Tween 20 can form interfacial layers that may sterically hamper the movement of pro-oxidants from the water to oil phases, thereby improving the oxidative stability. The change in POV and TRABS values in the NCPH- and ACPH-derived emulsions was more significant than in the Tween 20-loaded KO emulsions, which was possibly because of the antioxidant effect via the free radical scavenging activities of the NCPHs and ACPHs; this result agrees with the finding that hydrolysates in emulsions such as fish protein hydrolysates, rice dreg protein hydrolysate [8], and porcine bone protein hydrolysates [6] have antioxidant effects in water/oil emulsions. It has also been reported that antioxidative proteins can inhibit emulsion lipid oxidation through the interface effect and continuous phase effect during storage [32]. The interface of a protein-loaded O/W emulsion always has a higher degree of rigidity and continuity, which would likely prevent the penetration and diffusion of radicals into the lipid phase within the emulsion droplets [33]. Antioxidant protein hydrolysates in the continuous phase were thought to break the free radical chain and prevent the formation of peroxides by reacting with certain precursors of peroxide.

3. Materials and Methods

3.1. Chemicals

Commercial *Chlorella Pyrenoidosa* powder and Antarctic krill oil were obtained from Dalian Jianyang Biological Company (Dalian, China) and Liaoyu Group Co., Ltd. (Dalian, China), respectively. The neutral proteases (EINECS:253-457-5) and alkaline proteases (EINECS:232-752-2) were obtained from Yuanye Biotechnology Co., Ltd. (Shanghai, China). Ferrous chloride and ascorbic acid were obtained from Damao Chemical Reagent Factory (Tianjin, China). Sodium dodecyl sulfate (SDS), linoleic acid (stored at −20 °C), 1,1,3,3-tetraethoxypropane, trichloroacetic acid, Thiobarbituric acid (TBA), Nile Red, and Nile Blue were bought from Aladdin Industrial Co., Ltd. (Shanghai, China). Ammonium thiocyanate was bought from Sinopharm Group Reagent (Shanghai, China). Trypsin-EDTA, fetal bovine serum (FBS), and DMEM cell culture medium were bought from Invitrogen (Carlsbad, CA, USA). A superoxide dismutase (SOD) assay kit and reactive oxygen species (ROS) assay kit were bought from Nanjing Jiancheng Bioengineering Research Institute (Nanking, China).

3.2. Hydrolysates from Chlorella Protein

A total of 20 g Chlorella powder was dissolved in 2 L purified water (power: solution (*w/v*) = 1:100) to prepare a Chlorella powder solution. Before hydrolysis, the solution pH was adjusted to 7.5 (neutral proteases) and 9.0 (alkaline proteases), and the solution temperature was set at 45 °C (neutral proteases) and 50 °C (alkaline protease). Then, 20,000 U neutral protease and 20,000 U alkaline protease were added to the Chlorella powder solution for 5 h. Then, this process was stopped by performing incubation in boiling water for 10 min. The hydrolysate was observed by precipitation with 95% ethanol (hydrolysate: 95% ethanol (*v/v*) = 1:4), and the supernatant of the hydrolysates was then freeze-dried.

3.3. Determination of the Antioxidant Activity of Chlorella Protein Hydrolysates (CPHs)

The DPPH, O_2^-, HO·, and ABTS scavenging activities were measured, to represent the antioxidant activities of the CPHs and ascorbic acid (positive control) at 1.25, 2.5, 5, 10, and 20 mg/mL. The methods we used were in accordance with those of other reports, with small modifications [19,34–36].

3.3.1. DPPH Radical Scavenging Activity Assay

A total of 2 mL of CPHs or ascorbic acid was blended with 2 mL of DPPH (0.04 mg/mL) and kept in the dark for 30 min. Then, these solutions were centrifuged at 5000 r/min for 10 min; then, we measured the absorbance at 517 nm [34]. The calculation formula was as follows:

$$\text{DPPH radical scavenging activity } (\%) = \left(1 - \frac{(A_x - A_{x0})}{A_0}\right) \times 100\% \tag{1}$$

where A_x is the value of sample absorbance; A_{x0} is the value of the interference group absorbance (distilled water instead of DPPH); and A_0 is the absorbance of distilled water instead of the sample group.

3.3.2. Hydroxyl Radical (HO) Scavenging Activity

A total of 1 mL of CPHs or ascorbic acid was blended with 1 mL of salicylic acid at 9 mM, 1 mL of $FeSO_4$ at 9 mM, and 1 mL of H_2O_2 at 8.8 mM and was incubated at 37 °C for

30 min. Then, the absorbances of these mixtures were tested at 510 nm [36]. The calculation formula was as follows:

$$\text{HO radical scavenging activity } (\%) = \left(1 - \frac{(A_x - A_{x0})}{A_0}\right) \times 100\% \quad (2)$$

where A_x is the value of sample absorbance; A_{x0} is the value of the interference group absorbance (distilled water instead of H_2O_2); and A_0 is the absorbance of distilled water instead of the sample group.

3.3.3. Superoxide Anion Radical ($O_2{}^-$) Scavenging Activity

A total of 1 mL of CPHs or ascorbic acid was prepared and mixed with 1 mL of Tris-HCl at 50 mM and 0.6 mL of pyrogallol at 25 mM, and was incubated at 25 °C for 5 min. The reaction was stopped using HCl, and its absorbance was read at 299 nm [35]. The calculation formula was as follows:

$$O^{2-} \text{ radical scavenging activity } (\%) = \left(1 - \left(A_x - \frac{A_{x0}}{A_0}\right)\right) \times 100\% \quad (3)$$

where A_x is the value of sample absorbance; A_{x0} is the value of the interference group absorbance (distilled water instead of pyrogallol); and A_0 is the absorbance of distilled water instead of the sample group.

3.3.4. Determination of ABTS Scavenging Activity

The ABTS solutions were prepared with 7.4 mM ABTS and an equal volume of 2.45 mM potassium persulfate, kept in the dark for 15 h and diluted with PBS (pH 7.4) until the absorbance at 734 nm reached 0.70 ± 0.02. The 10 μL of CPHs, together with the 90 μL diluted ABTS solution, were incubated for 6 min in the dark and measured at 734 nm [19]. The calculation formula was as follows:

$$\text{ABTS radical scavenging activity } (\%) = \left(1 - \frac{(A_x - A_{x0})}{A_0}\right) \times 100\% \quad (4)$$

where A_x is the value of sample absorbance; A_{x0} is the value of the interference group absorbance (distilled water instead of ABTS); and A_0 is the absorbance of distilled water instead of the sample group.

3.4. Emulsifying Properties

The emulsification activity and the emulsion stability of CPHs on Antarctic krill oil were measured according to Pearce and Kinsella's method with modifications [37]. Each of 8 mL of 1.25 mg/mL, 2.5 mg/mL, 5 mg/mL, 10 mg/mL, and 20 mg/mL CPHs–distilled water solutions and 2 mL of Antarctic krill oil were mixed together and homogenized for 10 min at 13,500 rpm (T 10 basic ULTRA-TURRAX, IKA, Freiburg, Germany). Before and after the 10 min homogenization, 50 μL of the mixture sample from the middle layer of the emulsion was taken. Each sample was diluted 100-fold with 0.1% sodium dodecyl sulfate and shaken for 10 s. The absorbance of the sample was measured at 500 nm. The calculation formula was as follows:

$$\text{EAI } (m^2/g) = \frac{(2 \times 2.303 \times A \times D_F)}{l\varnothing C} \quad (5)$$

where A = A_{500}, D_F = dilution factor (100), l = passage path length of the cuvette (m), ∅ = oil fraction, and C = protein concentration in the aqueous phase (g/m^3);

$$\text{ESI (min)} = \frac{A_0 \times \Delta t}{\Delta A} \quad (6)$$

where $\Delta t = 10$ min and $\Delta A = A_0 - A_{10}$, A_0, and A_{10} are the absorbance of the sample at 0 min and 10 min after homogenization, respectively.

3.5. Foaming Properties

Foam expansion (FE) and foam stability (FS) were determined according to the method described by Shahidi and Synowiecki, with some adjustments [38]. Ten milliliters of protein hydrolysate solution (1.25 mg/mL, 2.5 mg/mL, 5 mg/mL, 10 mg/mL, and 20 mg/mL) were homogenized at 13,500 rpm for 1 min at room temperature. The solutions needed to be at standard conditions, and their volumes were recorded at 0 min and 10 min. The calculation formula was as follows:

$$\begin{aligned} \text{FE } (\%) &= \left(\frac{V_T}{V_o}\right) \times 100 \\ \text{FS } (\%) &= (V_t - V_o)/(V_T - V_o) \end{aligned} \tag{7}$$

where V_T is the total volume after homogenization; V_o is the original volume before homogenization; and V_t is the volume after standing at room temperature for 10 min.

3.6. Activity of SOD

MDA-MB-231 cells (1×10^6) from the American Type Culture Collection were cultured for 24 h and treated with CPHs to final concentrations of 0, 0.125, and 0.25, 0.5 mg/mL for 3 h. The cells were scraped and centrifuged at 1500 rpm/min (5 min) for collection. These cell pellets were washed and sonicated at 300 W to obtain the cell lysates. The SOD activity of the cell lysate was measured using a SOD kit, as stated in the manufacturer's manual (Nanjing Jiancheng Bioengineering Research Institute, Nanjing, China). The total protein content in the samples was measured using a BCA protein assay kit.

3.7. Reactive Oxygen Species (ROS) Level Determination

The ROS level was measured using an ROS kit, as stated in the manufacturer's manual (Nanjing Jiancheng Bioengineering Research Institute, Nanjing, China). MDA-MB-231 cells were incubated in DMEM culture medium containing 10% FBS for 24 h and then pretreated with CPHs to final concentrations of 0, 0.125, 0.25, and 0.5 mg/mL for 3 h. Afterward, the entire cell medium was freshly replaced. H_2O_2 was added to the cells and incubated for 3 h at a final concentration of 300 μM. Then, 100 μL of 2′-7′dichlorofluorescin diacetate (DCFH-DA,10 mM) was incubated with these cells for 30 min. The fluorescence of total ROS (T-ROS) was measured using fluorescence microscopy (Olympus IX81, Tokyo, Japan) (excitation wavelength: 485 nm, emission wavelength: 535 nm).

3.8. Lipid Peroxidation Inhibitory Activity Assay of CPHs

A total of 0.1 mL of linoleic acid together with 10 mL of 99.5% ethanol solution were added to CPHs (0, 1.25, 2.5, 10, 20 mg/mL) or 10 mg/mL ascorbic acid as a positive control in 10 mL of 0.2 M PBS (pH 7.2). The mixed solutions were placed in a 40 °C light-proof room for 0, 2, 4, or 6 days. TBA values were measured using the method of Ohkawa et al. [39]. The POV value was measured according to the Chinese National Standard GB 5009.227-2016 [40]. The calculation formula was as follows:

$$\text{Inhibition } (\%) = [\frac{A_0 - A_1}{A_0}] \times 100 \tag{8}$$

where A_0 is the absorbance of the control reaction (the addition of the hydrolysate is 0 mg) on the sixth day, and A_1 is the absorbance in the presence of the sample on that day.

3.9. Emulsion Preparation

A total of 1 mL of KO together with 9 mL of CPHs (0, 1.25, 2.5, 5, 10 mg/mL) or tween 20 (5 mg/mL) in distilled water were firstly dispersed at 13,500 rpm for 7 min using an IKA disperser (IKA® Works, Inc., Wilmington, NC, USA) to form primary emulsions.

These emulsions then underwent 20 min ultrasonication at 658 W in an ultrasonic crusher (SCIENTZ-IID, Ningbo, China), to form the final emulsions

3.10. Particle Size and Zeta Potential Measurements

Both particle sizes and zeta potentials were measured using a dynamic light scattering Zetasizer (Brookhaven Instruments Corporation, Holtsville, NY, USA) to reflect the physical condition of the emulsions. The emulsion samples were diluted 50 times and 1000 times with hyperpure water before the particle size and zeta potential measurements, to obtain a suitable intensity. The experiment was performed at room temperature in triplicates.

3.11. Confocal Laser Scanning Microscopy (CLSM)

CLSM was applied to reflect the microstructures of the CPH emulsions. The CLSM samples were prepared with different emulsions (1 mL) and 40 μL of Nile Red (0.1%, *w/v*) and Nile Blue (0.1%, *w/v*). A total of 10 μL of the CLSM sample was fixed on slides using nail polish and examined with a 100× magnification lens (excitation at 488 nm, excitation at 633 nm).

3.12. Oxidative Stability of CPH Emulsions

The oxidative stability of the CPH emulsions, the KO emulsions, and the Tween 20 emulsions was expressed by POVs and TRABS in an accelerated oxidation reaction (40 °C) for 6 days. The oil from their emulsions was extracted using a previously described hexane extraction method [41]. The POV and TRABS of the emulsions were sampled every 2 days for analysis. The POV value was measured. The PVs were determined as stated in the method of Undeland et al. [42]. TRABS was determined based on the method of the Chinese National Standard GB 5009, 181–2016 [43].

3.13. Statistical Analysis

The statistical analysis of each group was performed using SPSS 22 software (SPSS Inc., Chicago, IL, USA). One-way ANOVA with Tukey's test was used to analyze the homogeneity of variance, where $p < 0.05$ was considered significant. All the experiments were performed three parallel times, and the data are expressed as the SD ± means.

4. Conclusions

The present study showed that neutral protease protein hydrolysates (NCPHs) and alkaline protease protein hydrolysates (ACPHs) from *Chlorella pyrenoidosa* have antioxidant, emulsifying, and foaming activities. The NCPHs and ACPHs also induce SOD activities and mitigate H_2O_2-induced ROS levels in vitro. In addition, the NCPHs or ACPHs inhibited linoleic acid oxidation, and the NCPH- and ACPH-derived krill O/W emulsion remained physically stable for at least one month, where their POV and TRABS were lower than those of the KO and Tween 20-derived emulsions. Our study suggests that NCPHs and ACPHs have the potential to be applied in krill oil-in-water emulsions, as both emulsifiers and antioxidants.

Supplementary Materials: The following supporting information can be downloaded at: https://www.mdpi.com/article/10.3390/md20060345/s1, Figure S1: Hydroxyl (A) and ABTS (B) free radical scavenging activities of 0, 1.25, 2.5, 5, 10 and 20 mg/ml CPHs and VC.

Author Contributions: Conceptualization, Y.L.; data curation, Y.Q. and Q.W.; writing—original draft preparation, Y.Q.; writing—review and editing, Y.L. and J.W.; visualization, Y.N.; supervision, Y.L.; project administration, B.L. and H.W.; funding acquisition, F.Y. and H.Z. All authors have read and agreed to the published version of the manuscript.

Funding: This research was funded by [National Key R&D Program of China] grant number [2019YFD0902000], [General Program of the Educational Department of Liaoning Province] grant numbers [LJKZ0522 and LJKZ0539], and [Startup Foundation of Dalian Polytechnic University] grant number [6102072023].

Conflicts of Interest: The authors declare that they have no known competing financial interests or personal relationships that could have appeared to influence the work reported in this paper.

Abbreviations

Antarctic krill oil	KO
2,2′-azinobis (3-ethylbenzothiazoline-6-sulphonic acid)	ABTS
Chlorella pyrenoidosa	*C. pyrenoidosa*
Chlorella protein hydrolysate	CPHs
oil-in-water emulsions	O/W
1,1-diphenyl-2-picrylhydrazyl	DPPH
peroxide value	POV
eicosapentaenoic acid	EPA
docosahexaenoic acid	DHA
Maillard reaction products	MRP
thiobarbituric acid	TBA
reactive oxygen species	ROS
superoxide dismutase	SOD

References

1. Kohler, A.; Sarkkinen, E.; Tapola, N.; Niskanen, T.; Bruheim, I. Bioavailability of fatty acids from krill oil, krill meal and fish oil in healthy subjects–a randomized, single-dose, cross-over trial. *Lipids Health Dis.* **2015**, *14*, 19. [CrossRef] [PubMed]
2. Tou, J.C.; Jaczynski, J.; Chen, Y.-C. Krill for human consumption: Nutritional value and potential health benefits. *Nutr. Rev.* **2007**, *65*, 63–77. [CrossRef] [PubMed]
3. Wijendran, V.; Huang, M.-C.; Diau, G.-Y.; Boehm, G.; Nathanielsz, P.W.; Brenna, J.T. Efficacy of dietary arachidonic acid provided as triglyceride or phospholipid as substrates for brain arachidonic acid accretion in baboon neonates. *Pediatric Res.* **2002**, *51*, 265–272. [CrossRef] [PubMed]
4. Shen, Z.; Bhail, S.; Sanguansri, L.; Augustin, M.A. Improving the Oxidative Stability of Krill Oil-in-Water Emulsions. *J. Am. Oil Chem. Soc.* **2014**, *91*, 1347–1354. [CrossRef]
5. Schröder, A.; Berton-Carabin, C.; Venema, P.; Cornacchia, L. Interfacial properties of whey protein and whey protein hydrolysates and their influence on O/W emulsion stability. *Food Hydrocoll.* **2017**, *73*, 129–140. [CrossRef]
6. Liu, H.; Li, Y.; Diao, X.; Kong, B.; Liu, Q. Effect of porcine bone protein hydrolysates on the emulsifying and oxidative stability of oil-in-water emulsions. *Colloids Surf. A Physicochem. Eng. Asp.* **2018**, *538*, 757–764. [CrossRef]
7. Zhao, J.; Xiong, Y.L. Interfacial peptide partitioning and undiminished antioxidative and emulsifying activity of oxidatively stressed soy protein hydrolysate in an O/W emulsion. *LWT-Food Sci. Technol.* **2015**, *61*, 322–329. [CrossRef]
8. Zhao, Q.; Selomulya, C.; Wang, S.; Xiong, H.; Chen, X.D.; Li, W.; Peng, H.; Xie, J.; Sun, W.; Zhou, Q. Enhancing the oxidative stability of food emulsions with rice dreg protein hydrolysate. *Food Res. Int.* **2012**, *48*, 876–884. [CrossRef]
9. Shastik, E.; Li, L.; Liu, J. New methods for hydrogen production by marine microalga *Chlorella pyrenoidosa* in natural seawater. *Int. J. Hydrogen Energy* **2019**, *44*, 14707–14714. [CrossRef]
10. Singhal, R.; Basu, H.; Pimple, M.; Manisha, V.; Basan, M.; Reddy, A.V.R. Spectroscopic determination of U (VI) species sorbed by the Chlorella (*Chlorella pyrenoidosa*) fresh water algae. *J. Radioanal. Nucl. Chem.* **2013**, *298*, 587–592. [CrossRef]
11. He, M.; Li, L.; Liu, J.; Zhang, L. Improvement of H_2 photoproduction in *Chlorella pyrenoidosa* in artificial and natural seawater by addition of acetic acid and control of nutrients. *Algal Res.* **2015**, *10*, 104–109. [CrossRef]
12. Waghmare, A.G.; Salve, M.K.; LeBlanc, J.G.; Arya, S.S. Concentration and characterization of microalgae proteins from *Chlorella pyrenoidosa*. *Bioresour. Bioprocess.* **2016**, *3*, 16. [CrossRef]
13. Cherng, J.; Liu, C.; Shen, C.; Lin, H.; Shih, M. Beneficial effects of Chlorella-11 peptide on blocking LPS-induced macrophage activation and alleviating thermal injury-induced inflammation in rats. *Int. J. Immunopathol. Pharmacol.* **2010**, *23*, 811–820. [CrossRef]
14. Yamaguchi, N. Studies on Antioxidative Activities of Amino Compounds on Fats and Oils Part, I. Oxidation of methionine during course of autoxidation of linoleic acid. *J. Jpn. Soc. Food Sci. Technol.* **1971**, *18*, 313–318. [CrossRef]
15. Chen, Y.; Huang, F.; Xie, B.; Sun, Z.; McClements, D.J.; Deng, Q. Fabrication and characterization of whey protein isolates- lotus seedpod proanthocyanin conjugate: Its potential application in oxidizable emulsions. *Food Chem.* **2021**, *346*, 128680. [CrossRef]
16. Linke, A.; Hinrichs, J.; Kohlus, R. Impact of the powder particle size on the oxidative stability of microencapsulated oil. *Powder Technol.* **2020**, *364*, 115–122. [CrossRef]
17. Sivaraman, B.; Shakila, R.J.; Jeyasekaran, G.; Sukumar, D.; Manimaran, U.; Sumathi, G. Antioxidant activities of squid protein hydrolysates prepared with papain using response surface methodology. *Food Sci. Biotechnol.* **2016**, *25*, 665–672. [CrossRef]
18. Nalinanon, S.; Benjakul, S.; Kishimura, H.; Shahidi, F. Functionalities and antioxidant properties of protein hydrolysates from the muscle of ornate threadfin bream treated with pepsin from skipjack tuna. *Food Chem.* **2011**, *124*, 1354–1362. [CrossRef]

19. Wang, Z.; Liu, X.; Xie, H.; Liu, Z.; Rakariyatham, K.; Yu, C.; Shahidi, F.; Zhou, D. Antioxidant activity and functional properties of Alcalase-hydrolyzed scallop protein hydrolysate and its role in the inhibition of cytotoxicity in vitro. *Food Chem.* **2021**, *344*, 128566. [CrossRef]
20. Lawal, O.S. Functionality of African locust bean (*Parkia biglobossa*) protein isolate: Effects of pH, ionic strength and various protein concentrations. *Food Chem.* **2004**, *86*, 345–355. [CrossRef]
21. Wouters, A.G.B.; Rombouts, I.; Fierens, E.; Brijs, K.; Delcour, J.A. Relevance of the Functional Properties of Enzymatic Plant Protein Hydrolysates in Food Systems. *Compr. Rev. Food Sci. Food Saf.* **2016**, *15*, 786–800. [CrossRef]
22. Bowler, C.; Montagu, M.V.; Inze, D. Superoxide dismutase and stress tolerance. *Annu. Rev. Plant Physiol. Plant Mol. Biol.* **1992**, *43*, 83–116. [CrossRef]
23. Hu, X.M.; Wang, Y.M.; Zhao, Y.Q.; Chi, C.F.; Wang, B. Antioxidant Peptides from the Protein Hydrolysate of Monkfish (*Lophius litulon*) Muscle: Purification, Identification, and Cytoprotective Function on HepG2 Cells Damage by H_2O_2. *Mar. Drugs* **2020**, *18*, 153. [CrossRef]
24. Wu, R.; Wu, C.; Liu, D.; Yang, X.; Huang, J.; Zhang, J.; Liao, B.; He, H. Antioxidant and anti-freezing peptides from salmon collagen hydrolysate prepared by bacterial extracellular protease. *Food Chem.* **2018**, *248*, 346–352. [CrossRef] [PubMed]
25. Ko, S.-C.; Kim, D.; Jeon, Y.-J. Protective effect of a novel antioxidative peptide purified from a marine *Chlorella ellipsoidea* protein against free radical-induced oxidative stress. *Food Chem. Toxicol.* **2012**, *50*, 2294–2302. [CrossRef] [PubMed]
26. Sheih, I.C.; Fang, T.J.; Wu, T.K.; Lin, P.H. Anticancer and antioxidant activities of the peptide fraction from algae protein waste. *J. Agric. Food Chem.* **2010**, *58*, 1202–1207. [CrossRef] [PubMed]
27. Kang, K.-H.; Qian, Z.-J.; Ryu, B.; Karadeniz, F.; Kim, D.; Kim, S.-K. Antioxidant Peptides from Protein Hydrolysate of Microalgae Navicula incerta and their Protective Effects in Hepg2/CYP2E1 Cells Induced by Ethanol. *Phytother. Res.* **2012**, *26*, 1555–1563. [CrossRef] [PubMed]
28. Ejike, C.E.C.C.; Collins, S.A.; Balasuriya, N.; Swanson, A.K.; Mason, B.; Udenigwe, C.C. Prospects of microalgae proteins in producing peptide-based functional foods for promoting cardiovascular health. *Trends Food Sci. Technol.* **2017**, *59*, 30–36. [CrossRef]
29. Meshginfar, N.; Sadeghi Mahoonak, A.; Ghorbani, M.; Aalami, M. Effects of Protein Hydrolysate from Sheep Visceral on Oxidative Stability of Soybean Oil and Chicken Sausage. *J. Food Process. Preserv.* **2017**, *41*, e12875. [CrossRef]
30. Lam, R.S.; Nickerson, M.T. Food proteins: A review on their emulsifying properties using a structure-function approach. *Food Chem.* **2013**, *141*, 975–984. [CrossRef]
31. Padial-Dominguez, M.; Espejo-Carpio, F.J.; Perez-Galvez, R.; Guadix, A.; Guadix, E.M. Optimization of the Emulsifying Properties of Food Protein Hydrolysates for the Production of Fish Oil-in-Water Emulsions. *Foods* **2020**, *9*, 636. [CrossRef]
32. Faraji, H.; McClements, D.J.; Decker, E.A. Role of continuous phase protein on the oxidative stability of fish oil-in-water emulsions. *J. Agric. Food Chem.* **2004**, *52*, 4558–4564. [CrossRef]
33. Wong, B.T.; Zhai, J.; Hoffmann, S.V.; Aguilar, M.-I.; Augustin, M.; Wooster, T.J.; Day, L. Conformational changes to deamidated wheat gliadins and β-casein upon adsorption to oil–water emulsion interfaces. *Food Hydrocoll.* **2012**, *27*, 91–101. [CrossRef]
34. Shimada, K.; Fujikawa, K.; Yahara, K.; Nakamura, T. Antioxidative properties of xanthan on the autoxidation of soybean oil in cyclodextrin emulsion. *J. Agric. Food Chem.* **1992**, *40*, 945–948. [CrossRef]
35. Liu, J.; Wen, X.Y.; Zhang, X.Q.; Pu, H.M.; Kan, J.; Jin, C.H. Extraction, characterization and in vitro antioxidant activity of polysaccharides from black soybean. *Int. J. Biol. Macromol.* **2015**, *72*, 1182–1190. [CrossRef]
36. Halliwell, B.; Gutteridge, J.M.; Aruoma, O.I. The deoxyribose method: A simple "test-tube" assay for determination of rate constants for reactions of hydroxyl radicals. *Anal. Biochem.* **1987**, *165*, 215–219. [CrossRef]
37. Pearce, K.N.; Kinsella, J.E. Emulsifying properties of proteins: Evaluation of a turbidimetric technique. *J. Agric. Food Chem.* **1978**, *26*, 716–723. [CrossRef]
38. Shahidi, F.; Han, X.-Q.; Synowiecki, J. Production and characteristics of protein hydrolysates from capelin (*Mallotus villosus*). *Food Chem.* **1995**, *53*, 285–293. [CrossRef]
39. Ohkawa, H.; Ohishi, N.; Yagi, K. Assay for lipid peroxides in animal tissues by thiobarbituric acid reaction. *Anal. Biochem.* **1979**, *95*, 351–358. [CrossRef]
40. *GB 5009.227-2016*; The Chinese Food Safety Standards, Standards for Determination of Peroxide Value in Food. 2016.
41. Kavosi, M.; Mohammadi, A.; Shojaee-Aliabadi, S.; Khaksar, R.; Hosseini, S.M. Agriculture, Characterization and oxidative stability of purslane seed oil microencapsulated in yeast cells biocapsules. *J. Sci. Food Agric.* **2018**, *98*, 2490–2497. [CrossRef]
42. Undeland, I.; Hultin, H.O.; Richards, M.P. Added triacylglycerols do not hasten hemoglobin-mediated lipid oxidation in washed minced cod muscle. *J. Agric. Food Chem.* **2002**, *50*, 6847. [CrossRef]
43. *GB 5009.181-2016*; The Chinese Food Safety Standards, Standards for Determination of Malondialdehyde in Food. 2016.

marine drugs

MDPI

Article

Novel Antioxidant Collagen Peptides of Siberian Sturgeon (*Acipenser baerii*) Cartilages: The Preparation, Characterization, and Cytoprotection of H_2O_2-Damaged Human Umbilical Vein Endothelial Cells (HUVECs)

Yan Sheng [1], Yi-Ting Qiu [1], Yu-Mei Wang [1], Chang-Feng Chi [2,*] and Bin Wang [1,*]

[1] Zhejiang Provincial Engineering Technology Research Center of Marine Biomedical Products, School of Food and Pharmacy, Zhejiang Ocean University, Zhoushan 316022, China; 18223101235@163.com (Y.S.); qytdezh@icloud.com (Y.-T.Q.); wangym731@126.com (Y.-M.W.)

[2] National and Provincial Joint Laboratory of Exploration and Utilization of Marine Aquatic Genetic Resources, National Engineering Research Center of Marine Facilities Aquaculture, School of Marine Science and Technology, Zhejiang Ocean University, Zhoushan 316022, China

* Correspondence: chichangfeng@hotmail.com (C.-F.C.); wangbin@zjou.edu.cn (B.W.); Tel./Fax: +86-580-255-4818 (C.-F.C.); +86-580-255-4781 (B.W.)

Abstract: For making full use of aquatic by-products to produce high value-added products, Siberian sturgeon (*Acipenser baerii*) cartilages were degreased, mineralized, and separately hydrolyzed by five kinds of proteases. The collagen hydrolysate (SCH) generated by Alcalase showed the strongest 2,2-diphenyl-1-picrylhydrazyl radical (DPPH·) and hydroxide radical (HO·) scavenging activity. Subsequently, thirteen antioxidant peptides (SCP1-SCP3) were isolated from SCH, and they were identified as GPTGED, GEPGEQ, GPEGPAG, VPPQD, GLEDHA, GDRGAEG, PRGFRGPV, GEYGFE, GFIGFNG, PSVSLT, IELFPGLP, LRGEAGL, and RGEPGL with molecular weights of 574.55, 615.60, 583.60, 554.60, 640.64, 660.64, 885.04, 700.70, 710.79, 602.67, 942.12, 714.82, and 627.70 Da, respectively. GEYGFE, PSVSLT, and IELFPGLP showed the highest scavenging activity on DPPH· (EC_{50}: 1.27, 1.05, and 1.38 mg/mL, respectively) and HO· (EC_{50}: 1.16, 0.97, and 1.63 mg/mL, respectively), inhibiting capability of lipid peroxidation, and protective functions on H_2O_2-damaged plasmid DNA. More importantly, GEYGFE, PSVSLT, and IELFPGLP displayed significant cytoprotection on HUVECs against H_2O_2 injury by regulating the endogenous antioxidant enzymes of superoxide dismutase (SOD) and glutathione peroxidase (GSH-Px) to decrease the contents of reactive oxygen species (ROS) and malondialdehyde (MDA). Therefore, the research provided better technical assistance for a higher-value utilization of Siberian sturgeon cartilages and the thirteen isolated peptides—especially GEYGFE, PSVSLT, and IELFPGLP—which may serve as antioxidant additives for generating health-prone products to treat chronic diseases caused by oxidative stress.

Keywords: Siberian sturgeon (*Acipenser baerii*); cartilage; collagen peptide; antioxidant activity; cytoprotection

Citation: Sheng, Y.; Qiu, Y.-T.; Wang, Y.-M.; Chi, C.-F.; Wang, B. Novel Antioxidant Collagen Peptides of Siberian Sturgeon (*Acipenser baerii*) Cartilages: The Preparation, Characterization, and Cytoprotection of H_2O_2-Damaged Human Umbilical Vein Endothelial Cells (HUVECs). *Mar. Drugs* **2022**, *20*, 325. https://doi.org/10.3390/md20050325

Academic Editor: Hideki Kishimura

Received: 21 April 2022
Accepted: 12 May 2022
Published: 14 May 2022

1. Introduction

The balanced relationship between the endogenous antioxidant defense system and reactive oxygen species (ROS) will be broken under the toxic environment in the cells [1–3]. Excessive ROS can cause DNA mutation, enzyme inactivation, and membrane phospholipid oxidation, which further lead to oxidative stress, inducing cell necrosis or apoptosis, tissue injury, and pathologic transformations of the human body [4–6]. Such oxidative damage significantly increases the incidence of chronic diseases, including arthritis, hypertension, Alzheimer's disease, diabetes, and cardiovascular disease [7–10]. Many antioxidant chemical compounds can play highly effective functions to prevent and to cure those diseases and to clear away excessive ROS in the human body [11,12]. However, synthetic antioxidants have shown a potential toxicity risk and their applications are strictly regulated [13,14]. Therefore, researchers are focusing their research interests on natural active molecules and their derivatives, such as flavonoids, triterpenoid, quinones, and alkaloids [12,15–17]. Remarkably, antioxidant peptide (AP) originated from food proteins, which captured world-wide interest because of their advantages in environmental protection and in sustainability, and their small molecular weight (MW) and low toxic side effects [1,9,12].

Collagen and its derivatives, including gelatin, hydrolysate, and peptide, are traditionally produced from animal bones and skins, and they have served as multifunctional ingredients applied in food, cosmetics, photographic, and pharmaceuticals products. The global market volume of gelatin/collagen is expected to exceed 650 kilo-tones, which is approximately 4 billion US dollars by 2024 [18–21]. However, those products generated from mammalian resources have aroused the wide concern of customers because of the increasing number of infectious diseases and dietary restriction in Islam, Judaism and Hinduism [22,23]. Therefore, collagen and its derivatives from fish by-products are considered to be ideal substitutes due to good bioactivity, high nutrition, weak antigenicity, excellent moisture retention, and good biocompatibility properties [18,24–26].

Recently, collagen peptides from aquatic organism drew great interest from the food, medicine, and cosmetics industries because of their multiple functions, including free radical scavenging activity, lipid peroxidation inhibition ability, cytoprotection, and ultraviolet damage protection [21,24,27,28]. For example, bioactive peptides from collagen hydrolysates of giant croaker swim bladders [29], sea cucumber [30], and redlip croaker scales [11] could significantly accelerate the proliferation of HUVECs, RAW264.7, and HepG2 cells, and protect them against the oxidative damage of H_2O_2 by increasing the activities of superoxide dismutase (SOD) catalase (CAT) and glutathione peroxidase (GSH-Px) and reducing the levels of ROS and malondialdehyde (MDA). Gelatin peptides from Pacific cod had a significant protective effect on ultraviolet-A (UVA) damaged cells and skins by up-regulating the levels of SOD, CAT, and GSH-Px [31–33]. Similarly, collagen peptides from silver carp skins showed a stronger beneficial effect than casein derived peptides and tea poly-phenols on alleviating the UV-caused unusual lesions of skin compositions and antioxidant indices in the serum and in the skins [34]. In addition, collagen peptides from the croceine croaker swim bladders showed a favorable anti-fatigue function in mice by increasing antioxidase activities to reduce ROS damage, enhancing the lactic dehydrogenase activity to get rid of excessive lactic acid to further alleviate the development of physical fatigue [35].

Sturgeon, belonging to the family Acipenseridae, is the common name of 27 kinds of cartilaginous fish, and its farmed production in China is approximately 4.4 million tons accounting for nearly 80% of world production [36,37]. In the receiving process of sturgeon eggs, cartilage, which accounts for 10% of the sturgeon's weight, becomes a by-product. Therefore, active substances in sturgeon cartilage, such as chondroitin sulfate [38], collagen [39,40], and anti-inflammatory peptides [41], were studied constantly to replace shark cartilage, which is used in health and functional products. The Siberian sturgeon, *Acipenser baerii* Brandt, inhabits large Siberian rivers from the Ob to the Kolyma and Lake Baikal, and it is one of the important breeding varieties in China. In this experiment, antioxidant collagen peptides from the cartilage of the Siberian sturgeon (*A. baerii*) were prepared and identified. Moreover, their protective function on H_2O_2 injured HUVECs was evaluated.

2. Results and Discussion

2.1. Preparation of Collagen Hydrolysate of Siberian Sturgeon Cartilage (SCH)

The effects of five kinds of proteases on the DPPH· and HO· scavenging rates of collagen hydrolysates of Siberian sturgeon cartilage are presented in Figure 1. At 10.0 mg/mL, the DPPH· and HO· scavenging rates of collagen hydrolysate generated by Alcalase were $47.43 \pm 1.86\%$ and $72.22 \pm 2.11\%$, which were observably stronger than the rates of collagen hydrolysates produced using papain, flavorzyme, trypsin, and pepsin, respectively

($p < 0.05$). Compared with microbial fermentation, chemical degradation, and solvent extraction, enzymatic hydrolysis is one of the most popular and useful ways to generate bioactive hydrolysates from protein resources due to its easy manipulation, high efficiency, and eco-friendly features [1,42,43]. In addition, the specificity of protease is the very key property determining the MW, amino acid sequence, and bioactivity of the prepared hydrolysates because of their different cleavage sites [1,11]. In addition, multiple endonuclease enzymes, exonuclease enzymes, and their combinations are generally selected to degrade different proteins to generate active hydrolysates [1,9]. The present results supported the previous reports that the selectivity of enzymes significantly affected the peptide component and the bioactivities of prepared hydrolysates [1,14]. In consequence, the collagen hydrolysate of Siberian sturgeon cartilage prepared using Alcalase was named SCH and selected for further experimentation.

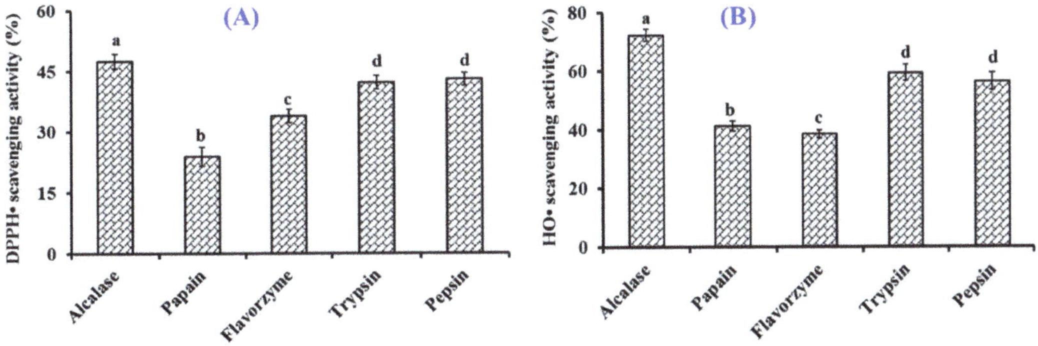

Figure 1. Effects of Alcalase, papain, pepsin, flavorzyme, and trypsin on radical scavenging activity of collagen hydrolysates from Siberian sturgeon (*Acipenser baerii*) cartilages. (**A**) 2,2-diphenyl-1-picrylhydrazyl radical (DPPH·) scavenging activity; (**B**) hydroxide radical (HO·) scavenging activity. All data are presented as the mean ± SD of triplicate results. $^{a-d}$ Values with different letters indicate significant difference ($p < 0.05$).

2.2. *Purification of APs from SCH*

2.2.1. Fractionation of SCH by Ultrafiltration

Using 3.0 kDa ultrafiltration membranes, SCH was fractionated into two peptide components (SCH-1 and SCH-2) and their radical scavenging rates are shown in Figure 2. At 5.0 mg/mL, the DPPH· and HO· scavenging rates of SCH-1 were 38.52 ± 1.69% and 45.37 ± 1.97%, which were significantly stronger than those activities of SCH and SCH-2 ($p < 0.05$). The changes of amino acid composition and MW could significantly modulate the bioactivity of peptides, and their average MWs could adversely affect the antioxidant capability of enzymatic hydrolysates [44,45]. The current result agreed well with the previous finding that peptide components with smaller MWs from skipjack roe [46–48], skate cartilage [49], *Bacillus amyloliquefaciens* [50], *Tolithes ruber* [51], croceine croaker muscle [13], and Tilapia skin [31] possessed the highest antioxidant activity. Then, SCH-1 was chosen for further purification.

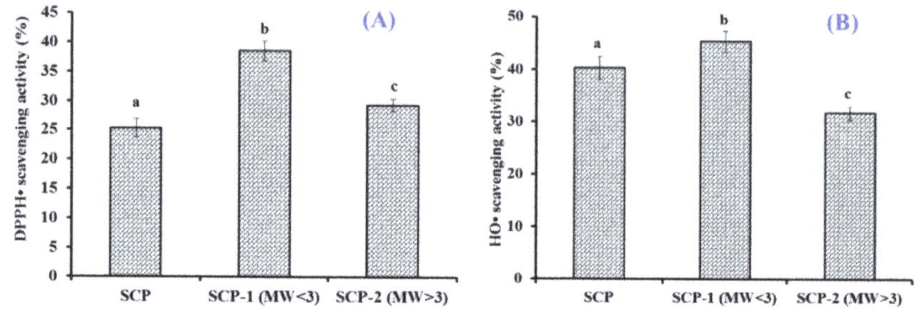

Figure 2. Radical scavenging activity of SCH and its two fractions by ultrafiltration. (**A**) DPPH· scavenging activity; (**B**): HO· scavenging activity. All data are presented as the mean ± SD of triplicate results. [a–c] Values with different letters indicate a significant difference ($p < 0.05$).

2.2.2. Gel Filtration Chromatography (GFC)

Figure 3A showed that three peptide subfracitons (SCH-1a, SCH-1b, and SCH-1c) were isolated from SCH-1 based on their MWs. At 5.0 mg/mL, the DPPH· and HO· scavenging rates of SCH-1b were 56.64 ± 2.69% and 66.79 ± 2.65%, which were significantly higher than those of SCH, SCH-1, and other subfracitons ($p < 0.05$) (Figure 3B). As a kind of size exclusion chromatography, GFC is generally applied to either fractionate active ingredients or to remove an impurity with a particular size range from a complex mixture of components [1,9,52]. Therefore, GFC is frequently employed to isolate peptides with different MWs from marine protein hydrolysates [1,47,53]. In the experiment, the MW of SCH-1b was bigger than that of SCH-1c, but its radical scavenging rates were significantly higher than those of SCH-1c ($p < 0.05$), which suggested that the bioactivities of APs are not only influenced by MW but also amino acid composition and sequence [1,42].

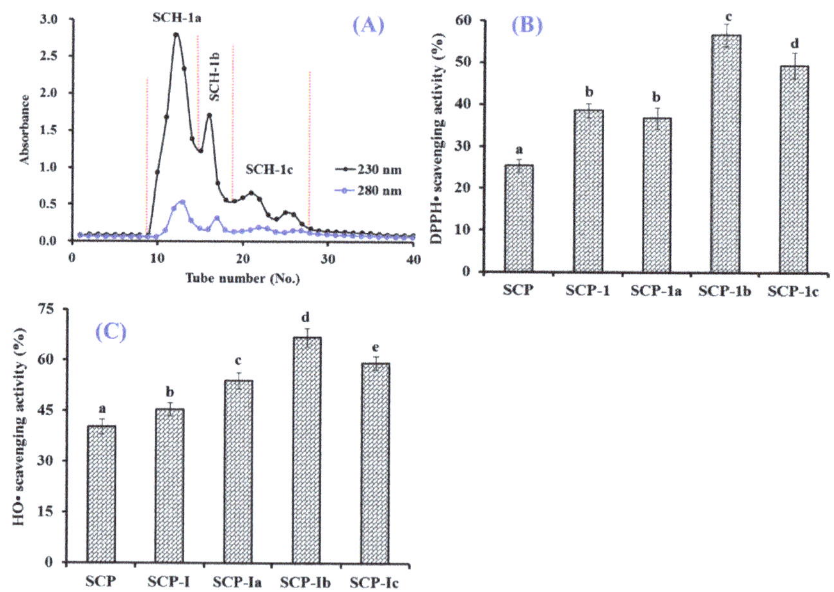

Figure 3. Chromatogram map of SCH-1 on a Sephadex G-25 column (**A**) and the scavenging activity of SCH-1 and its fractions (SCH-1a, SCH-1b, and SCH-1c) on DPPH· (**B**) and HO· (**C**). All data are presented as the mean ± SD of triplicate results. [a–e] Values with different letters indicate significant difference ($p < 0.05$).

2.2.3. RP-HPLC Separation of SCH-1b

SCH-1 with high radical scavenging activity was further purified by RP-HPLC and its chromatogram is shown in Figure 4. On the chromatographic peaks of SCH-1, thirteen peptide peaks with retention times of 4.58 min (SCP1), 8.98 min (SCP2), 10.73 min (SCP3), 13.01 min (SCP4), 18.03 min (SCP5), 21.02 min (SCP6), 21.75 min (SCP7), 24.81 min (SCP8), 33.85 min (SCP9), 39.79 min (SCP10), 42.52 min (SCP11), 44.18 min (SCP12), and 45.62 min (SCP13), respectively, were purified from SCH-1b (Table 1). Based on the hydrophobic and the hydrophilic properties, RP-HPLC employing an ODSC18 column can effectively isolate APs with high purity from different protein hydrolysates of aquatic resources, such as croaker (*Otolithes ruber*) [51], tuna [46,54], red stingray [55], Pacific Cod [32,33], shortclub cuttlefish [56], *Euphausia superba* [57], and mackerel (*Scomber japonicus*) [58]. Then, thirteen peptides (SCP1 to SCP13) were corrected and lyophilized for further structure identification.

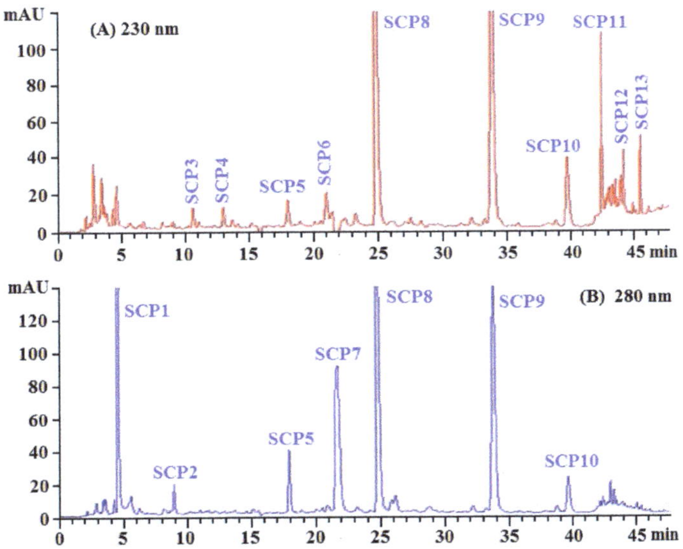

Figure 4. Elution profile of the subfraction (SCH-1b) by RP-HPLC using a linear gradient of acetonitrile (0.06% trifluoroacetic acid) at 230 nm (**A**) and 280 nm (**B**).

Table 1. Retention time, amino acid sequences, and molecular mass of thirteen APs (SCP1- SCP13) from collagen hydrolysate of Siberian sturgeon cartilage.

	Retention Time (min)	Amino Acid Sequence	Determined Mass/Theoretical Mass (Da)
SCP1	4.58	GPTGED	574.55/574.54
SCP2	8.98	GEPGEQ	615.60/615.59
SCP3	10.73	GPEGPAG	583.60/583.59
SCP4	13.01	VPPQD	554.60/554.59
SCP5	18.03	GLEDHA	640.64/640.65
SCP6	21.02	GDRGAEG	660.64/660.63
SCP7	21.75	PRGFRGPV	885.04/885.02
SCP8	24.81	GEYGFE	700.70/700.69
SCP9	33.85	GFIGFNG	710.79/710.78
SCP10	39.79	PSVSLT	602.67/602.68
SCP11	42.52	GIELFPGLP	942.12/942.11
SCP12	44.18	LRGEAGL	714.82/714.81
SCP13	45.62	RGEPGL	627.70/627.69

2.3. Determination of Amino Acid Sequences of Thirteen Isolated APs (SCP1 to SCP13)

Using a Protein Sequencer and an ESI/MS, the amino acid sequences and the MWs of thirteen isolated APs (SCP1 to SCP13) were determined and the results are shown in Table 1. The sequences of SCP1 to SCP13 were identified as Gly-Pro-Thr-Gly-Glu-Asp (GPTGED, SCP1), Gly-Glu-Pro-Gly-Glu-Gln (GEPGEQ, SCP2), Gly-Pro-Glu-Gly-Pro-Ala-Gly (GPEGPAG, SCP3), Val-Pro-Pro-Gln-Asp (VPPQD, SCP4), Gly-Leu-Glu-Asp-His-Ala (GLEDHA, SCP5), Gly-Asp-Arg-Gly-Ala-Glu-Gly (GDRGAEG, SCP6), Pro-Arg-Gly-Phe-Arg-Gly-Pro-Val (PRGFRGPV, SCP7), Gly-Glu-Tyr-Gly-Phe-Glu (GEYGFE, SCP8), Gly-Phe-Ile-Gly-Phe-Asn-Gly (GFIGFNG, SCP9), Pro-Ser-Val-Ser-Leu-Thr (PSVSLT, SCP10), Gly-Ile-Glu-Leu-Phe-Pro-Gly-Leu-Pro (GIELFPGLP, SCP11), Leu-Arg-Gly-Glu-Ala-Gly-Leu (LRGEAGL, SCP12), and Arg-Gly-Glu-Pro-Gly-Leu (RGEPGL, SCP13) with MWs of 574.55, 615.60, 583.60, 554.60, 640.64, 660.64, 885.04, 700.70, 710.79, 602.67, 942.12, 714.82, and 627.70 Da, respectively, and their determined MWs were well consistent with their theoretical mass (Table 1).

2.4. Antioxidant Activity of Thirteen Isolated APs (SCP1 to SCP13)

2.4.1. Radical Scavenging Activity of Thirteen Isolated APs (SCP1 to SCP13)

Figure 5A shows that the DPPH· scavenging rates of SCP8, SCP10, and SCP11 were 77.03 ± 2.08%, 80.09 ± 2.15%, and 71.1 ± 2.14%, respectively, which were significantly higher than those of ten other isolated collagen APs but still lower than that (95.37 ± 3.25%) of ascorbic acid. In addition, the half clearance concentrations (EC_{50} values) of SCP8, SCP10, and SCP11 were 1.27, 1.05, and 1.38 mg/mL, respectively, which were significantly less than those of APs from skipjack tuna milt (GRVPRV: 4.13 mg/mL; AQRPR 1.80 mg/mL) [59], loach (PSYV: 17.0 mg/mL) [60], Antarctic krill (NVPDM: 4.88 mg/mL; NGPDPRPSQQ: 7.05 mg/mL; TFPIYDPQ: 2.15 mg/mL) [61], and hairtail muscle (QNDER: 4.95 mg/mL) [62].

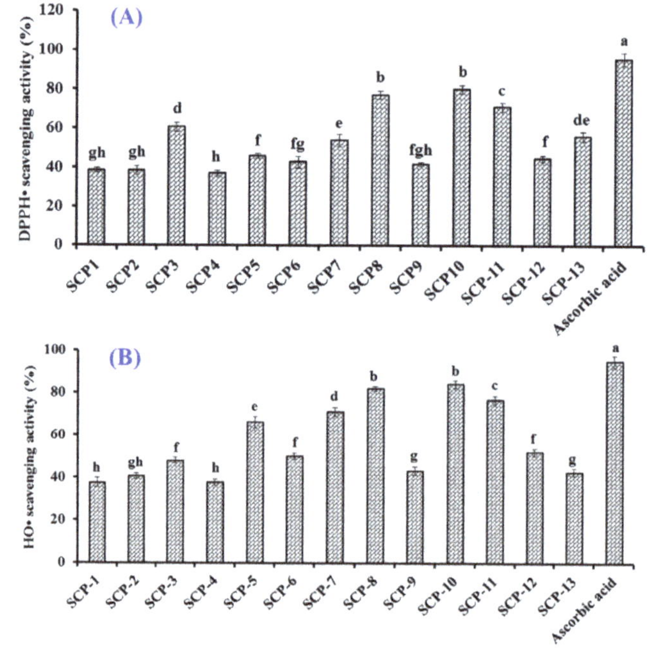

Figure 5. DPPH· (**A**) and HO· (**B**) scavenging rates of thirteen isolated APs (SCP1–SCP13) from collagen hydrolysate of Siberian sturgeon cartilages. All data are presented as the mean ± SD of triplicate results. [a–h] Values with different letters indicate significant difference ($p < 0.05$).

Figure 5B showed that the HO· scavenging rates of SCP8, SCP10, and SCP11 were 81.94 ± 1.05%, 84.11 ± 1.82%, and 76.78 ± 1.92%, respectively, which were significantly higher than those of ten other isolated collagen APs but still lower than that (94.84 ± 2.79%) of ascorbic acid. The EC_{50} values of SCP8, SCP10, and SCP11 on HO· were 1.16, 0.97, and 1.63 mg/mL, respectively, which were significantly less than those of APs from skipjack tuna milts (GRVPRV: 5.78 mg/mL; AQRPR 2.80 mg/mL) [59] and roes (SGE: 2.76 mg/mL; QAEP: 2.10 mg/mL) [48], miiuy croaker muscle (NFWWP: 2.39 mg/mL; YFLWP: 2.47 mg/mL) [63], Antarctic krill (NVPDM: 1.84 mg/mL; NWDDMRIVAV: 2.61 mg/mL) [61], *Misgurnus anguillicaudatus* (PSYV: 2.64 mg/mL) [60], and grass carp skin (VGGRP: 2.06 mg/mL; PYSFK: 2.28 mg/mL) [64]. The present results suggested that SCP8, SCP10, and SCP11 could effectively scavenge excess HO· to inhibit the oxidative stress in cells and biological tissues.

MW can significantly affect the antioxidant abilities of APs because a smaller size is beneficial to them in getting into cells or into tissues and playing their roles [50,65,66]. In the study, thirteen isolated APs (SCP1 to SCP13) range from pentapeptides to nonapeptides and their MWs range from 554.60 to 942.12 Da, respectively, which are very helpful for them to approach and to effectively scavenge excess free radicals.

Hydrophobic and aromatic amino acids, such as Leu, Ile, Tyr, Pro, and Phe, play key roles in the activity of APs. These two kinds of amino acids are able to improve the peptides' solubility in lipids, which further facilitate the combination between APs and free radicals and promote the antioxidant capabilities of APs [1,9,50]. Leu, Thr, Ala, Ile, and Val were reported to play key roles in the antioxidant capabilities of HFGBPFH, ILGATIDNSK, GADIVA, and GAEGFIF, respectively [61,67,68]. Aromatic amino acids could restrain the extension of the radical-mediated peroxide domino effect by changing free radicals into more stable phenoxy radicals [63,69]. Pro residue in sequences of LDEPDPL and PHH was beneficial to their antioxidant activity because Pro residue could improve the flexibility of peptides and directly scavenge singlet oxygen by its pyrrolidine ring [59,70,71]. Therefore, Tyr and Phe in SCP8, Phe and Ile in SCP10, and Ile, Leu, Phe, and Pro in SCP11 should play key roles for their antioxidant activities.

Hydrophilic amino acids are the key factor for the scavenging abilities of APs on mental ions and hydroxide radicals [48]. Glu/Gln, Asp/Asn, and Lys residues had strong positive impacts on the antioxidant activities of QDHKA, AEHNH, LDEPDPLI, AEDKKLIQ, and NTDGSTDYGILQINSR [48,72,73]. Gly residue in WMGPY, EMGPA, GADIVA, and GAEGFIF could increase the flexibility of peptide skeleton and directly neutralize ROS by acting as a single hydrogen donor [25,74]. Therefore, Gly and Glu in SCP8, Gly and Asn in SCP10, and Gly and Glu in SCP11 were important to their antioxidant capabilities.

2.4.2. Lipid Peroxidation Inhibition Ability

Compared with the blank control group, the absorbance values of the SCP8, SCP10, and SCP11 groups at 500 nm were significantly decreased when the temperature was kept at 40 °C for 7 days in the linoleic acid system (Figure 6). More importantly, the inhibiting capabilities of SCP10 drew near the variation trend of glutathione (GSP). Lipid oxidation is a very complex chemical reaction, which is affected by multiple factors. Therefore, lipid peroxidation inhibition assay was generally applied to compare and to analyze the antioxidant abilities of peptides from marine protein resources, such as Antarctic krill [61], channel catfish [75], miiuy croaker [63], and croceine croaker [13]. These results suggested that SCP8, SCP10, and SCP11 have significant protective ability on unsaturated fatty acid against peroxidation.

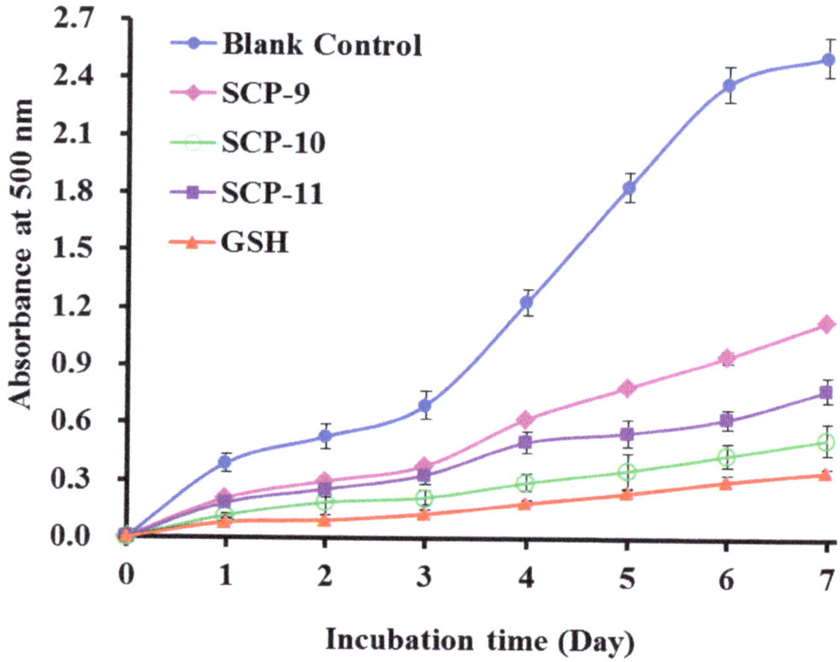

Figure 6. Lipid peroxidation inhibition capability of three isolated APs (SCP8, SCP10, and SCP11) from collagen hydrolysate of Siberian sturgeon cartilages. All data are presented as the mean ± SD of triplicate results.

2.4.3. Protective Activity of SCP8, SCP10, and SCP11 against H_2O_2-damaged Plasmid DNA

The protective abilities of SCP8, SCP10, and SCP11 on plasmid DNA (pBR322DNA) against H_2O_2 damage were determined and presented in Figure 7. Plasmid DNA keeps the supercoiled (SC) form under normal conditions (Figure 7, lane 6), but the supercoiled (SC) form will translate into a relaxed open circular (OC) form when free radicals split one phosphodiester chain of pBR322 DNA. Moreover, the open circular (OC) form will turn into the linear (LIN) form when excess free radicals split the second breakage near the first splitting breakage. In this experiment, the plasmid DNA strands was split by HO·, produced from the chemical reaction of $FeSO_4$ and H_2O_2, and converted into the OC and the LIN forms [61,76]. Lane 5 indicated that most of the SC forms of plasmid DNA were mutated to LIN forms, which suggested that the chemical reaction generated excessive HO·, which further broke the double-strand of pBR322 DNA. Lane 2 to Lane 4 displayed that the content of SC form of pBR322 DNA was obvious more than that of the model group (Lane 5), which suggested that SCP8, SCP10, and SCP11 have a remarkable effect on protecting plasmid DNA against oxidative damage by scavenging superfluous HO·, and this result agreed well with the previous finding that SCP8, SCP10, and SCP11 could effectively scavenge HO· to protect biomolecules. In addition, SCP8, SCP10, and SCP11 may serve as a radical scavenger in health products to prevent and to treat these degenerative diseases caused by free radicals.

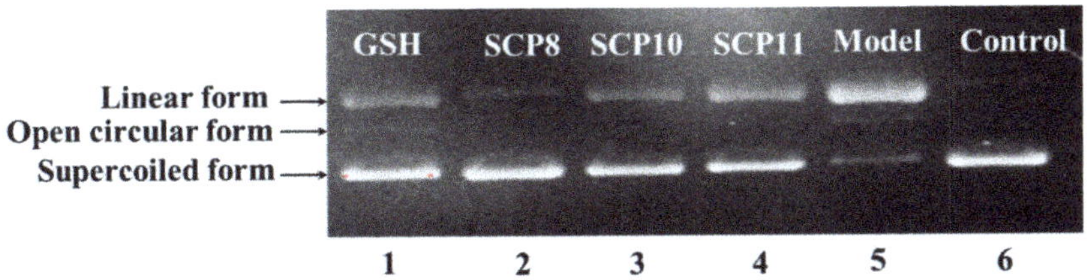

Figure 7. The protective effects of SCP8, SCP10, and SCP11 on the H_2O_2-damaged plasmid DNA (pBR322DNA). Lane 1, DNA + $FeSO_4$ + H_2O_2 + GSH (200 μM); Lane 2, DNA + $FeSO_4$ + H_2O_2 + SCP8 (200 μM); Lane 3, DNA + $FeSO_4$ + H_2O_2 + SCP10 (200 μM); Lane 4, DNA + $FeSO_4$ + H_2O_2 + SCP11 (200 μM); Lane 5, pBR322DNA + $FeSO_4$ + H_2O_2; Lane 6, the native pBR322DNA.

2.4.4. Cytoprotection of SCP8, SCP10, and SCP11 on H_2O_2-Induced HUVECs

Effects of H_2O_2, SCP8, SCP10, and SCP11 on the Viability of HUVECs

To establish the cell model of oxidative damage, HUVECs were treated with different concentrations of H_2O_2 (0~600 μM). Figure 8A indicated that the viability of HUVECs showed a significant downward trend at the H_2O_2 concentrations, which increased from 0 to 600 μM and dropped to 49.06 ± 1.96% at the concentration of 200 μM. Therefore, the H_2O_2 concentration of 200 μM was chosen to establish the cell model of oxidative damage [66].

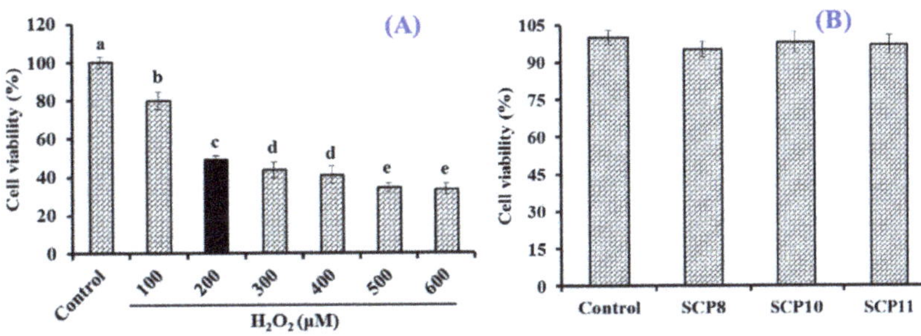

Figure 8. Effects of H_2O_2 concentration (**A**) and isolated peptides (SCP8, SCP10, and SCP11) (**B**) on the viability of HUVECs. All data are presented as the mean ± SD of triplicate results. [a–e] Values with different letters indicate significant difference ($p < 0.05$).

The Effects of SCP8, SCP10, and SCP11 at 200 μM on the viability of HUVECs were studied by the MTT method and the data is shown in Figure 8B. No significant difference was found between the blank control and the peptide groups, which indicated that SCP8, SCP10, and SCP11 had no significant cytotoxicity to HUVECs. Therefore, the concentration of 200 μM was determined for the subsequent cytoprotection experiment of SCP8, SCP10, and SCP11.

Effect of SCP8, SCP10, and SCP11 on the Cell Viability and the ROS Level of H_2O_2-Injured HUVECs

As shown in Figure 9A, the HUVEC viability of the SCP10 group was 69.36 ± 2.97% at 200 μM, which was significantly higher than those of the model (49.06 ± 1.96%), SCP8 (62.4 ± 2.87%), and SCP11 (57.59 ± 3.21%) groups ($p < 0.05$), and it was lower than that of the positive control (86.03 ± 3.57%) ($p < 0.001$) (Figure 9A). Figures 9B and 10 show the effects of SCP8, SCP10, and SCP11 on the ROS level of H_2O_2-injured HUVECs. The ROS levels of the SCP8, SCP10, and SCP11 groups were significantly decreased from 445.5 ± 14.57% to 302.2 ± 16.8%, 269.8 ± 11.5%, and 317.6 ± 6.4% for the control group, respectively ($p < 0.001$). These data indicated that SCP8, SCP10, and SCP11 could significantly scavenge ROS to protect HUVECs against H_2O_2 injury.

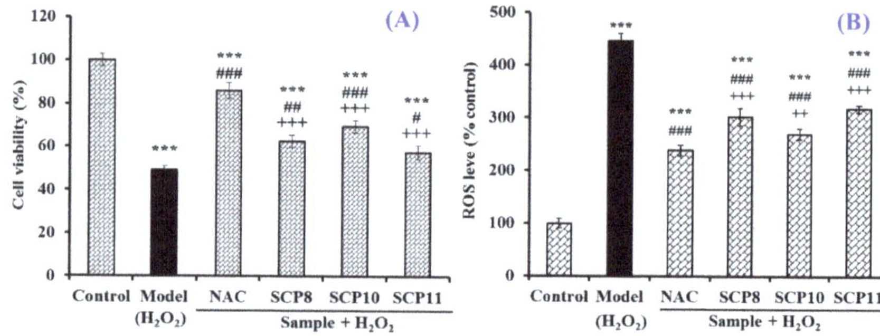

Figure 9. Effects of SCP8, SCP10, and SCP11 on the cell viability (**A**) and ROS level (**B**) of H_2O_2-injured HUVECs. N-Acetyl-L-Cysteine (NAC) was used as the positive control. All data are presented as the mean ± SD of triplicate results. *** $p < 0.001$ vs. blank group; ### $p < 0.001$, ## $p < 0.01$ and # $p < 0.05$ vs. model group; +++ $p < 0.001$, ++ $p < 0.01$ vs. NAC + H_2O_2 group.

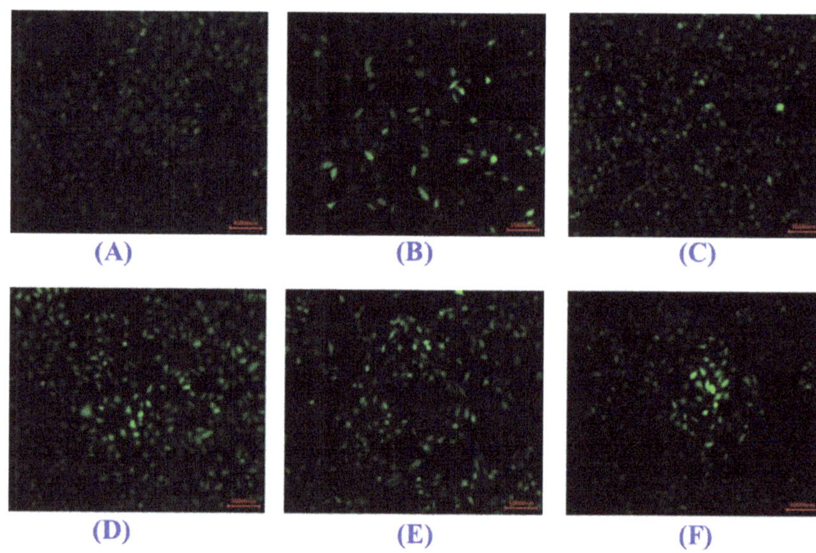

Figure 10. Determination of ROS contents in HUVECs by DCFH-DA staining. (**A**) Control; (**B**) H_2O_2-induced cell model; (**C**) Positive control (NAC); (**D**) SCP8; (**E**) SCP10; (**F**) SCP11. The scale bar was 50,000 nm.

Effects of SCP8, SCP10, and SCP11 on the Levels of Antioxidases and MDA of H_2O_2-Injured HUVECs

As shown in Figure 11A, the activity of SOD in the SCP10 group was 165.1 ± 11.2 U/mg prot, which was significantly higher than those in the model (107.8 ± 7.3 U/mg prot) and the SCP8 (147.2 ± 12.6 U/mg prot) and SCP11 (121.9 ± 10.8 U/mg prot) groups ($p < 0.001$), respectively. Similarly, the activity of GSH-Px in the SCP10 group (55.77 ± 2.48 U/mg prot) was significantly higher than those in the model (41.74 ± 2.36 U/mg prot) and the SCP8 (51.46 ± 2.65 U/mg prot) and the SCP11 (46.8 ± 1.82 U/mg prot) groups ($p < 0.001$), respectively (Figure 11B). However, the activity of antioxidases in the SCP8, SCP10, and SCP11 groups was significantly lower than those in the positive control group ($p < 0.05$). In addition, SCP8, SCP10, and SCP11 could significantly reduce the MDA contents of H_2O_2-injured HUVECs. Compared with the model group (10.84 ± 0.72 nmol/mg prot), the MDA contents of the SCP8, SCP10, and SCP11 groups were gradually reduced to 8.22 ± 0.45, 7.37 ± 0.69, and 9.07 ± 0.84 nmol/mg prot at 200 μM, respectively ($p < 0.05$) (Figure 11C). Nonetheless, the MDA contents of the SCP8, SCP10, and SCP11 groups were significantly higher than that (6.05 ± 0.54 nmol/mg prot) of the positive control group.

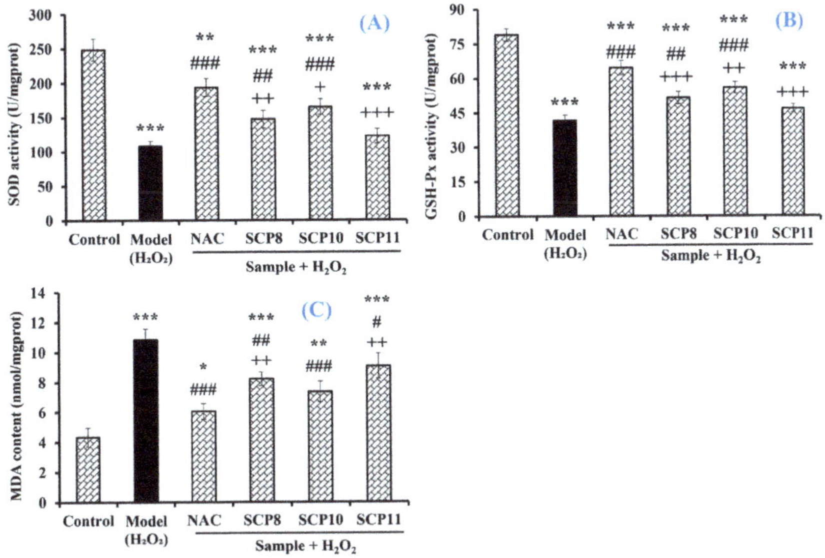

Figure 11. Effects of SCP8, SCP10, and SCP11 on the levels of SOD (**A**), GSH-Px (**B**), and MDA (**C**) in H_2O_2-injured HUVECs. All data are presented as the mean ± SD ($n = 3$). *** $p < 0.001$, ** $p < 0.01$ and * $p < 0.05$ vs. blank group; ### $p < 0.001$, ## $p < 0.01$, and # $p < 0.05$ vs. model group; +++ $p < 0.001$ and ++ $p < 0.01$ and + $p < 0.05$ vs. NAC+H_2O_2 group.

In an abnormal environment, excess ROS generated in cells can induce DNA mutations, loss of protein structures, and lipid peroxidation of cell membrane [4,8,24]. Those oxidative stress states are closely linked to many chronic diseases, including neurodegenerative disorders, cardiovascular disease, diabetes mellitus, inflammation, etc. [10,12,52]. Therefore, excess ROS must be eliminated promptly and efficiently by endogenous antioxidant defense systems to decrease such oxidative damage [1,53]. Presently, some bioactive peptides show remarkable protection on cells and tissues by alleviating the oxidative and the inflammatory responses. For example, LCGEC could suppress the apoptosis of HaCaT cells by altering the Nrf2 pathway [47]. To decrease the contents of ROS and MDA, FWKVV, FMPLH, and FPYLRH could significantly up-regulate the levels of SOD and GSH-Px in H_2O_2-injured HUVECs [66,77]. By regulating the NF-κB/caspase pathways and enhancing antioxidase activities, EVSGPGLSPN could protect PC12 cells against H_2O_2-induced neurotoxicity [78].

In addition, small natural products have been identified as being capable of directly interacting with the Cys residues of Keap1 and thus resulting in the dissociation of Keap1 from Nrf2, which finally promotes Nrf2 nuclear accumulation and activates the Nrf2 pathway [79,80]. Moreover, a number of peptides have been identified to be capable of binding to Keap1, especially the Glu residues that form electrostatic interactions with R380, R415, and R483 and the Asp residue that forms an intramolecular interaction to stabilize the β-hairpin conformation of the structure [81]. The binding site of Keap1 in the Kelch domain can be divided into five subcysts, P1-P5, which can combine with the Neh2 domain of Nrf2 to promote its ubiquitination [82]. The five subcysts are P1 (Arg415, Ile461, Gly423, Phe478, Arg483, Ser508), P2 (Ser363, Arg380, Asn382, Asp422), P3 (Gly509, Ser555, Ala556, Gly571, Ser602, Gly603), P4 (Tyr525, Gln530, Tyr572), and P5 (Tyr334, Phe577), respectively. Wang et al. reported that the Glu residue of peptide EDYGA from the soft-shelled turtle could directly bind to the Arg415 residue on the Kelch domain of

Keap1 to form a hydrogen bond [81]. Similarly, the Glu residues in an amino acid sequence of RDPEER from watermelon seed could combine with Asn382, Arg380, and Tyr334 on the Kelch domain of Keap1 to form hydrogen bonds [83]. Tonolo et al. found that the Ser residues in the amino acid sequence of APSFSDIPNPIGSENSE from fermented milk could bind to Arg415 and Ser363 residues on the Kelch domain of Keap1 to form a hydrogen bond to activate the Nrf2 pathway [84]. The Thr residues in the amino acid sequence of NTVPAKSCQAQPTTM could bind to the Ser602 residue in the Kelch domain of Keap1 to form a hydrogen bond [81]. Furthermore, Li et al. reported that the Thr residue of the peptide VTSALVGPR from the urechis unicinctus visceral could bind to Gly423 on the Kelch domain of Keap1 to form a hydrogen bond and to activate the Nrf2 pathway [85]. The EAMAPKHK from fermented rubbing cheese could regulate the Nrf2 pathway through its Pro residue combining with Asp422 on the Kelch domain of Keap1 to form a hydrogen bond [86]. In addition, the Gly residue in an amino acid sequence of PVLGPVR could combine with Ile461 on the Kelch domain of Keap1 to form a hydrogen bond [86]. Then, those amino acid residues in the amino acid sequences of APs occupy the active site of Nrf2 in the Kelch domain of Keap1, competitively inhibit Nrf2 binding, promote Nrf2 into the nucleus, further activate the Keap1/Nrf2 signal pathway, and protect cells from oxidative stress.

According to the introduced literature, we speculated that Gly and Glu in SCP8 (GEYGFE), Pro and Ser in SCP10 (PSVSLT), and Glu, Pro, and Gly in SCP11 (IELFPGLP) should play key roles in protecting HUVECs against H_2O_2 injury by regulating the endogenous antioxidant defense systems (Nrf2 pathway) to scavenge excess ROS, and their mechanism of action will be explored in our future studies.

3. Materials and Methods

3.1. Materials and Chemical Reagents

Cartilages of Siberian sturgeon (*A. baerii*) were kindly provided by Thousand Island Lake Sturgeon Technology Co., Ltd. (Hangzhou, China). HUVECs were purchased from the Cell Bank of Type Culture Collection of the Chinese Academy of Sciences (Shanghai, China). 3-[4,5-dimethylthiazol-2-yl]-2,5 diphenyl tetrazolium bromide (MTT), trypsin, Alcalase, NAC, DPPH, papain, and pepsin were purchased from Sigma-Aldrich Trading Co., Ltd. (Shanghai, China). Flavorzyme and Sephadex G-25 was purchased from Shanghai Source Poly Biological Technology Co., Ltd. (Shanghai, China). Collagen peptides of SCP1 to SC13 with a purity higher than 98% were synthesized in Shanghai Apeptide Co., Ltd. (Shanghai, China).

3.2. Preparation of Collagen Hydrolysate from Siberian Sturgeon Cartilages

The Siberian sturgeon cartilages were thawed, broken, homogenized, and degreased using the method described by Luo et al. [37]. In short, the cartilage was cut into approximately 0.5 cm^2 pieces, homogenized, added into a NaOH solution (0.1 M) with a cartilage/solution ratio of 1:8 (w/v) and uninterruptedly stirred for 6 h, and the NaOH solution was substituted every three hours. Subsequently, the degreased cartilages were rinsed using cold tap water three times and demineralized using EDTA-2Na (0.5 M) with a cartilage/solution ratio of 1:8 (w/v) for two days, and the EDTA-2Na solution was changed every 12 h. The pretreated cartilage was rinsed using cold tap water three times.

Pretreated cartilages were suspended in a buffer solution to prepare the 10% (w/v) sample slurry. After that, the mixed solution was separately hydrolyzed for 6.5 h with 3.0% dose of Alcalase (pH 9.0, 50 °C), papain (pH 7.0, 50 °C), trypsin (pH 8.0, 37.0 °C), flavorzyme (pH 7.5, 45 °C), and pepsin (pH 2.0, 37.0 °C), respectively. The collagen hydrolysate solutions were put in a 95 °C water bath for 15 min to inactivate proteases, centrifuged at 6000× g for 20 min, dialyzed, and lyophilized. The activities of the prepared collagen hydrolysates were evaluated using DPPH· and HO· scavenging assays [45]. Then, the collagen hydrolysate produced using Alcalase revealed the maximum activity among the five hydrolysates, and it was named SCH.

3.3. Purification of APs from SCH

APs were prepared from SCH according to the following designed isolated process (Figure 12).

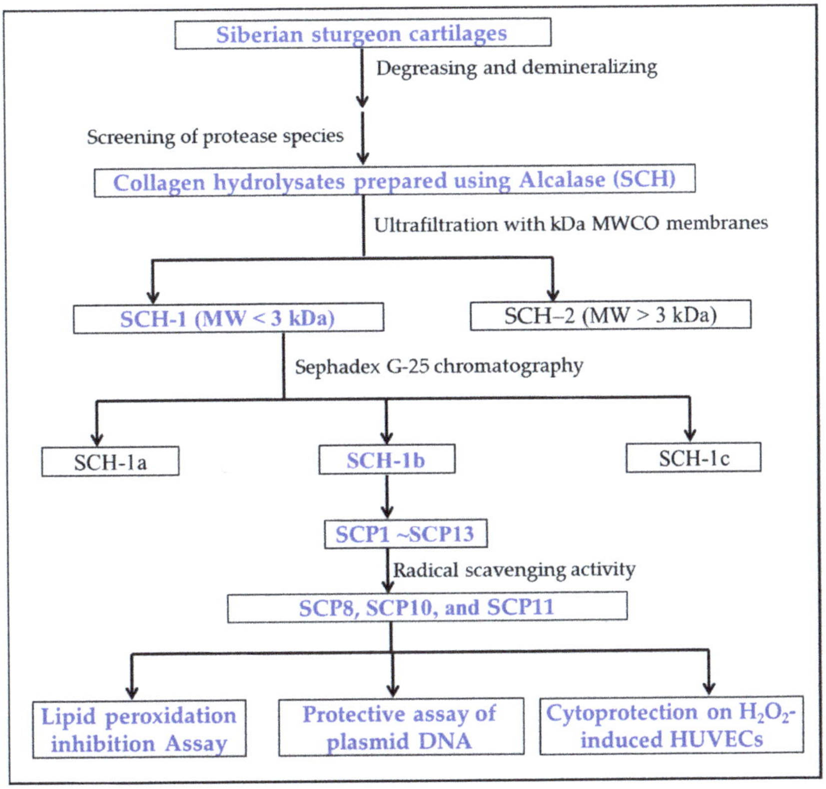

Figure 12. The flow chart of preparation and activity evaluation of APs from collagen hydrolysate (SCH) of Siberian sturgeon cartilages.

The SCH solution was fractionated using a 3 kDa MW cut-off ultrafiltration membrane and two resulting components, defined as SCH-1 (MW < 3 kDa), and SCH-2 (MW > 3 kDa) were collected, dialyzed, freeze-dried, and their radical scavenging activity was detected.

A total of 10 mL of SCH-1 solutions (50.0 mg/mL) were injected into the chromatography column of Sephadex G-25 (2.6 cm × 150 cm) and washed out by phosphate buffer solution (PBS, pH 7.2), with a flow rate of 1.0 mL/min. The effluent solution was collected every 2 min and measured at 230 and 280 nm. Finally, three peptide components (SCH-1a, SCH-1b, and SCH-1c) were enriched, desalted, freeze-dried, and their radical scavenging activity was detected.

The SCH-1b (20 μL, 100.0 μg/mL) was pre-treated with a 0.22 μm microporous membrane and purified by a HPLC column of Waters Symmetry C18 (4.6 × 250 mm, 5 μm) using a gradient of acetonitrile containing 0.06% trifluoroacetic acid. The sample was isolated with a flow velocity of 0.8 mL/min and monitored at 230 and 280 nm. In the end, thirteen APs (SCP1 to SCP13) were purified from SCH-1b on the basis of the chromatographic peaks.

3.4. Analysis of Sequences and MWs of Thirteen APs (SCP1 to SCP13)

The N-terminal amino-acid sequences of thirteen APs (SCP1 to SCP13) were determined by the Edman degradation method using an Applied Biosystems 494 protein sequencer (Foster City, CA, USA). The MWs of thirteen APs (SCP1 to SCP13) were measured by a Q-TOF MS coupled to an electrospray ionization (ESI) source.

3.5. Radical Scavenging, Lipid Peroxidation Inhibition, and Plasmid DNA Protective Assays

3.5.1. Radical Scavenging Assays

The DPPH· and the HO· scavenging assays were performed on the previous methods, and the EC_{50} value was set as the AP dose, resulting in a 50% decrease of the initial radical concentration [14,45].

DPPH· Scavenging Activity

Two milliliters of samples consisting of distilled water and different concentrations of the analytes were placed in cuvettes, and 500 μL of an ethanolic solution of DPPH (0.02%) and 1.0 mL of ethanol were added. A control sample containing the DPPH solution without the sample was also prepared. In the blank, the DPPH solution was substituted with ethanol. The antioxidant activity of the sample was evaluated using the inhibition percentage of the DPPH radical with the following equation:

$$\text{DPPH radical scavenging activity (\%)} = (A0 + A' - A)/A0 \times 100\% \quad (1)$$

where A is the absorbance rate of the sample, A0 is the control group absorbance, and A′ is the blank absorbance.

HO· Scavenging Activity

A total of 1.0 mL of a 1.87 mM 1,10-phenanthroline solution and 2.0 mL of the sample were added to a screw-capped tube and mixed. Then, 1.0 mL of a $FeSO_4{\cdot}7H_2O$ solution (1.87 mM) was added to the mixture. The reaction was initiated by adding 1.0 mL of H_2O_2 (0.03%, v/v). After incubating at 37 °C for 60 min in a water bath, the absorbance of the reaction mixture was measured at 536 nm against a reagent blank. The reaction mixture without any antioxidant was used as the negative control, and a mixture without H_2O_2 was used as the blank. The hydroxyl radical scavenging activity (HRSA) was calculated using the following formula:

$$\text{HRSA (\%)} = [(As - An)/(Ab - An)] \times 100\% \quad (2)$$

where As, An, and Ab are the absorbance values determined at 536 nm of the sample, negative control, and blank after the reaction, respectively.

3.5.2. Lipid Peroxidation Inhibition Assay

Lipid peroxidation inhibition assays were operated on the reported methods [11,14]. Briefly, a sample (5.0 mg) was dissolved in 10 mL of 50 mM PBS (pH 7.0) and added to 0.13 mL of a solution of linoleic acid and 10 mL of 99.5% ethanol. Then, the total volume was adjusted to 25 mL with deionized water. The mixture was incubated in a conical flask with a screw cap at 40 °C in a dark room, and the degree of oxidation was evaluated by measuring ferric thiocyanate values. The reaction solution (100 μL) incubated in the linoleic acid model system was mixed with 4.7 mL of 75% ethanol, 0.1 mL of 30% ammonium thiocyanate, and 0.1 mL of 20 mM ferrous chloride solution in 3.5% HCl. After 3 min, the thiocyanate value was measured at 500 nm, following color development with $FeCl_2$ and thiocyanate at different intervals during the incubation period at 40 °C.

3.5.3. Protective Assay on Plasmid DNA

The protective effects of SCP8, SCP10, and SCP11, on supercoiled plasmid DNA (pBR322) were measured using the previous method [11]. In brief, 15 μL of reaction mixtures containing 5 μL of PBS (10 mM, pH 7.4), 2 μL of $FeSO_4$ (1.0 mM), 1μL of pBR322 (0.5 μg), 5 μL of the peptide (SCP8, SCP10, or SCP11, respectively), and 2 μL of H_2O_2 (1.0 mM) were incubated at 37 °C. After 0.5 h incubation, the reaction was terminated by adding 2 μL of a loading buffer containing glycerol (50%, *v*/*v*), ethylenediaminetetraacetic acid (40 mM), and bromophenol blue (0.05%). The resulted reaction mixtures were subsequently electrophoresed on 1% agarose gel containing 0.5 μg/mL EtBr for 50 min (60 V), and the DNA in the agarose gel was photographed under ultraviolet light.

3.6. Protective Function of SCP8, SCP10, and SCP11 on H_2O_2-Injured HUVECs

3.6.1. Cell Culture and Viability Determination

The HUVECs were cultured according to the described method by Cai et al. [66] and Wang et al. [77]. In brief, HUVECs with the density of 1.0 × 10^5 cells/well were seeded into a 96-well plate containing 100 μL of culture media. After incubated for 24 h, 20 μL of SCP8, SCP10, and SCP11 solutions dissolved in the DMEM medium were separately added in the sample groups with the final concentration of 200 μg/mL. In addition, peptide was substituted by PBS (pH 7.2) in the control group. After incubated for 24 h, 20 μL of MTT was added into the plate and OD490 nm was measured after 4 h. The cell viability was calculated on the basis of the following formula:

$$\text{Cell viability (\%)} = (OD_{\text{sample}}/OD_{\text{control}}) \times 100. \tag{3}$$

3.6.2. Protection of SCP8, SCP10, and SCP11 on H_2O_2-Injured HUVECs

HUVECs with the density of 1.0 × 10^5 cells/well were seeded into a 96-well plate containing 100 μL of culture media. After 24 h, the supernatant in the HUVECs wells was aspirated and H_2O_2 was added, and its final concentrations, respectively, reached 0, 100, 200, 300, 400, 500, and 600 μM. After 24 h, cell viability was determined according to the above method and the H_2O_2 concentration that induced cell viability by approximately 50% was chosen to establish the oxidative damage model of HUVECs [66,77].

After culturing for 24 h, the supernatant in the HUVECs wells was wiped off. Subsequently, 100 μL of the peptide samples at the final concentrations of 200 μM were joined in the protection groups. After 8 h, the peptide sample was cleared and H_2O_2 at 200 μM was put in the model and the peptide sample groups and then treated for 24 h. A total of 100 μL of NAC (1.5 mM) was used as the positive control group. The blank control group used 20 μL PBS instead of the peptide solution.

3.6.3. Determination of ROS, MDA, and Antioxidases

The levels of ROS in the blank control, model, and sample groups were measured on the reported method and expressed as a percentage of the of blank control [66].

The activity of SOD and GSH-Px and the content of MDA were measured using assay kits in accordance with the protocols of the Nanjing Jiancheng Bioengineering Institute Co., Ltd. (Nanjing, China), and the levels of SOD and GSH-Px were indicated as U/mg prot.

3.7. Statistical Analysis

The data are expressed as the mean ± standard deviation (SD, $n = 3$). An ANOVA test was used to analyze the differences between the means of each group, using SPSS 19.0 (Statistical Program for Social Sciences, SPSS Corporation, Chicago, IL, USA). A Duncan's test was used to determine the significance between different groups ($p < 0.05$, $p < 0.01$, or $p < 0.001$).

4. Conclusions

In the study, thirteen APs were isolated from the collagen hydrolysate of Siberian sturgeon cartilages produced using Alcalase and identified as GPTGED, GEPGEQ, GPEGPAG, VPPQD, GLEDHA, GDRGAEG, PRGFRGPV, GEYGFE, GFIGFNG, PSVSLT, IELFPGLP, LRGEAGL, and RGEPGL, respectively. Among them, GEYGFE, PSVSLT, and IELFPGLP showed the highest radical scavenging activity, lipid peroxidation inhibiting capability, and protection on H_2O_2-injured HUVECs and on plasmid DNA. Therefore, this research provides free technical support for higher-valued utilizing fish by-products. More importantly, thirteen isolated collagen APs, especially GEYGFE, PSVSLT, and IELFPGLP, may act as antioxidant additives for generating health products to treat chronic diseases caused by oxidative stress. Moreover, the antioxidant mechanism of GEYGFE, PSVSLT, and IELFPGLP will be systematically researched in our follow-up study.

Author Contributions: Y.S.: conceptualization, data curation, and formal analysis. Y.-T.Q.: investigation, methodology, validation, and writing—original draft. Y.-M.W.: conceptualization, data curation, and formal analysis. C.-F.C.: investigation, methodology, and validation. B.W.: resources, funding acquisition, supervision, and writing—review and editing. All authors have read and agreed to the published version of the manuscript.

Funding: This work was funded by the National Natural Science Foundation of China (No. 82073764) and the Ten-thousand Talents Plan of Zhejiang Province (No. 2019R52026).

Institutional Review Board Statement: Not applicable.

Informed Consent Statement: Not applicable.

Data Availability Statement: Data are contained within the article.

Conflicts of Interest: The authors declare no conflict of interest.

Abbreviations

DPPH·, 2,2-diphenyl-1-picrylhydrazyl radical; HO·, hydroxide radical; ROS, reactive oxygen species; AP, antioxidant peptide; MW, molecular weight; SCH, Collagen hydrolysate of Siberian Sturgeon Cartilage; GFC, Gel Filtration Chromatography; SCP1, Gly-Pro-Thr-Gly-Glu-Asp (GPTGED); SCP2, Gly-Glu-Pro-Gly-Glu-Gln (GEPGEQ); SCP3, Gly-Pro-Glu-Gly-Pro-Ala-Gly (GPEGPAG); SCP4, Val-Pro-Pro-Gln-Asp (VPPQD); SCP5, Gly-Leu-Glu-Asp-His-Ala (GLEDHA); SCP6, Gly-Asp-Arg-Gly-Ala-Glu-Gly (GDRGAEG) SCP7, Pro-Arg-Gly-Phe-Arg-Gly-Pro-Val (PRGFRGPV); SCP8, Gly-Glu-Tyr-Gly-Phe-Glu (GEYGFE); SCP9, Gly-Phe-Ile-Gly-Phe-Asn-Gly (GFIGFNG); SCP10, Pro-Ser-Val-Ser-Leu-Thr (PSVSLT); SCP11, Gly-Ile-Glu-Leu-Phe-Pro-Gly-Leu-Pro (GIELFPGLP); SCP12, Leu-Arg-Gly-Glu-Ala-Gly-Leu (LRGEAGL); SCP13, Arg-Gly-Glu-Pro-Gly-Leu (RGEPGL); GSP, glutathione; SC, supercoiled; OC, open circular; LIN, linear; HUVECs, Human umbilical vein endothelial cells; MTT, 3-(4,5-Dimethylthiazol-2yl)-2,5-diphenyltetrazolium bromide.

References

1. Sila, A.; Bougatef, A. Antioxidant peptides from marine by-products: Isolation, identification and application in food systems. *J. Funct. Foods* **2016**, *21*, 10–26. [CrossRef]
2. Vliet, A.; Janssen, H.; Anathy, V. Oxidative stress in chronic lung disease: From mitochondrial dysfunction to dysregulated redox signaling. *Mol. Asp. Med.* **2018**, *63*, 59–69. [CrossRef] [PubMed]
3. Caballero, E.P.; Mariz, P.N.; Rigazio, C.S.; Santamaría, M.H.; Corral, R.S. Honokiol attenuates oxidative stress-dependent heart dysfunction in chronic Chagas disease by targeting AMPK/NFE2L2/SIRT3 signaling pathway. *Free Radic. Biol. Med.* **2020**, *156*, 113–124. [CrossRef] [PubMed]
4. Cabello, V.C.; Simon, F.; Trollet, C.; Santibañez, J.F. Oxidative stress in disease and aging: Mechanisms and therapies. *Oxid. Med. Cell. Longev.* **2016**, *6*, 4310469.
5. Deng, Z.; Yu, H.; Yang, Z.; Hu, L.; Liu, Q.; Wang, Y.; Wei, H.K.; Peng, J. Gly-Pro-Ala peptide and FGSHF3 exert protective effects in DON-induced toxicity and intestinal damage via decreasing oxidative stress. *Food Res. Int.* **2021**, *139*, 109840. [CrossRef] [PubMed]
6. Wang, Y.Z.; Zhao, Y.Q.; Wang, Y.M.; Zhao, W.H.; Wang, P.; Chi, C.F. Antioxidant peptides from Antarctic Krill (*Euphausia superba*) hydrolysate: Preparation, identification and cytoprotection on H_2O_2-induced oxidative stress. *J. Funct. Foods* **2021**, *86*, 104701. [CrossRef]
7. Chi, C.F.; Hu, F.Y.; Wang, B.; Li, T.; Ding, G.F. Antioxidant and anticancer peptides from protein hydrolysate of blood clam (*Tegillarca granosa*) muscle. *J. Funct. Foods* **2015**, *15*, 301–313. [CrossRef]
8. Liguori, I.; Russo, G.; Curcio, F.; Bulli, G.; Aran, L.; Della, M.D.; Gargiulo, G.; Testa, G.; Cacciatore, F.; Bonaduce, D.; et al. Oxidative stress, aging, and diseases. *Clin. Interv. Aging* **2018**, *13*, 757–772. [CrossRef]
9. Wen, C.; Zhang, J.; Zhang, H.; Duan, Y.; Ma, H. Plant protein-derived antioxidant peptides: Isolation, identification, mechanism of action and application in food systems: A review. *Trends Food Sci. Technol.* **2020**, *105*, 308–322. [CrossRef]
10. Uchida, D.; Takaki, A.; Oyama, A.; Adachi, T.; Wada, N.; Onishi, H.; Okada, H. Oxidative stress management in chronic liver diseases and hepatocellular carcinoma. *Nutrients* **2020**, *12*, 1576. [CrossRef]

11. Wang, W.Y.; Zhao, Y.Q.; Zhao, G.X.; Chi, C.F.; Wang, B. Antioxidant peptides from collagen hydrolysate of redlip croaker (*Pseudosciaena polyactis*) scales: Preparation, characterization, and cytoprotective effects on H_2O_2-damaged HepG2 cells. *Mar. Drugs* **2020**, *18*, 156. [CrossRef] [PubMed]
12. Lv, R.; Dong, Y.; Bao, Z.; Zhang, S.; Lin, S.; Sun, N. Advances in the activity evaluation and cellular regulation pathways of food-derived antioxidant peptides. *Trends Food Sci. Technol.* **2022**, *122*, 171–186. [CrossRef]
13. Chi, C.F.; Hu, F.Y.; Wang, B.; Ren, X.J.; Deng, S.G.; Wu, C.W. Purification and characterization of three antioxidant peptides from protein hydrolyzate of croceine croaker (*Pseudosciaena crocea*) muscle. *Food Chem.* **2015**, *168*, 662–667. [CrossRef] [PubMed]
14. Zhao, W.H.; Luo, Q.B.; Pan, X.; Chi, C.F.; Sun, K.L.; Wang, B. Preparation, identification, and activity evaluation of ten antioxidant peptides from protein hydrolysate of swim bladders of miiuy croaker (*Miichthys miiuy*). *J. Funct. Foods* **2018**, *47*, 503–511. [CrossRef]
15. Hritcu, L.; Ionita, R.; Postu, P.A.; Gupta, G.K.; Turkez, H.; Lima, T.C.; Carvalho, C.U.S.; De Sousa, D.P. Antidepressant flavonoids and their relationship with oxidative stress. *Oxid. Med. Cell. Longev.* **2017**, *2017*, 5762172. [CrossRef]
16. Macáková, K.; Afonso, R.; Saso, L.; Mladěnka, P. The influence of alkaloids on oxidative stress and related signaling pathways. *Free Radic. Biol. Med.* **2019**, *134*, 429–444. [CrossRef]
17. Ikram, M.; Jo, M.H.; Choe, K.; Khan, A.; Ahmad, S.; Saeed, K.; Kim, M.W.; Kim, M.O. Cycloastragenol, a triterpenoid saponin, regulates oxidative stress, neurotrophic dysfunctions, neuroinflammation and apoptotic cell death in neurodegenerative conditions. *Cells* **2021**, *10*, 2719. [CrossRef]
18. Liu, D.; Nikoo, M.; Boran, G.; Zhou, P.; Regenstein, J.M. Collagen and gelatin. *Annu. Rev. Food Sci. Technol.* **2015**, *6*, 527–557. [CrossRef]
19. Grand View Research. (June 2016). Gelatin Market Size Expected to Reach $4.08 Billion by 2024. Available online: http://www.grandviewresearch.com/pressrelease/global-gelatin-market (accessed on 13 June 2016).
20. Nurilmala, M.; Hizbullah, H.H.; Karnia, E.; Kusumaningtyas, E.; Ochiai, Y. Characterization and antioxidant activity of collagen, gelatin, and the derived peptides from yellowfin tuna (*Thunnus albacares*) skin. *Mar. Drugs* **2020**, *18*, 98. [CrossRef]
21. Al, N.S.; Dayah, A.A.; Hasan, I.; Daghmash, R. Cosmetic, biomedical and pharmaceutical applications of fish gelatin/hydrolysates. *Mar. Drugs* **2021**, *19*, 145.
22. Uddin, S.M.K.; Hossain, M.A.M.; Sagadevan, S.; Amin, M.A.; Johan, M.R. Halal and kosher gelatin: Applications as well as detection approaches with challenges and prospects. *Food Biosci.* **2021**, *44*, 101422. [CrossRef]
23. Qiu, Y.T.; Wang, Y.M.; Yang, X.R.; Zhao, Y.Q.; Chi, C.F.; Wang, B. Gelatin and antioxidant peptides from gelatin hydrolysate of skipjack tuna (*Katsuwonus pelamis*) scales: Preparation, identification and activity evaluation. *Mar. Drugs* **2019**, *17*, 565. [CrossRef] [PubMed]
24. Felician, F.F.; Xia, C.; Qi, W.; Xu, H. Collagen from marine biological sources and medical applications. *Chem Biodivers.* **2018**, *15*, 1700557. [CrossRef] [PubMed]
25. Zhang, L.; Zhao, G.X.; Zhao, Y.Q.; Qiu, Y.T.; Chi, C.F.; Wang, B. Identification and active evaluation of antioxidant peptides from protein hydrolysates of skipjack tuna (*Katsuwonus pelamis*) head. *Antioxidants* **2019**, *8*, 318. [CrossRef] [PubMed]
26. Zhang, J.B.; Zhao, Y.Q.; Wang, Y.M.; Chi, C.F.; Wang, B. Eight peptides from collagen hydrolysate fraction of Spanish mackerel (*Scomberomorous niphonius*) skin: Isolation, identification, and antioxidant activity in vitro. *Mar. Drugs* **2019**, *17*, 224. [CrossRef] [PubMed]
27. Park, S.H.; Jo, Y.J. Static hydrothermal processing and fractionation for production of a collagen peptide with anti-oxidative and anti-aging properties. *Process Biochem.* **2019**, *83*, 176–182. [CrossRef]
28. Ahmed, M.; Verma, A.K.; Patel, R. Collagen extraction and recent biological activities of collagen peptides derived from sea-food waste: A review. *Sustain. Chem. Pharm.* **2020**, *18*, 100315. [CrossRef]
29. Zheng, J.; Tian, X.; Xu, B.; Yuan, F.; Gong, J.; Yang, Z. Collagen peptides from swim bladders of giant croaker (*Nibea japonica*) and their protective effects against H_2O_2-induced oxidative damage toward human umbilical vein endothelial cells. *Mar. Drugs* **2020**, *18*, 430. [CrossRef]
30. Li, Y.; Li, J.; Lin, S.J.; Yang, Z.S.; Jin, H.X. Preparation of antioxidant peptide by microwave-assisted hydrolysis of collagen and its protective effect against H_2O_2-induced damage of RAW264.7 cells. *Mar. Drugs* **2019**, *17*, 642. [CrossRef]
31. Sun, L.; Zhang, Y.; Zhuang, Y. Antiphotoaging effect and purification of an antioxidant peptide from tilapia (*Oreochromis niloticus*) gelatin peptides. *J. Funct. Foods* **2013**, *5*, 154–162. [CrossRef]
32. Chen, T.; Hou, H. Protective effect of gelatin polypeptides from pacific cod (*Gadus Macrocephalus*) against UV irradiation-induced damages by inhibiting inflammation and improving transforming growth factor-β/smad signaling pathway. *J. Photochem. Photobiol. B* **2016**, *162*, 633–640. [CrossRef] [PubMed]
33. Chen, T.; Hou, H.; Fan, Y.; Wang, S.; Chen, Q.; Si, L.; Li, B. Protective effect of gelatin peptides from pacific cod skin against photoaging by inhibiting the expression of MMPs via MAPK signaling pathway. *J. Photochem. Photobiol. B* **2016**, *165*, 34–41. [CrossRef] [PubMed]
34. Zhang, L.; Zheng, Y.; Cheng, X.; Meng, M.; Luo, Y.; Li, B. The anti-photoaging effect of antioxidant collagen peptides from silver carp (*Hypophthalmichthys molitrix*) skin is preferable to tea polyphenols and casein peptides. *Food Funct.* **2017**, *8*, 698–1707. [CrossRef]

35. Zhao, Y.Q.; Zeng, L.; Yang, Z.S.; Huang, F.F.; Ding, G.F.; Wang, B. Anti-Fatigue effect by peptide fraction from protein hydrolysate of croceine croaker (*Pseudosciaena crocea*) swim bladder through inhibiting the oxidative reactions including DNA damage. *Mar. Drugs* **2016**, *14*, 221. [CrossRef]
36. Gui, M.; Song, J.; Zhang, L.; Wang, S.; Wu, R.; Ma, C. Chemical characteristics and antithrombotic effect of chondroitin sulfates from sturgeon skull and sturgeon backbone. *Carbohyd. Polym.* **2015**, *123*, 454–460. [CrossRef]
37. Luo, Q.B.; Chi, C.F.; Yang, F.; Zhao, Y.Q.; Wang, B. Physicochemical properties of acid- and pepsin-soluble collagens from the cartilage of Siberian sturgeon. *Environ. Sci. Pollut. Res.* **2018**, *25*, 31427–31438. [CrossRef]
38. Wang, T.; Zhang, S.; Ren, S.; Zhang, X.; Yang, F.; Chen, Y.; Wang, B. Structural characterization and proliferation activity of chondroitin sulfate from the sturgeon, *Acipenser schrenckii*. *Int. J. Biol. Macromol.* **2020**, *164*, 3005–3011. [CrossRef]
39. Zhu, L.; Li, J.; Wang, Y.; Sun, X.; Li, B.; Poungchawanwong, S.; Hou, H. Structural feature and self-assembly properties of type II collagens from the cartilages of skate and sturgeon. *Food Chem.* **2020**, *331*, 127340. [CrossRef]
40. Lai, C.S.; Tu, C.W.; Kuo, H.C.; Sun, P.P.; Tsai, M.L. Type II Collagen from cartilage of *Acipenser baerii* promotes wound healing in human dermal fibroblasts and in mouse skin. *Mar. Drugs* **2020**, *18*, 511. [CrossRef]
41. Yuan, L.; Chu, Q.; Wu, X.; Yang, B.; Zhang, W.; Jin, W.; Gao, R. Anti-inflammatory and antioxidant activity of peptides from ethanol-soluble hydrolysates of sturgeon (*Acipenser schrenckii*) cartilage. *Front. Nutr.* **2021**, *8*, 689648. [CrossRef]
42. Qiao, Q.Q.; Luo, Q.B.; Suo, S.K.; Zhao, Y.Q.; Chi, C.F.; Wang, B. Preparation, characterization, and cytoprotective effects on HUVECs of fourteen Novel Angiotensin-I-Converting Enzyme inhibitory peptides from protein hydrolysate of tuna processing by-products. *Front. Nutr.* **2022**, *9*, 868681. [CrossRef] [PubMed]
43. Zheng, S.L.; Luo, Q.B.; Suo, S.K.; Zhao, Y.Q.; Chi, C.F.; Wang, B. Preparation, identification, molecular docking study and protective function on HUVECs of Novel ACE Inhibitory Peptides from protein hydrolysate of Skipjack tuna muscle. *Mar. Drugs* **2022**, *20*, 176. [CrossRef]
44. Chi, C.; Hu, F.; Li, Z.; Wang, B.; Luo, H. Influence of different hydrolysis processes by trypsin on the physicochemical, antioxidant, and functional properties of collagen hydrolysates from *Sphyrna lewini*, *Dasyatis akjei*, and *Raja porosa*. *J. Aquat. Food Prod. Technol.* **2016**, *25*, 616–632. [CrossRef]
45. Li, Z.; Wang, B.; Chi, C.; Luo, H.; Gong, Y.; Ding, G. Influence of average molecular weight on antioxidant and functional properties of collagen hydrolysates from *Sphyrna lewini*, *Dasyatis akjei* and *Raja porosa*. *Food Res. Int.* **2013**, *51*, 283–293. [CrossRef]
46. Intarasirisawat, R.; Benjakula, S.; Wu, J.; Visessanguan, W. Isolation of antioxidative and ACE inhibitory peptides from protein hydrolysate of skipjack (*Katsuwana pelamis*) roe. *J. Funct. Foods* **2013**, *5*, 1854–1862. [CrossRef]
47. Han, J.; Huang, Z.; Tang, S.; Lu, C.; Wan, H.; Zhou, J. The novel peptides ICRD and LCGEC screened from tuna roe show antioxidative activity via Keap1/Nrf2-ARE pathway regulation and gut microbiota modulation. *Food Chem.* **2020**, *327*, 127094. [CrossRef] [PubMed]
48. Wang, J.; Wang, Y.M.; Li, L.Y.; Chi, C.F.; Wang, B. Twelve antioxidant peptides from protein hydrolysate of Skipjack tuna (*Katsuwonus pelamis*) roe prepared by flavourzyme: Purification, sequence identification, and activity evaluation. *Front. Nutr.* **2022**, *8*, 813780. [CrossRef]
49. Pan, X.; Zhao, Y.Q.; Hu, F.Y.; Wang, B. Preparation and identification of antioxidant peptides from protein hydrolysate of skate (Raja porosa) cartilage. *J. Funct. Foods* **2016**, *25*, 220–230. [CrossRef]
50. Rahman, M.S.; Hee, C.Y.; Seok, C.Y.; Alam, M.B.; Han, L.S.; Cheol, Y.J. A novel antioxidant peptide, purified from bacillus amyloliquefaciens, showed strong antioxidant potential via Nrf2 mediated heme oxygenase-1 expression. *Food Chem.* **2018**, *239*, 502–510. [CrossRef]
51. Nazeer, R.A.; Kumar, N.S.S.; Ganesh, R.J. In vitro and in vivo studies on the antioxidant activity of fish peptide isolated from the croaker (*Otolithes ruber*) muscle protein hydrolysate. *Peptides* **2012**, *35*, 261–268. [CrossRef]
52. Hu, X.M.; Wang, Y.M.; Zhao, Y.Q.; Chi, C.F.; Wang, B. Antioxidant peptides from the protein hydrolysate of monkfish (*Lophius litulon*) muscle: Purification, identification, and cytoprotective function on HepG2 cells damage by H_2O_2. *Mar. Drugs* **2020**, *18*, 153. [CrossRef] [PubMed]
53. Sridhar, K.; Inbaraj, B.S.; Chen, B.H. Recent developments on production, purification and biological activity of marine peptides. *Food Res. Int.* **2021**, *147*, 110468. [CrossRef] [PubMed]
54. Chi, C.F.; Hu, F.Y.; Wang, B.; Li, Z.R.; Luo, H.Y. Influence of amino acid compositions and peptide profiles on antioxidant capacities of two protein hydrolysates from Skipjack tuna (*Katsuwonus pelamis*) dark muscle. *Mar. Drugs* **2015**, *13*, 2580–2601. [CrossRef] [PubMed]
55. Pan, X.Y.; Wang, Y.M.; Li, L.; Chi, C.F.; Wang, B. Four antioxidant peptides from protein hydrolysate of red stingray (*Dasyatis akajei*) cartilages: Isolation, identification, and in vitro activity evaluation. *Mar. Drugs* **2019**, *17*, 263. [CrossRef] [PubMed]
56. Sudhakar, S.; Nazeer, R.A. Preparation of potent antioxidant peptide from edible part of shortclub cuttlefish against radical mediated lipid and DNA damage. *LWT Food Sci. Technol.* **2015**, *64*, 593–601. [CrossRef]
57. Fernando, I.P.S.; Park, S.Y.; Han, E.J.; Kim, H.S.; Kang, D.S.; Je, J.Y.; Ahn, C.B.; Ahn, G. Isolation of an antioxidant peptide from krill protein hydrolysates as a novel agent with potential hepatoprotective effects. *J. Funct. Foods* **2020**, *67*, 103889. [CrossRef]
58. Bashir, K.M.I.; Sohn, J.H.; Kim, J.S.; Choi, J.S. Identification and characterization of novel antioxidant peptides from mackerel (*Scomber japonicus*) muscle protein hydrolysates. *Food Chem.* **2020**, *323*, 126809. [CrossRef]

59. Wang, Y.M.; Li, X.Y.; Wang, J.; He, Y.; Chi, C.F.; Wang, B. Antioxidant peptides from protein hydrolysate of skipjack tuna milt: Purification, identification, and cytoprotection on H_2O_2 damaged human umbilical vein endothelial cells. *Process Biochem.* **2022**, *113*, 258–269. [CrossRef]
60. You, L.; Zhao, M.; Regenstein, J.M.; Ren, J. Purification and identification of antioxidative peptides from loach (Misgurnus anguillicaudatus) protein hydrolysate by consecutive chromatography and electrospray ionization-mass spectrometry. *Food Res. Int.* **2010**, *43*, 1167–1173. [CrossRef]
61. Zhang, S.Y.; Zhao, G.X.; Suo, S.K.; Wang, Y.M.; Chi, C.F.; Wang, B. Purification, identification, activity evaluation, and stability of antioxidant peptides from alcalase hydrolysate of Antarctic Krill (*Euphausia superba*) proteins. *Mar. Drugs* **2021**, *19*, 347. [CrossRef]
62. Ahn, C.B.; Cho, Y.S.; Je, J.Y. Purification and anti-inflammatory action of tripeptide from salmon pectoral fin byproduct protein hydrolysate. *Food Chem.* **2015**, *168*, 151–156. [CrossRef] [PubMed]
63. He, Y.; Pan, X.; Chi, C.F.; Sun, K.L.; Wang, B. Ten new pentapeptides from protein hydrolysate of miiuy croaker (*Miichthys miiuy*) muscle: Preparation, identification, and antioxidant activity evaluation. *LWT* **2019**, *105*, 1–8. [CrossRef]
64. Cai, L.; Wu, X.; Zhang, Y.; Li, X.; Ma, S.; Li, J. Purification and characterization of three antioxidant peptides from protein hydrolysate of grass carp (*Ctenopharyngodon idella*) skin. *J. Funct. Foods* **2015**, *16*, 234–242. [CrossRef]
65. Tonolo, F.; Moretto, L.; Grinzato, A.; Fiorese, F.; Folda, A.; Scalcon, V. Fermented soy-derived bioactive peptides selected by a molecular docking approach show antioxidant properties involving the Keap1/Nrf2 pathway. *Antioxidants* **2020**, *9*, 1306. [CrossRef]
66. Cai, S.Y.; Wang, Y.M.; Zhao, Y.Q.; Chi, C.F.; Wang, B. Cytoprotective effect of antioxidant pentapeptides from the protein hydrolysate of swim bladders of miiuy croaker (*Miichthys miiuy*) against H_2O_2-mediated human umbilical vein endothelial cell (HUVEC) injury. *Int. J. Biol. Macromol.* **2019**, *20*, 5425. [CrossRef]
67. Rajapakse, N.; Mendis, E.; Jung, W.K.; Je, J.Y.; Kim, S.K. Purification of a radical scavenging peptide from fermented mussel sauce and its antioxidant properties. *Food Res. Int.* **2005**, *38*, 175–182. [CrossRef]
68. Chen, H.; Wang, S.; Zhou, A.; Miao, J.; Liu, J.; Benjakul, S. A novel antioxidant peptide purified frecom defatted round scad (*Decapterus maruadsi*) protein hydrolysate extends lifespan in *Caenorhabditis elegans*. *J. Funct. Foods* **2020**, *68*, 103907. [CrossRef]
69. Sheih, I.C.; Wu, T.K.; Fang, T.J. Antioxidant properties of a new antioxidative peptide from algae protein waste hydrolysate in different oxidation systems. *Bioresour. Technol.* **2009**, *100*, 3419–3425. [CrossRef]
70. Saito, K.; Jin, D.H.; Ogawa, T.; Muramoto, K.; Hatakeyama, E.; Yasuhara, T.; Nokihara, K. Antioxidative properties of tripeptide libraries prepared by the combinatorial chemistry. *J. Agric. Food Chem.* **2003**, *51*, 3668–3674. [CrossRef]
71. Chang, O.K.; Ha, G.E.; Han, G.S.; Seol, K.H.; Kim, H.W.; Jeong, S.G.; Oh, M.H.; Park, B.Y.; Ham, J.S. Novel antioxidant peptide derived from the ultrafiltrate of ovomucin hydrolysate. *J. Agric. Food Chem.* **2013**, *61*, 7294–7300. [CrossRef]
72. Memarpoor, Y.M.; Asoodeh, A.; Chamani, J. A novel antioxidant and antimicrobial peptide from hen egg white lysozyme hydrolysates. *J. Funct. Foods* **2012**, *4*, 278–286. [CrossRef]
73. Zheng, Z.; Si, D.; Ahmad, B.; Li, Z.; Zhang, R. A novel antioxidative peptide derived from chicken blood corpuscle hydrolysate. *Food Res. Int.* **2018**, *106*, 410–419. [CrossRef] [PubMed]
74. Yang, X.R.; Zhao, Y.Q.; Qiu, Y.T.; Chi, C.F.; Wang, B. Preparation and characterization of gelatin and antioxidant peptides from gelatin hydrolysate of Skipjack tuna (*Katsuwonus pelamis*) bone stimulated by in vitro gastrointestinal digestion. *Mar. Drugs* **2019**, *17*, 78. [CrossRef] [PubMed]
75. Theodore, A.E.; Raghavan, S.; Kristinsson, H.G. Antioxidative activity of protein hydrolysates prepared from alkaline-aided channel catfish protein isolates. *J. Agric. Food Chem.* **2008**, *56*, 7459–7466. [CrossRef] [PubMed]
76. Zhao, G.X.; Yang, X.R.; Wang, Y.M.; Zhao, Y.Q.; Chi, C.F.; Wang, B. Antioxidant peptides from the protein hydrolysate of Spanish Mackerel (*Scomberomorous niphonius*) muscle by in vitro gastrointestinal digestion and their in vitro activities. *Mar. Drugs* **2019**, *17*, 531. [CrossRef] [PubMed]
77. Wang, Y.Z.; Wang, Y.M.; Pan, X.; Chi, C.F.; Wang, B. Antioxidant mechanisms of the oligopeptides (FWKVV and FMPLH) from muscle hydrolysate of miiuy croaker against oxidative damage of HUVECs. *Oxid. Med. Cell. Longev.* **2021**, *2021*, 9987844. [CrossRef]
78. Liu, C.; Guo, Y.; Zhao, F. Potential mechanisms mediating the protective effects of a peptide from walnut (*Juglans mandshurica* Maxim) against hydrogen peroxide induced neurotoxicity in PC12 cells. *Food Funct.* **2019**, *10*, 3491–3501. [CrossRef]
79. Lu, M.C.; Ji, J.A.; Jiang, Z.Y.; You, Q.D. The Keap1-Nrf2-ARE pathway as a potential preventive and therapeutic target: An update. *Med. Res. Rev.* **2016**, *36*, 924–963. [CrossRef]
80. Wells, G. Peptide and small molecule inhibitors of the Keap1-Nrf2 protein-protein interaction. *Biochem. Soc. Trans.* **2015**, *43*, 674–679. [CrossRef]
81. Wang, N.; Wang, W.; Sadiq, F.A.; Wang, S.; Caiqin, L.; Jianchang, J. Involvement of Nrf2 and Keap1 in the activation of antioxidant responsive element (ARE) by chemopreventive agent peptides from soft-shelled turtle. *Process Biochem.* **2020**, *92*, 174–181. [CrossRef]
82. Bello, M.; José, A.M.G. Molecular recognition between potential natural inhibitors of the Keap1-Nrf2 complex. *Int. J. Biol. Macromol.* **2017**, *105*, 981–992. [CrossRef] [PubMed]
83. Wen, C.T.; Zhang, J.X.; Zhang, H.H.; Duan, Y.Q.; Ma, H.L. Study on the structure–activity relationship of watermelon seed antioxidant peptides by using molecular simulations. *Food Chem.* **2021**, *2021*, 364. [CrossRef] [PubMed]

84. Tonolo, F.; Fiorese, F.; Moretto, L.; Folda, A.; Scalcon, V.; Grinzato, A.; Ferro, S.; Arrigoni, G.; Bindoli, A.; Feller, E.; et al. Identification of new peptides from fermented milk showing antioxidant properties: Mechanism of action. *Antioxidants.* **2020**, *9*, 2. [CrossRef] [PubMed]
85. Li, J.; Lu, J.; Asakiya, C.; Huang, K.; Zhou, X.; Liu, Q.; He, X. Extraction and identification of three new urechis unicinctus visceral peptides and their antioxidant activity. *Mar. Drugs* **2022**, *20*, 293. [CrossRef]
86. Wei, G.Q.; Zhao, Q.; Wang, D.D.; Fan, Y.Z.; Shi, Y.; Huang, A.X. Novel ACE inhibitory, antioxidant and α-glucosidase inhibitory peptides identified from fermented rubing cheese through peptidomic and molecular docking. *LWT Food Sci. Technol.* **2022**, *2022*, 159. [CrossRef]

marine drugs

MDPI

Article

Monkfish Peptides Mitigate High Fat Diet-Induced Hepatic Steatosis in Mice

Jiena Ye [1,†], Xiaoxiao Tian [1,†], Qiongfen Wang [2], Jiawen Zheng [1], Yanzhuo Yang [1], Baogui Xu [1], Shuai Zhang [1], Falei Yuan [1,*] and Zuisu Yang [1,*]

1 Zhejiang Provincial Engineering Technology Research Center of Marine Biomedical Products, School of Food and Pharmacy, Zhejiang Ocean University, Zhoushan 316022, China; z20105500018@zjou.edu.cn (J.Y.); z18095135044@zjou.edu.cn (X.T.); jwzheng1996@163.com (J.Z.); z20105500026@zjou.edu.cn (Y.Y.); z19105500022@zjou.edu.cn (B.X.); zhangxj_hys@163.com (S.Z.)

2 Zhoushan Institute for Food and Drug Control, Zhoushan 316000, China; wqf6512@aliyun.com

* Correspondence: yuanfalei@zjou.edu.cn (F.Y.); yzs@zjou.edu.cn (Z.Y.)

† These authors contributed equally to this work.

Abstract: Non-alcoholic fatty liver disease (NAFLD) is a hepatic metabolic syndrome usually accompanied by fatty degeneration and functional impairment. The aim of the study was to determine whether monkfish peptides (LPs) could ameliorate high-fat diet (HFD)-induced NAFLD and its underlying mechanisms. NAFLD was induced in mice by giving them an HFD for eight weeks, after which LPs were administered in various dosages. In comparison to the HFD control group: body weight in the LP-treated groups decreased by 23–28%; triacylglycerol levels in the blood decreased by 16–35%; and low-density lipoproteins levels in the blood decreased by 23–51%. Additionally, we found that LPs elevated the activity of hepatic antioxidant enzymes and reduced the inflammatory reactions within fatty liver tissue. Investigating the effect on metabolic pathways, we found that in LP-treated mice: the levels of phospho-AMP-activated protein kinase (p-AMPK), and phospho-acetyl CoA carboxylase (p-ACC) in the AMP-activated protein kinase (AMPK) pathway were up-regulated and the levels of downstream sterol regulatory element-binding transcription factor 1 (SREBP-1) were down-regulated; lipid oxidation increased and free fatty acid (FFA) accumulation decreased (revealed by the increased carnitine palmitoyltransferase-1 (CPT-1) and the decreased fatty acid synthase (FASN) expression, respectively); the nuclear factor erythroid-2-related factor 2 (Nrf2) antioxidant pathway was activated; and the levels of heme oxygenase-1 (HO-1) and nicotinamide quinone oxidoreductase 1 (NQO1) were increased. Overall, all these findings demonstrated that LPs can improve the antioxidant capacity of liver to alleviate NAFLD progression mainly through modulating the AMPK and Nrf2 pathways, and thus it could be considered as an effective candidate in the treatment of human NAFLD.

Keywords: monkfish peptides; NAFLD; the AMPK/Nrf2 pathway; lipid metabolism

Citation: Ye, J.; Tian, X.; Wang, Q.; Zheng, J.; Yang, Y.; Xu, B.; Zhang, S.; Yuan, F.; Yang, Z. Monkfish Peptides Mitigate High Fat Diet-Induced Hepatic Steatosis in Mice. *Mar. Drugs* **2022**, *20*, 312. https://doi.org/10.3390/md20050312

Academic Editors: Bin Wang and Chang-Feng Chi

Received: 9 April 2022
Accepted: 2 May 2022
Published: 5 May 2022

1. Introduction

Non-alcoholic fatty liver disease (NAFLD) refers to a clinicopathological syndrome characterized by inflammation of the liver lobule and hepatic parenchymal steatosis. NAFLD can range from simple steatosis to more severe liver diseases, such as steatohepatitis, fibrosis, and even liver cancer [1]. The occurrence of NAFLD worldwide is between 14% and 24% of liver diseases, yet the underlying mechanism of the condition remains unclear [2]. HFD provides a high amount of saturated fatty acids, especially palmitic acid (C16:0). The excess of palmitic acid generates an increase in the hepatic inflammatory response [3]. With a lack of clinical intervention options, diet regulation remains the most effective means of managing NAFLD [4].

Recent research has focused largely on the effects of mitochondrial dysfunction, insulin resistance, obesity, and changes to the gut microbiome on the development of NAFLD. Mitochondrial dysfunction is involved in the progression of NAFLD, which changes the homeostasis of fatty liver, thereby producing higher levels of malondialdehyde (MDA) and reactive oxygen species (ROS) [5,6]. When oxidative stress occurs, nuclear factor erythroid-2-related factor 2 (Nrf2) combines with antioxidant redox elements to protect cells against stress. Together, they regulate the expression of downstream genes such as heme oxygenase-1 (HO-1) and nicotinamide quinone oxidoreductase 1 (NQO1) [7,8]. Both liraglutide and tetrahydrocurcumin ameliorated NAFLD by increasing the mRNA levels of Nrf2, HO-1, GCLM, and NQO1 [9,10]. The body's antioxidant defense enzymes include catalase (CAT), glutathione peroxidase (GSH-Px), and superoxide dismutase (SOD). Decreasing these enzymes can also lead to oxidative stress.

Insulin resistance breaks down the adipose tissue, which in turn releases more free fatty acids (FFA), adipokines, and inflammatory factors to the liver and adipose tissue. Much attention has been paid to reducing the level of FFA in the treatment of NAFLD [11]. AMP-activated protein kinase (AMPK) is recognized as a major energy-related protein kinase that mediates the development of liver dysfunction [11]. Acetyl CoA carboxylase (ACC) is the target molecule of AMPK. ACC catalyzes the production of malonyl-CoA by prompting the synthesis and elongation of fatty acids as well as inhibiting the oxidation of fatty acids through the inhibition of carnitine palmitoyltransferase-1 (CPT-1) [12]. AMPK phosphorylation can induce ACC phosphorylation and inhibit ACC activity. ACC enters a negative feedback loop that increases the content of CPT-1 and oxidizes fatty acids, thus reducing fatty acid content in the liver [13]. The activation of AMPK weakens the proteolytic process of sterol regulatory element-binding proteins (SREBP)-1c and leads to accelerated fatty acid oxidation, thereby eliminating the abnormal accumulation of FFA. Liensinine significantly ameliorated HFD-triggered hepatic oxidative stress and dyslipidemia by mediating Nrf2/AMPK signaling, and dimethyl fumarate similarly mitigated NAFLD progression by mediating Nrf2, SREBP-1c, and nuclear factor-κB (NF-κB) signaling [14,15]. Excessive dietary fat directly enhances hepatic lipid synthesis and inflammatory responses [16,17]. Obesity is closely related to NAFLD, because it is characterized by liver-neutral lipid accumulation [18,19]. One of the morphological features of steatosis is the accumulation of lipid droplets in hepatic parenchymal cells.

Bioactive peptides, generally composed of three to twenty amino acid residues, are known for their antihypertensive and antilipemic properties [20]. Milk is recognized as a major source of bioactive peptides and fish proteins may be another important source [21]. Although it has been shown that protein hydrolysates from yellow catfish alleviate mouse NAFLD through inhibiting lipid metabolism, the underlying mechanisms have yet to be studied [22]. Herring milt protein hydrolysates attenuate insulin resistance from excessive fat consumption [23]. Fish protein hydrolysates can regulate lipid metabolism and improve dyslipidemia in Zucker rats [24,25]. Every year, approximately 12% of aquatic products worldwide are used for non-food purposes [24]. Monkfish meat has traditionally been considered a low-value food. Monkfish peptides (LPs) have been found to have strong antioxidant activities and fat absorption capabilities [26–28]. However, the regulatory effects of LPs on NAFLD, and the underlying molecular mechanisms are still unclear. Thus, in the current study, we tested the protective effects of LPs against high-fat diet-induced NAFLD in mice. We also sought to determine whether the protective effects of LPs involve the AMPK and Nrf2 signaling pathways.

2. Results

2.1. Identification and Protein Analysis of LPs

LPs with a molecular weight of less than 1 kDa were harvested, and 198 mg of LPs were prepared from 100 g of the fish meat. The total yield was 0.198%. Using database alignment, the corresponding sequences were found in the protein database of the Lophiiformes species in the National Center for Biotechnology Information (NCBI). As shown in Supplementary Table S1, database matching obtained 98 low molecular weight peptides that consisted of 17 heptapeptides, 31 octapeptides, 26 nonapeptides, 13 decapeptides, 9 undecapeptides, and 2 dodecapeptides. There were 96 peptides with two charges and 2 peptides with one charge. A total of 3276 free peptides were identified by de novo sequencing, and the results did not overlap with the data obtained through the database comparison method. The shortest free peptide identified through de novo sequencing was a tetrapeptide and the longest was an octapeptide. Amino acid local confidence (ALC) is the confidence level of de novo sequencing data. Generally, ALC > 80% is adequately reliable. Accordingly, Supplementary Table S2 lists 66 free peptides with ALC > 80% identified by the de novo sequencing results. They had a distribution ranging from tetrapeptide to nonapeptide, including 13 tetrapeptides, 32 pentapeptides, 13 hexapeptides, 4 heptapeptides, and 4 nonapeptides. Additionally, 39 polypeptides had two charges and 27 polypeptides had one charge. Supplementary Table S3 lists the types of proteins. Each of these proteins plays a different role in organisms. For example, the protein nicotinamide adenine dinucleotide (NADH) dehydrogenase is an enzyme located in the inner membrane of mitochondria that catalyzes the transfer of electrons from NADH to coenzyme Q. This enzyme is an "entry enzyme" of oxidative phosphorylation in the mitochondria [29]. ATPase, also known as adenosine triphosphatase, catalyzes the hydrolysis of adenosine triphosphate (ATP) to adenosine diphosphate (ADP) and a phosphate ion. Cytochrome c oxidase transfers the electron of a respiratory substrate directly to molecular oxygen (i.e., with automatic oxidation) through the cytochrome system. This shows that there is an abundance of low-molecular-weight peptides in LPs, of which tetrapeptides and pentapeptides account for most. These protein types also show that LPs are likely to have good antioxidant activity, which is consistent with the results of previous studies [27].

2.2. *LPs Lowered Body Weight and Liver Weight*

As shown in Figure 1A, after seven days of adaptive feeding, the mice in the experimental groups were fed with a high-fat diet (HFD) for eight weeks. The average body weight of mice in the HFD group increased 82% more than that of the normal diet (ND) group. From Week 9 onward, all groups were fed normal diets (Figure 1D) during which the average weight of all the experimental groups decreased (LP-50, 24%, LP-100, 23%, LP-200, 28%, and silibinin (SIL) 32%). After another four weeks of intervention, the average liver weight and liver weight index of the HFD group, calculated as the percentage of liver weight divided by body weight, was higher than that of the ND group by 51% and 34% ($p < 0.01$ Figure 1B,C). Meanwhile the average liver weight and liver weight indexes of the SIL, LP-50, LP-100, and LP-200 groups decreased by 32%, 17%, 29%, and 34%, and 19%, 13%, 22%, and 25%, respectively, as compared with the HFD group ($p < 0.01$ Figure 1B,C).

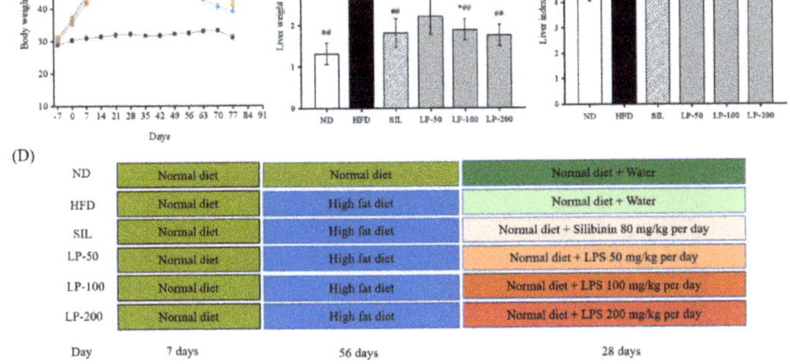

Figure 1. (**A**): Effects of LPs on the alterations of body weight. (**B**): Effects of LPs on the alterations of liver weight. (**C**): Effects of LPs on the liver index (Liver weight/Body weight × 100) of mice with non-alcoholic fatty liver disease (NAFLD). (**D**): Research schedule of NAFLD mice. Values are presented as means ± SD. Values with different labels are significantly different in the groups (* $p < 0.05$, ** $p < 0.01$ vs. ND group, # $p < 0.05$, ## $p < 0.01$ vs. HFD group).

2.3. Effects of LPs on Blood Lipids

The results of the blood lipid indexes found in the serum are shown in Figure 2. Compared to the ND group serum, total cholesterol (TC) levels increased by a substantial 68% in the HFD group ($p < 0.01$, Figure 2A). Meanwhile the SIL and LPs-treated groups (LP-50, LP-100, and LP-200) decreased by 30%, 16%, 29%, and 35%, respectively, in contrast to the HFD group ($p < 0.05$, Figure 2A). There was no significant difference between the LP-200 group and the ND group, and the repair effect was the best between them. The changes in triacylglycerol (TG) and low-density lipoproteins (LDL)-c levels in the serum were the same. In comparison with the ND group, the TG and LDL-c concentrations in the HFD group increased by 91% and 137%, respectively ($p < 0.01$, Figure 2B,C). Compared with the HFD group, the concentration of TG decreased in the SIL, LP-50, LP-100, and LP-200 groups by 42%, 13%, 29%, and 45%, respectively. Furthermore, the concentration of LDL-c decreased in the SIL, LP-50, LP-100, and LP-200 groups by 47%, 23%, 41%, and 51%, respectively ($p < 0.05$, Figure 2B,C). The concentrations of TG and LDL-c in the SIL group and the LP-200 group were not significantly different from the ND group. Compared with the ND group, the concentration of high-density lipoproteins (HDL)-c in each experimental group decreased significantly ($p < 0.05$, Figure 2D). Compared with the HFD group, the level of HDL-c in the LP-50 group was not significantly different, and the level of HDL-c in the SIL, LP-100, and LP-200 groups increased by 46%, 9%, 23%, and 50%, respectively ($p < 0.05$, Figure 2D). The FFA levels in the serum of the HFD group were twice the amount of that in the ND group ($p < 0.01$, Figure 2E). The FFA levels in the serum decreased in the SIL, LP-50, LP-100, and LP-200 by 61%, 28%, 43%, and 62%, respectively, compared to the HFD group ($p < 0.01$, Figure 2E). There was no significant difference between the LP-200 group and the ND group, and the repair effect was the best in the LP-200 group. Thus, it can be concluded that the LP-200 group is most effective in regulating blood lipid levels.

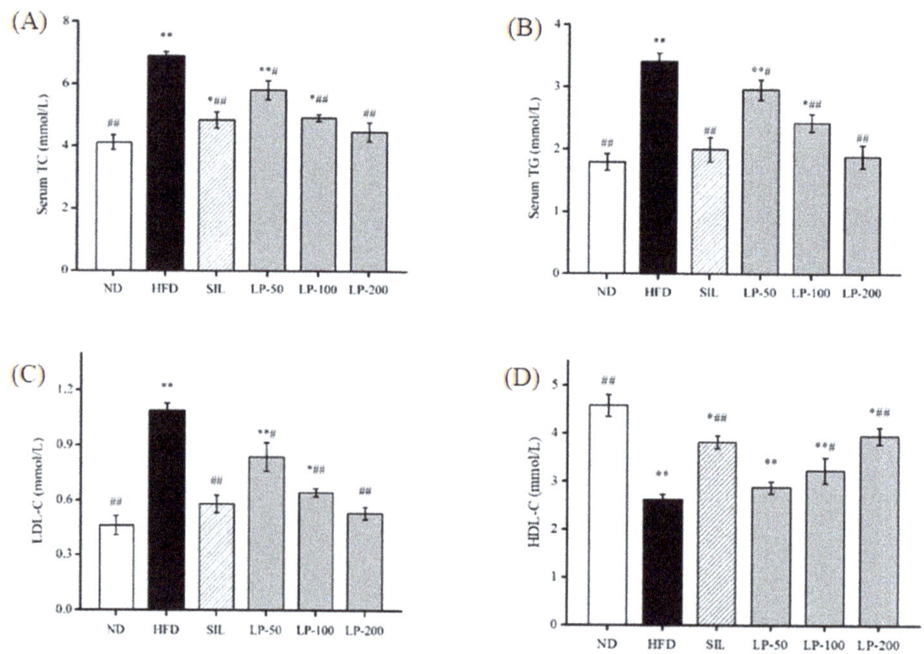

Figure 2. *Cont.*

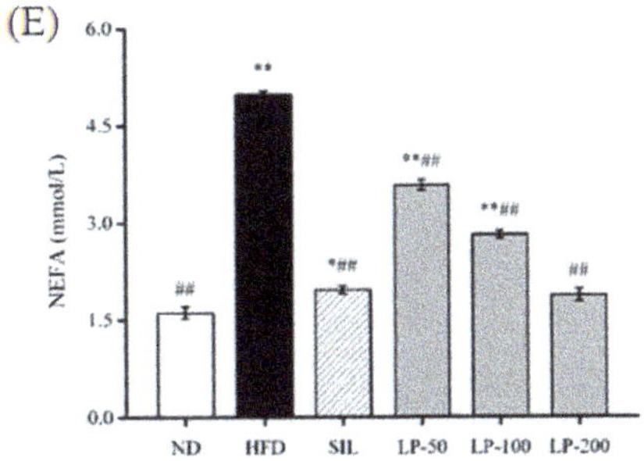

Figure 2. Effects of LPs on plasma total cholesterol (TC) (**A**), triacylglycerol (TG) (**B**), low-density lipoprotein (LDL-c) (**C**), high-density lipoprotein (HDL-c), (**D**) and free fatty acids (FFA) (**E**). Values are presented as means ± SD. Values with different labels are significantly different in the groups (* $p < 0.05$, ** $p < 0.01$ vs. ND group, # $p < 0.05$, ## $p < 0.01$ vs. HFD group).

2.4. *Effects of LPs on Aspartate Aminotransferase (AST) and Alanine Aminotransferase (ALT)*

An increase in aspartate aminotransferase (AST) and alanine aminotransferase (ALT) activity in the blood is usually interpreted as a marker for lesions [30]. The ALT and AST levels in the HFD group increased by 105% and 93%, respectively, indicating that an HFD gave rise to liver injuries ($p < 0.01$, Figure 3). Compared with the HFD group, ALT contents in the serum of the SIL, LP - 50, LP-100, and LP-200 groups decreased by 52%, 20%, 37%, and 55%, respectively, and the concentration of AST in the SIL, LP-50, LP-100, and LP-200 decreased by 47%, 12%, 31%, and 44%, respectively ($p < 0.01$, Figure 3). Although no statistical significance was found among the SIL, LP-200, and ND groups, AST levels in the LP-50 and the LP-100 groups were significantly higher than baseline, a trend similarly followed by ALT levels. The ALT levels of LP-50 and LP-100 were significantly higher than those of the ND group ($p < 0.01$ Figure 3B), and so were the levels in the SIL group ($p < 0.05$ Figure 3B). The LP-200 group did not show any significant difference.

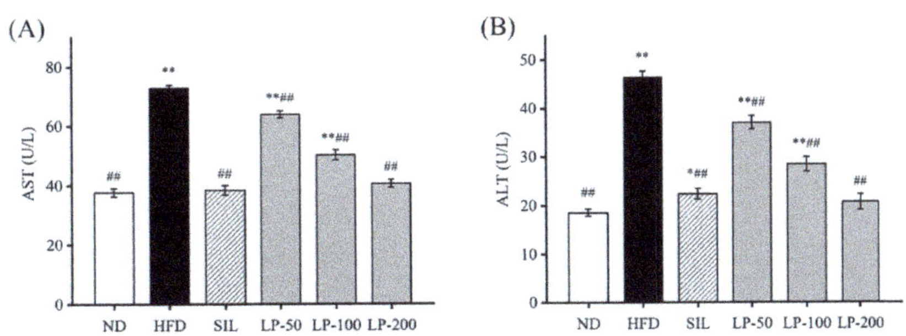

Figure 3. Effects of LPs on the levels of aspartate aminotransferase (AST) (**A**) and alanine aminotransferase (ALT) (**B**). Values with different labels are significantly different in the groups (* $p < 0.05$, ** $p < 0.01$ vs. ND group, ## $p < 0.01$ vs. HFD group).

2.5. *Effects of LPs on Antioxidant Capacity*

The antioxidant capacity of liver tissues in different groups is shown in Table 1. The levels of total antioxidant capacity (T-AOC), CAT, SOD, and GSH-Px in the HFD group were significantly lower than those in the ND group ($p < 0.01$). The levels of these same indicators in the SIL and LPs-treated groups were significantly lower than those in the HFD group ($p < 0.01$). There was no significant difference between the SIL, LP-200, and ND groups. The MDA level in the HFD group was significantly higher than that in the ND group. Compared with the HFD group, the MDA content in the SIL, LP-100, and LP-200 groups significantly decreased ($p < 0.05$).

Table 1. Effects of LPs on Antioxidant Capacities in Liver.

Groups	T-AOC (U/mg prot)	CAT (U/mg prot)	SOD (U/mg prot)	MDA (nmol/mg prot)	GSH-Px (U/mg prot)
ND	$5.22 \pm 0.07^{\#\#}$	$126.11 \pm 1.37^{\#\#}$	$121.42 \pm 0.97^{\#\#}$	$5.02 \pm 0.28^{\#\#}$	$140.12 \pm 1.63^{\#\#}$
HFD	$2.14 \pm 0.47^{**}$	$50.26 \pm 1.33^{**}$	$58.13 \pm 1.01^{**}$	$9.03 \pm 0.99^{**}$	$67.78 \pm 1.67^{**}$
SIL	$5.10 \pm 0.13^{\#\#}$	$123.03 \pm 1.04^{\#\#}$	$111.79 \pm 1.05^{**,\#\#}$	$5.44 \pm 0.14^{\#}$	$163.83 \pm 2.39^{**,\#\#}$
LP-50	$3.75 \pm 0.13^{**,\#}$	$73.22 \pm 1.13^{**,\#\#}$	$76.27 \pm 0.88^{**,\#\#}$	$7.66 \pm 0.68^{*}$	$88.64 \pm 2.27^{**,\#\#}$
LP-100	$4.38 \pm 0.17^{**,\#\#}$	$95.55 \pm 1.76^{**,\#\#}$	$97.24 \pm 0.84^{**,\#\#}$	$6.16 \pm 0.18^{*,\#}$	$109.07 \pm 1.12^{**,\#\#}$
LP-200	$5.07 \pm 0.15^{\#\#}$	$126.04 \pm 1.97^{\#\#}$	$113.10 \pm 0.47^{**,\#\#}$	$4.92 \pm 0.69^{\#}$	$135.41 \pm 2.04^{*,\#\#}$

The data are expressed as the mean ± SD (n = 8 per group). ** $p < 0.01$ vs. ND group. ## $p < 0.01$ vs. HFD group. * $p < 0.05$ vs. ND group. # $p < 0.05$ vs. HFD group. Groups: ND = normal control; HFD = HFD control; SIL = HFD + silibinin; LP-50 = HFD + 50 LP mg/kg; LP-100 = HFD + 100 LP mg/kg; LP-200 = HFD + 200 LP mg/kg.

2.6. Effects of LPs on the Level of Inflammatory Factors

To determine the effects of LPs on inflammation, we examined the levels of IL-6, IL-1β, TNF-α, and IFN-γ in the blood. The concentration of TNF-α in the HFD group increased 94% in comparison with the ND group ($p < 0.01$, Figure 4A). The concentration of TNF-α in the SIL, LP-50, LP-100, and LP-200 groups decreased by 42%, 18%, 36%, and 45%, respectively, compared to the HFD group levels ($p < 0.01$, Figure 4A). There was no significant difference between the LP-200 group and the ND group. The concentration of IL-6 in each experimental group significantly increased in comparison to the ND group ($p < 0.05$, Figure 4B). The concentration of IL-6 in the SIL, LP-50, LP-100, and LP-200 groups decreased by 38%, 14%, 26%, and 39%, respectively, compared with the HFD group ($p < 0.01$, Figure 4B). The concentrations of IL-1β and IFN-γ in the HFD group were significantly higher than those in the ND group ($p < 0.01$, Figure 4C,D). Compared with the HFD group, IL-1β levels in the SIL, LP-50, LP-100, and LP-200 groups showed significant decreases of 46%, 16%, 40%, and 45%, respectively, and as did the levels of IFN-γ in these groups with decreases of 45%, 17%, 42%, and 51%, respectively ($p < 0.01$, Figure 4C,D). From these results, it can be concluded that the SIL group and the LP-200 group were the best at inhibiting the inflammatory response of mice with NAFLD.

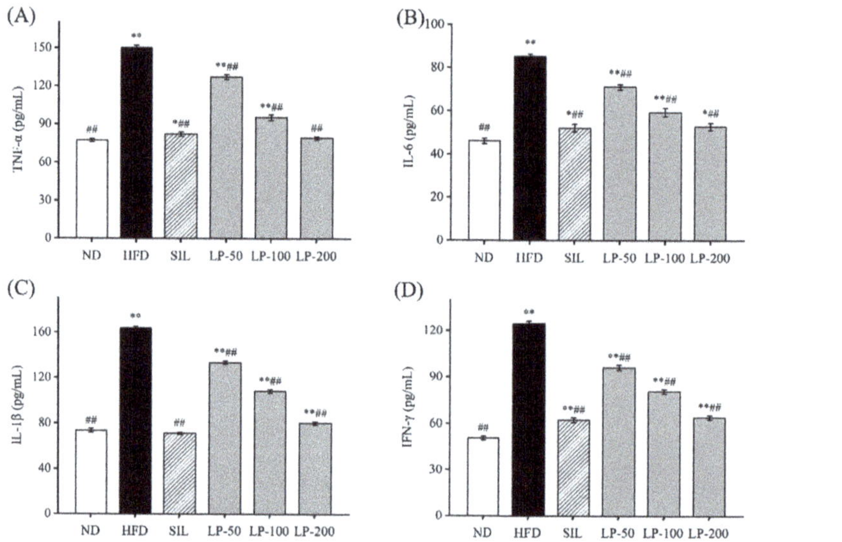

Figure 4. Effects of LPs on the level of inflammatory factors: TNF-α (**A**), IL-6 (**B**), IL-1β (**C**), and IFN-γ (**D**). Data are presented as means ± SD. Values with different labels are significantly different among the groups (* $p < 0.05$, ** $p < 0.01$ vs. ND group, ## $p < 0.01$ vs. HFD group).

2.7. Effects of LPs on Hepatic Histopathology

The results of the histopathological examination of the liver tissue are shown in Figure 5. The liver volume of the HFD group was enlarged, and white particles could be seen on the surface. In the SIL group and LPs groups, the size of the liver shrank, and the white particles of fat decreased (Figure 5A). Hematoxylin and eosin (H&E) staining revealed hypertrophy of the liver cells in the HFD group. The fat tissue was mainly composed of lipid droplets, and the hepatocyte cords were disordered. Compared with the HFD group, the LP-50 and LP-100 groups had fewer lipid droplets. The SIL and LP-200 groups greatly inhibited the accumulation of lipid droplets, attenuating the swelling and disorder of hepatocytes (Figure 5B). The oil red O staining and transmission electron microscopy (TEM) results were consistent with those of the H&E staining. In the ND group, there were no obvious lipid droplets in the hepatocytes. In contrast, there were many red lipid droplets in the model group. The numbers of these droplets in the LPs groups decreased, especially in the LP-200 group (Figure 5C). Hepatic steatosis is related to changes in the mitochondria of hepatocytes [31]. The results show that the electron density of lipid droplets was low, meaning the content of saturated fatty acids was high, and that the structure of hepatocytes in the model group was fuzzy with a blurry boundary. In the normal group, the amount of endoplasmic reticulum was reduced, and there were a large number of round lipid droplets of different sizes. After the intervention of SIL and LPs, the swelling degree of liposomes was reduced, the changes in the mitochondria and endoplasmic reticulum were significantly reduced, and the number of lipid droplets was significantly reduced. The electron density of liposomes was higher than that of the model group (Figure 5D). Livers also increased in size during HFD intervention and H&E staining showed macrovesicular steatosis, ballooning, and inflammation. According to the NAS scoring standard, the structural changes in the liver tissue in 10 visual fields were observed under a microscope, and the results in Figure 5E were obtained, which shows the NAS score: livers showed an average NAS score of 4.8. Quantitative analysis of oil red O staining showed that the fat area in the HFD group was 20%, while that in the LPs groups decreased to 14%, 11%, and 5%, respectively (Figure 5F).

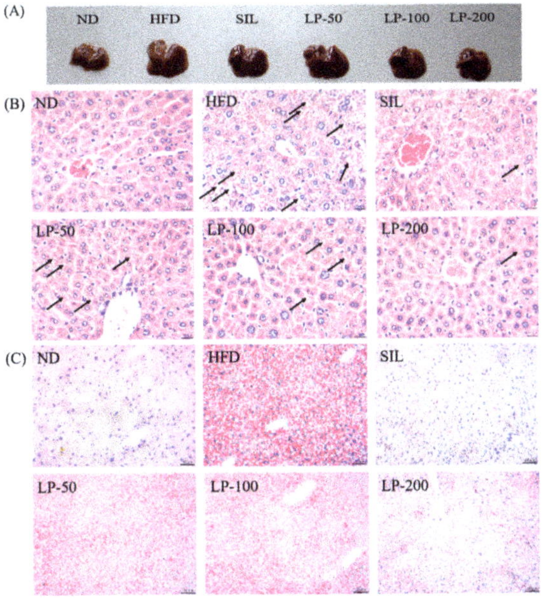

Figure 5. *Cont.*

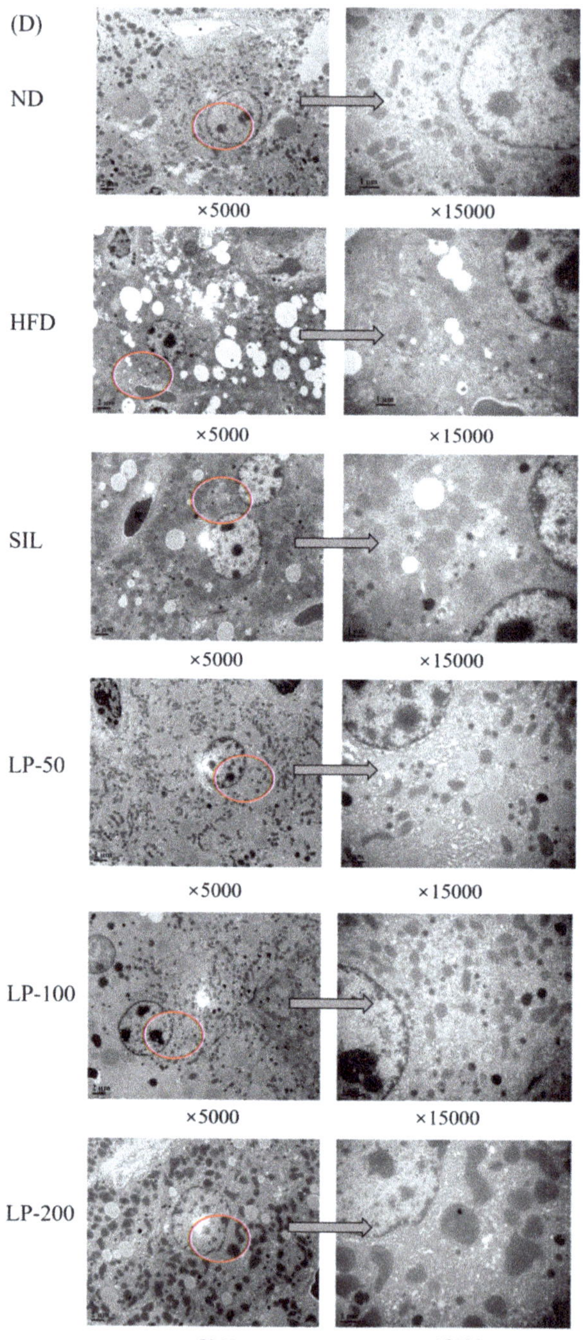

Figure 5. *Cont.*

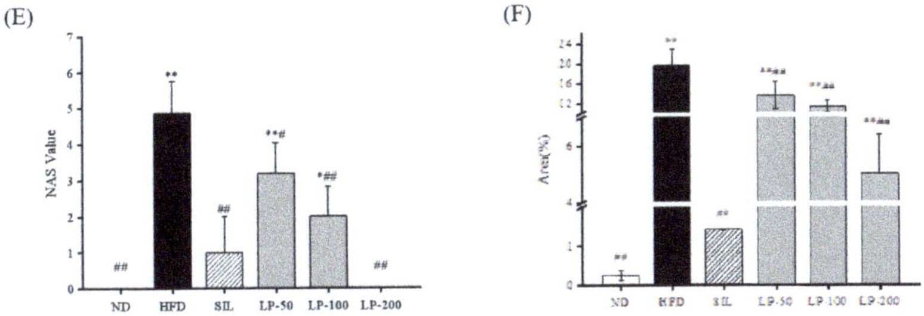

Figure 5. Micrograph (**A**), hematoxylin and eosin (H&E) staining (×400, scale bars of images are 20 μm) (**B**), oil red O staining (×200, scale bars of images are 50 μm) (**C**), transmission electron microscopy (×5000, scale bars of images are 2 μm; ×15,000, scale bars of images are 1 μm) (**D**) Histopathological analysis was performed using the NAFLD activity score (NAS) value for each group (**E**), and oil droplets were analyzed by Image J (**F**). Data are presented as means ± SD. Values with different labels are significantly different among the groups (* $p < 0.05$, ** $p < 0.01$ vs. ND group, # $p < 0.05$, ## $p < 0.01$ vs. HFD group).

2.8. *Effects of LPs on the Protein Expressions of AMPK Pathways*

To clarify the molecular mechanism of LPs inhibiting the abnormal development of FFA, we examined the expression level of the AMPK pathway-related proteins. The phosphorylation level of the AMPK and ACC proteins in the HFD group was much lower than that in the ND group ($p < 0.01$, Figure 6). The expression of the sterol regulatory element-binding transcription factor 1 (SREBP-1) protein downstream was significantly up-regulated, resulting in a significant increase in fatty acid synthase (FASN) expression compared with the ND group ($p < 0.01$, Figure 6), as well as a significant decrease in the CPT-1 protein ($p < 0.01$). After the intervention of SIL and LPs, the phosphorylation levels of AMPK and ACC were significantly enhanced compared with the HFD group ($p < 0.01$, Figure 6), and the expression of the SREBP-1 protein down-stream was downregulated. Thus, the content of the FASN protein was decreased and the protein content of CPT-1 was increased. The expression of peroxisome proliferator-activated receptor alpha (PPARα) in the HFD group was significantly decreased ($p < 0.01$, Figure 6), and its expression was significantly upregulated by SIL and LPs ($p < 0.01$, Figure 6). These results show that LPs can inhibit the abnormal accumulation of FFA by regulating the synthesis of lipid metabolism-related proteins, thus increasing lipid β oxidation and reducing fatty acid synthesis.

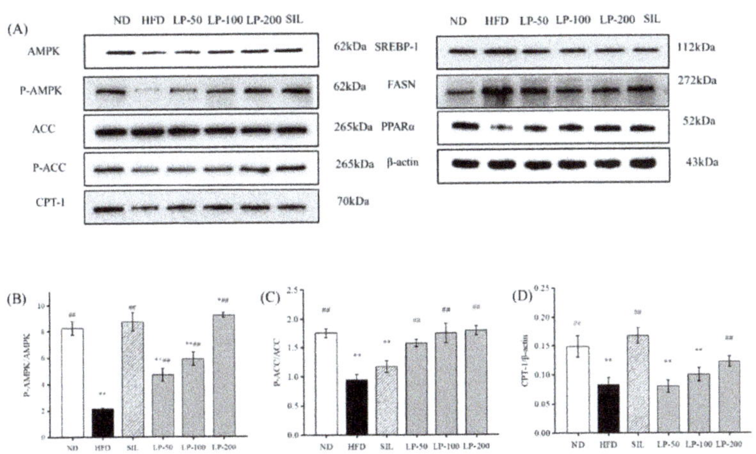

Figure 6. *Cont.*

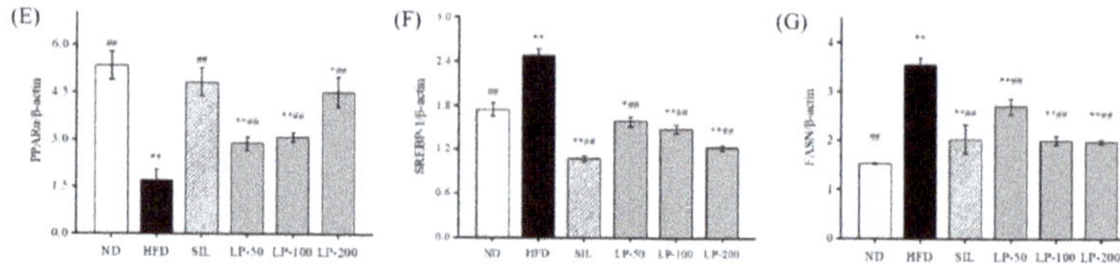

Figure 6. Effects of LPs on the AMP-activated protein kinase (AMPK) pathway-related proteins: (**A**) Western blot analysis of AMPK, phospho-AMP-activated protein kinase (p-AMPK), acetyl CoA carboxylase (ACC), p-ACC, carnitine palmitoyltransferase-1 (CPT-1), sterol regulatory element-binding transcription factor 1 (SREBP-1), fatty acid synthase (FASN), peroxisome proliferator-activated receptor alpha (PPARα), and β-actin. The expressions of p-AMPK (**B**), p-ACC (**C**), CPT-1 (**D**), PPARα (**E**), SREBP-1 (**F**), and FASN (**G**). Values are presented as means ± SD. Values with different labels are significantly different among the groups (* $p < 0.05$, ** $p < 0.01$ vs. ND group, ## $p < 0.01$ vs. HFD group).

2.9. *Effects of LPs on the Expressions of Hepatic Nrf2 Pathway Proteins*

Studies have shown that upregulation of Nrf2 expression in the liver can improve NAFLD [32–34]. Therefore, we can speculate that LPs mitigate hepatic oxidative stress through the Nrf2 pathway. The expression levels of Nrf2, downstream HO-1, and NQO1 in the HFD group were significantly lower than the levels of those indicators in the ND group ($p < 0.01$, Figure 7). Compared with the HFD group, Nrf2 expression was significantly increased after SIL and LPs intervention ($p < 0.01$, Figure 7), and the expression levels of HO-1 and NQO1 in the SIL and LP-200 groups significantly increased ($p < 0.05$, Figure 7).

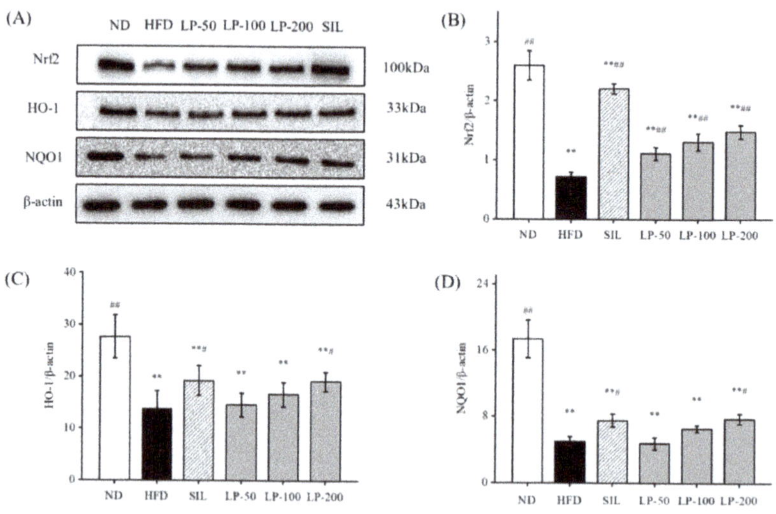

Figure 7. Effects of LPs on the Nrf2 pathway-related proteins: (**A**) Western blot analysis of Nrf2, HO-1, NQO1, and β-actin. The expressions of Nrf2 (**B**), HO-1 (**C**), and NQO1 (**D**). Values are presented as means ± SD. Values with different labels are significantly different among the groups (** $p < 0.01$ vs. ND group, # $p < 0.05$, ## $p < 0.01$ vs. HFD group).

3. Discussion

In this study, we investigated the effects of LPs on liver metabolism. We found that LPs were able to lower body weight in LP-50, LP-100, and LP-200 groups by 24, 23, and 28 percent; to lower TG levels by 13, 29, and 45 percent; to lower LDL-c levels by 23, 41, and 51 percent; and to lower FFA levels by 28, 43, and 62 percent. After the administration of LPs, the markers for liver lesions were decreased, antioxidant capacities were enhanced, and inflammation inhibited. Upon further investigation, we found the mechanism of action to be via AMPK and Nrf2 pathways.

The conventional hypothesis regarding the pathogenesis of NAFLD is the "second hit" theory proposed by Day and James in 1998 [35]. In this theory, the "first strike" is liver fat deposition and hepatocyte fatty change in response to various lipid metabolism disorders. Insulin resistance (IR) is considered to be the central link of the first strike. The accumulation of fat in the liver is also related to a high-calorie diet, sedentary lifestyle, and possible genetic predisposition. The "second hit" follows, which mainly includes the effects of oxidative stress, lipid peroxidation, mitochondrial dysfunction, and increased production of serum endotoxin and inflammatory factors. This "second hit" increases the liver's susceptibility to inflammatory necrosis and fibrosis, in turn accelerating the progression of NAFLD. Inflammation damage can also lead to non-alcoholic steatohepatitis, liver fibrosis, cirrhosis, and even liver cancer.

In recent years, marine active peptides have received growing attention due to their anti-hypertensive and anti-oxidative properties [36]. Mendisa et al. isolated bioactive peptides from squid and found them to inhibit lipid peroxidation by using a linoleic acid model [37]. In this study, functions of LPs were studied in a murine model of NAFLD, induced by an HFD. Excessive intake of fat leads to disorders of lipid metabolism in the liver, which can result in the clinical features of NAFLD such as fatty degeneration with increased serum FFA level and dyslipidemia [38,39]. As shown in Figures 1B and 2, the liver index of the LPs and SIL groups decreased significantly compared with the HFD control group ($p < 0.05$). The TG, TC, LDL-C, and FFA levels significantly increased in the HFD group, and decreased in the experimental groups. AST and ALT are markers generally used for identifying liver lesions and dysfunctions and also can be used as indicators of NAFLD [40]. The levels of AST and ALT in the HFD group significantly increased ($p < 0.01$), indicating that liver damage had occurred in the HFD mice. The AST and ALT levels in the LPs group, however, significantly decreased ($p < 0.05$), suggesting that the effect of NAFLD on the liver was somewhat mitigated by the peptides.

Oxidative stress plays a critical role in the progression of NAFLD as the excess of reactive oxygen species directly induces lipid peroxidation [41]. MDA accumulation is used as a marker for oxidative stress as it is one of the major products of lipid peroxidation, and the markers of the endogenous antioxidant system that counteract this stress are T-AOC, GSH, SOD, and CAT [42]. Table 1 shows a significantly higher level of MDA in the HFD group compared to the ND group ($p < 0.01$), while T-AOC, GSH, SOD, and CAT levels were significantly decreased ($p < 0.05$). The level of MDA in the LPs group was improved. Based on these data, we determined that the protective effects of LPs in NAFLD are due to partially enhancing the endogenous antioxidant system and reducing the MDA level in hepatocytes, thus protecting the liver from excessive reactive oxygen species.

Inflammatory cytokines, also important regulators, are often overexpressed in NAFLD [43]. For example, IL-6 inhibits fat decomposition and promotes fat storage in NAFLD, while TNF-α inhibits the transport of lipids and lipoproteins, leading to an accumulation of lipids in liver cells [44]. In addition, TNF-α also mediates superoxide formation and lipid peroxidation, triggering a cascade of cytokine responses [45]. By examining the levels of TNF-α, IL-1β, and IL-6 in mice during our study, we found LPs to have an inhibitory effect on the HFD-induced inflammation.

H&E staining is a more intuitive approach to analyzing the characteristics of NAFLD, and oil red O staining can be used to show the accumulation of fat in liver tissues. Additionally, in this study, the alterations the in morphology of the liver cell mitochondria were observed by transmission electron microscopy. Figure 5 shows liver tissue from the HFD group in which yellow coloration, white fat granules, disordered arrangement of hepatocyte cords, fat vacuoles, and lipid accumulation can be seen. Compared with the HFD group, liver samples from the LPs group appeared ruddy and smooth, with neater hepatic cords, and a reduced amount of fat.

AMPK is a critical protein in energy regulation and p-AMPK reduces lipid synthesis through accelerating fatty acid β-oxidation. The AMPK-signaling pathway further affects liver lipid metabolism via downstream targets such as CPT-1 and FAS [46]. The FASN level is regulated by the inhibition of SREBP1 expression in response to AMPK phosphorylation, resulting in a decrease in lipid synthesis. AMPK also regulates lipid metabolism by adjusting the ACC and CPT-1 pathways, with previous studies having shown the role of PPAR-α in elevating fatty acid oxidation through the induction of CPT-1 expression [47]. The results of Figure 6 show that the HFD group had significantly reduced levels of p-AMPK, p-ACC, PPAR-α, and CPT-1, and significantly increased SREBP-1 and FASN content ($p < 0.05$). Notably, HFD generates mitochondrial dysfunction, and active PPAR-α negatively interferes with NF-κB activation [48]. Thus, liver PPAR-α downregulation in obesity also has a pro-inflammatory connotation. These outcomes indicate that in the HFD group, β-oxidation of fat in the liver was decreased and fatty acid synthesis was increased, leading to lipid accumulation in liver cells, eventually causing NAFLD. It can be seen that LPs altered the homeostasis of hepatic lipids and up-regulated the expression of the p-AMPK protein. A significant increase in PPAR-α and CPT-1 expression, and a significant decrease in the SREBP-1 and FASN content were seen in the LPs groups in a dose-dependent manner ($p < 0.05$). Thus, it can be said that LPs can effectively improve lipid metabolism in mice affected by NAFLD by decreasing fat synthesis, increasing fat oxidation, and inhibiting fat production. Recent studies demonstrated that AMPK regulated Nrf2 nuclear translocation to induce HO-1 gene expression [49]. Nrf2 plays a pivotal role in cellular defenses against oxidative stress by regulating the gene expression of antioxidant and detoxication enzymes [50].

Next, we measured the expression of Nrf2 and its associated pathways. As shown in Figure 7, regardless of the dosage, LPs are able to significantly increase the level of Nrf2. As well as this, the levels of HO-1 and NQO1 in mouse liver are increased. This indicates that AMPK affects the expression of HO-1 by regulating Nrf2. Therefore, LPs may ameliorate high-fat diet-related oxidative damage by activating the AMPK pathway to modulate the Nrf2-mediated antioxidant pathway.

4. Materials and Methods

4.1. Preparation of Monkfish Muscle Peptides

Monkfish (*Lophius litulon*) with an approximate body length of 39.21 ± 1.71 cm was purchased from a local market in Zhoushan, Zhejiang Province. Fish muscle peptides were obtained following an already described procedure [22]. Briefly, tissue fat was removed by adding 95% ethanol extraction followed by centrifugation. The precipitate was subsequently washed with distilled water and centrifuged again. The defatted monkfish meat was digested with neutral protease (E/S, 2000 U/g) at 45 °C for five hours. The hydrolysate was separated using a 1000 Da ultrafiltration membrane, and a peptide solution with a molecular weight of 1000 Da or less was collected. Free amino acids were removed by a 150 Da ultrafiltration membrane and were vacuum freeze-dried to obtain LPs with a molecular weight less than 1000 Da. Ultra-high pressure liquid chromatography and mass spectrometry (UPLC-MS) were performed. PEAKS studio was used to analyze the spectrum information, and the NCBI database was used for comparison and de novo sequencing analysis to obtain the structural composition of <1 kDa peptide.

4.2. Animals and Treatments

Six weeks old male ICR mice were provided by the Experimental Animal Center of Zhejiang Province. The Experimental Animal Ethics Committee of Zhejiang Ocean University approved the procedures for the use of the laboratory animals (Certificate Number SCXK ZHE2014-0001). Mice were housed in an animal facility at a room temperature of 20–25 °C and had free access to water and food. After seven days of adaptive feeding, the mice were randomly divided into the following six groups (48 in total, $n = 8$ per group): ND, HFD, HFD with silibinin (SIL, 80 mg/kg/day), HFD with LP-50 (50 mg/kg/day), HFD with LP-100 (100 mg/kg/day), and HFD with LP-200 (200 mg/kg/day). The HFD used was purchased from Research Diets, Inc. (New Brunswick, NJ, USA) (Product #D12492). NAFLD was induced by continuous feeding for eight weeks. Both LPs and silibinin were administered by intragastric needle feeding. After four weeks of intervention, the mice were fasted for sixteen hours before euthanization. Plasma was collected by centrifuging the blood at 4 °C and 4000 r/min for 10 min. The livers were acutely dissected and weighed.

4.3. Determination of the Serum Lipid Index, AST, ALT, and Liver Oxidative Stress Index

Serum was collected and analyzed for TC, FFA, LDL, TG, HDL, AST, ALT, MDA, CAT, T-AOC, GSH-Px, and SOD with the aid of detection kits according to the manufacturer's instructions (Nanjing Jiancheng Biotechnology Research Institute, Nanjing, China).

4.4. Pro-Inflammatory Factors Analysis

The levels of hepatic TNF-α, IL-6, IL-Iβ, and IFN-γ were determined by Quantikine ELISA kits (Elabscience Biotechnology, Inc., Wuhan, China). The 96-well plates were coated with primary antibodies before the reference standards and test samples were added. After rinsing the plates, a biotinylated antibody was applied. A peroxidase-conjugated streptavidin was then added, and the concentrations of the primary antibodies were detected using Tetramethylbenzidine through analyzing OD at λ max = 450 nm.

4.5. Histopathological Examination of the Liver

Liver tissues were harvested and fixed overnight in 4% paraformaldehyde and then embedded in paraffin. Four-millimeter paraffin sections were subsequently made and stained with H&E. Photomicrographs were taken under an optical microscope (Biological microscope CX31, Olympus, Tokyo, Japan). TEM was performed to examine the detailed information of the liver injuries. Oil Red O staining was carried out according to the method used by Shen et al. [51]. Fresh liver sections were then taken and stained with an analytical kit (Nanjing Jiancheng Biotech, Nanjing, China). TEM procedure was determined according to Huang et al. [52].

4.6. Western Blotting

The liver tissue was homogenized using ultrasound and then lysed in a RIPA buffer. The procedure of Western blotting as described by Tang et al. was used to differentiate the protein molecules [53]. The protein concentration was measured using the bicinchoninic acid (BCA) method (KeyGENbio, Nanjing, China). Protein extracts were loaded onto 12% SDS-polyacrylamide gel and subsequently transferred onto a PVDF membrane. After incubating with primary and secondary antibodies, protein bands were visualized with enhanced chemiluminescence (ECL). Western blotting bands were imaged and quantitated with the FluorChem FC3 software (3.4.0.728, ProteinSimple, Waltham, MA, USA). All antibodies were purchased from Affinity (Affinity Biosciences, Cincinnati, OH, USA).

4.7. Statistical Analysis

Data were presented as mean ± standard deviation (SD) (n = 8). For comparing data in different groups, an ANOVA analysis was performed by the SPSS 19.0 software (IBM, Armonk, NY, USA). A probability value of less than 5% was considered statistically significant.

5. Conclusions

According to the results of our experiment, we hypothesize that LPs act by resisting the second attack of NAFLD pathogenesis (including oxidative stress, lipid peroxidation, and increased production of inflammatory factors), so as to assist in repairing liver function (Figure 8). We previously found that LPs had a high antioxidant activity and could effectively scavenge DPPH, hydroxyl, ABTS, and superoxide anion radicals, and protect RAW264.7 cells from H_2O_2-induced injury. LPs can be used as raw materials for natural antioxidants [26]. In order to provide a theoretical basis for the stable development and application of LPs and related products, we systematically analyzed the composition of LPs and identified the corresponding proteins using both database search and de novo sequencing methods. In the field of drug discovery, these functional proteins can be used as the lead compound for further modification and screening of active peptide analogues.

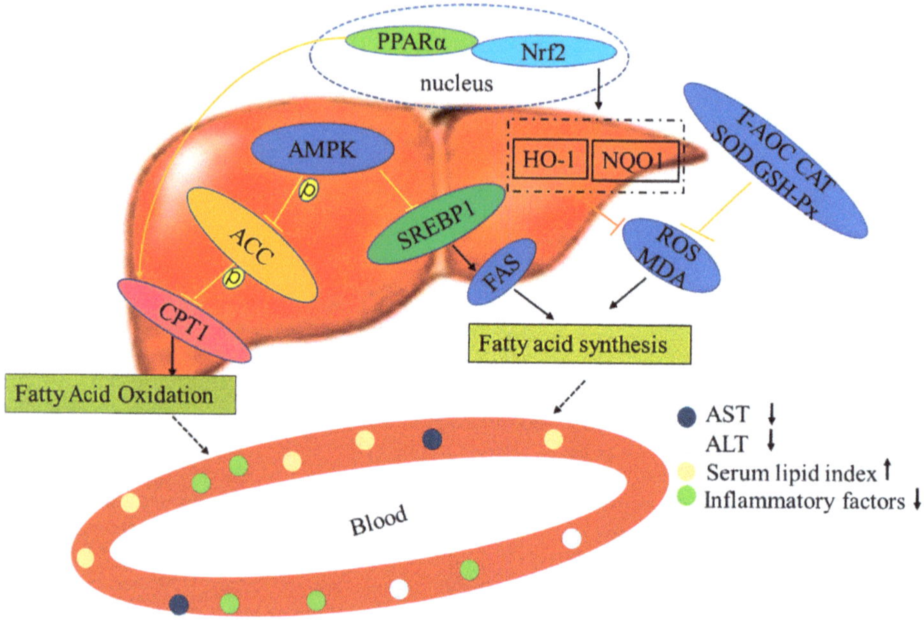

Figure 8. Mechanisms of LPs on alleviating NAFLD.

Supplementary Materials: The following supporting information can be downloaded at: https://www.mdpi.com/article/10.3390/md20050312/s1, Table S1: The free peptide was obtained by database search, Table S2: Free peptides with ALC% over 80 in de novo sequencing, Table S3: Source proteins of the identified peptides in Low Molecular Weight Monkfish (*Lophius litulon*) Peptides.

Author Contributions: Conceptualization, J.Y., X.T. and Z.Y.; data curation, J.Y., X.T., Z.Y., S.Z., Q.W. and F.Y.; methodology, J.Y., X.T., J.Z. and B.X.; writing—original draft preparation, J.Y. and X.T.; writing—review and editing, J.Y., X.T., Y.Y. and F.Y.; funding acquisition, Z.Y. and F.Y. All authors have read and agreed to the published version of the manuscript.

Funding: This study was supported by the Zhejiang Provincial Public Welfare Technology Research Program (LGN21D060002), Fundamental Research Funds for the Provincial Universities of Zhejiang Province (2021JZ011), and National Science Foundation (81773629).

Institutional Review Board Statement: The Experimental Animal Ethics Committee of Zhejiang Ocean University approved the procedures for the use of the laboratory animals (Certificate Number SCXK ZHE2014-0001, approval date 1 March 2019).

Informed Consent Statement: Not applicable.

Data Availability Statement: Not applicable.

Acknowledgments: The authors are indebted to Xiaoxia Jiang for her generous technical support. The authors have no conflict of interest to disclose.

Conflicts of Interest: The authors declare no conflict of interest.

References

1. Kwon, M.; Lim, S.-J.; Joung, E.-J.; Lee, B.; Oh, C.-W.; Kim, H.-R. Meroterpenoid-rich fraction of an ethanolic extract from *Sargassum serratifolium* alleviates obesity and non-alcoholic fatty liver disease in high fat-fed C57BL/6J mice. *J. Funct. Foods* **2018**, *47*, 288–298. [CrossRef]
2. Xu, L.; Yan, L.; Tao, W. Pilose antler peptide attenuates high-fat-diet-induced liver injury. *Toxicol. Mech. Methods* **2018**, *28*, 279–285. [CrossRef] [PubMed]
3. Echeverría, F.; Valenzuela, R.; Espinosa, A.; Bustamante, A.; Álvarez, D.; Gonzalez-Mañan, D.; Ortiz, M.; Soto-Alarcon, S.A.; Videla, L.A. Reduction of high-fat diet-induced liver proinflammatory state by eicosapentaenoic acid plus hydroxytyrosol supplementation: Involvement of resolvins RvE1/2 and RvD1/2. *J. Nutr. Biochem.* **2019**, *63*, 35–43. [CrossRef] [PubMed]
4. Polyzos, S.A.; Kountouras, J.; Mantzoros, C.S. Obesity and nonalcoholic fatty liver disease: From pathophysiology to therapeutics. *Metabolism* **2019**, *92*, 82–97. [CrossRef]
5. Rolo, A.P.; Teodoro, J.S.; Palmeira, C.M. Role of oxidative stress in the pathogenesis of nonalcoholic steatohepatitis. *Free Radic. Biol. Med.* **2012**, *52*, 59–69. [CrossRef]
6. Xu, M.; Ge, C.; Qin, Y.; Gu, T.; Lv, J.; Wang, S.; Ma, Y.; Lou, D.; Li, Q.; Hu, L.; et al. Activated TNF-α/RIPK3 signaling is involved in prolonged high fat diet-stimulated hepatic inflammation and lipid accumulation: Inhibition by dietary fisetin intervention. *Food Funct.* **2019**, *10*, 1302–1316. [CrossRef]
7. Lee, J.M.; Johnson, J.A. An important role of Nrf2-ARE pathway in the cellular defense mechanism. *J. Biochem. Mol. Biol.* **2004**, *37*, 139–143. [CrossRef]
8. Nguyen, T.; Nioi, P.; Pickett, C.B. The Nrf2-antioxidant response element signaling pathway and its activation by oxidative stress. *J. Biol. Chem.* **2009**, *284*, 13291–13295. [CrossRef]
9. Han, X.; Ding, C.; Zhang, G.; Pan, R.; Liu, Y.; Huang, N.; Hou, N.; Han, F.; Xu, W.; Sun, X. Liraglutide ameliorates obesity-related nonalcoholic fatty liver disease by regulating Sestrin2-mediated Nrf2/HO-1 pathway. *Biochem. Biophys. Res. Commun.* **2020**, *525*, 895–901. [CrossRef]
10. Gao, F.; Chen, M.; Yu, J.; Xu, L.; Yu, L.; Jiang, H.; Gu, Z. Tetrahydrocurcumin protects against nonalcoholic fatty liver disease by improving lipid metabolism and redox homeostasis. *J. Funct. Foods* **2022**, *89*, 104957. [CrossRef]
11. Kim, S.; Hong, J.; Jeon, R.; Kim, H.S. Adzuki bean ameliorates hepatic lipogenesis and proinflammatory mediator expression in mice fed a high-cholesterol and high-fat diet to induce nonalcoholic fatty liver disease. *Nutr. Res.* **2016**, *36*, 90–100. [CrossRef] [PubMed]
12. Brownsey, R.W.; Boone, A.N.; Elliott, J.E.; Kulpa, J.E.; Lee, W.M. Regulation of acetyl-CoA carboxylase. *Biochem. Soc. Trans.* **2006**, *34*, 223–227. [CrossRef] [PubMed]
13. Wu, Y.; Zhou, F.; Jiang, H.; Wang, Z.; Hua, C.; Zhang, Y. Chicory (*Cichorium intybus* L.) polysaccharides attenuate high-fat diet induced non-alcoholic fatty liver disease via AMPK activation. *Int. J. Biol. Macromol.* **2018**, *118*, 886–895. [CrossRef] [PubMed]
14. Liang, L.; Ye, S.; Jiang, R.; Zhou, X.; Zhou, J.; Meng, S. Liensinine alleviates high fat diet (HFD)-induced non-alcoholic fatty liver disease (NAFLD) through suppressing oxidative stress and inflammation via regulating TAK1/AMPK signaling. *Int. Immunopharmacol.* **2022**, *104*, 108306. [CrossRef]
15. Vanani, A.R.; Kalantari, H.; Mahdavinia, M.; Rashno, M.; Khorsandi, L.; Khodayar, M.J. Dimethyl fumarate reduces oxidative stress, inflammation and fat deposition by modulation of Nrf2, SREBP-1c and NF-kappaB signaling in HFD fed mice. *Life Sci.* **2021**, *283*, 119852. [CrossRef] [PubMed]
16. Cani, P.D.; Amar, J.; Iglesias, M.A.; Poggi, M.; Knauf, C.; Bastelica, D.; Neyrinck, A.M.; Fava, F.; Tuohy, K.M.; Chabo, C.; et al. Metabolic endotoxemia initiates obesity and insulin resistance. *Diabetes* **2007**, *56*, 1761–1772. [CrossRef]
17. Yang, J.; Bindels, L.B.; Segura Munoz, R.R.; Martínez, I.; Walter, J.; Ramer-Tait, A.E.; Rose, D.J. Disparate Metabolic Responses in Mice Fed a High-Fat Diet Supplemented with Maize-Derived Non-Digestible Feruloylated Oligo- and Polysaccharides Are Linked to Changes in the Gut Microbiota. *PLoS ONE* **2016**, *11*, e0146144. [CrossRef]
18. Ley, R.E.; Turnbaugh, P.J.; Klein, S.; Gordon, J.I. Microbial ecology: Human gut microbes associated with obesity. *Nature* **2006**, *444*, 1022–1023. [CrossRef]
19. Turnbaugh, P.J.; Ley, R.E.; Mahowald, M.A.; Magrini, V.; Mardis, E.R.; Gordon, J.I. An obesity-associated gut microbiome with increased capacity for energy harvest. *Nature* **2006**, *444*, 1027–1031. [CrossRef]
20. Kitts, D.D.; Weiler, K. Bioactive Proteins and Peptides from Food Sources. Applications of Bioprocesses used in Isolation and Recovery. *Curr. Pharm. Des.* **2003**, *9*, 1309–1323.
21. Möller, N.P.; Scholz-Ahrens, K.E.; Roos, N.; Schrezenmeir, J. Bioactive peptides and proteins from foods: Indication for health effects. *Eur. J. Nutr.* **2008**, *47*, 171–182. [CrossRef] [PubMed]
22. Kim, M.R.; Kim, J.W.; Park, J.B.; Hong, Y.K.; Ku, S.K.; Choi, J.S. Anti-obesity effects of yellow catfish protein hydrolysate on mice fed a 45% kcal high-fat diet. *Int. J. Mol. Med.* **2017**, *40*, 784–800. [CrossRef] [PubMed]
23. Wang, Y.; Gagnon, J.; Nair, S.; Sha, S. Herring Milt Protein Hydrolysate Improves Insulin Resistance in High-Fat-Diet-Induced Obese Male C57BL/6J Mice. *Mar. Drugs* **2019**, *17*, 456. [CrossRef] [PubMed]
24. Drotningsvik, A.; Mjøs, S.A.; Pampanin, D.M.; Slizyte, R.; Carvajal, A.; Remman, T.; Høgøy, I.; Gudbrandsen, O.A. Dietary fish protein hydrolysates containing bioactive motifs affect serum and adipose tissue fatty acid compositions, serum lipids, postprandial glucose regulation and growth in obese Zucker fa/fa rats. *Br. J. Nutr.* **2016**, *116*, 1336–1345. [CrossRef] [PubMed]

25. Wergedahl, H.; Liaset, B.; Gudbrandsen, O.A.; Lied, E.; Espe, M.; Muna, Z.; Mørk, S.; Berge, R.K. Fish protein hydrolysate reduces plasma total cholesterol, increases the proportion of HDL cholesterol, and lowers acyl-CoA:cholesterol acyltransferase activity in liver of Zucker rats. *J. Nutr.* **2004**, *134*, 1320–1327. [CrossRef]
26. Tian, X.; Zheng, J.; Xu, B.; Ye, J.; Yang, Z.; Yuan, F. Optimization of Extraction of Bioactive Peptides from Monkfish (*Lophius litulon*) and Characterization of Their Role in H(2)O(2)-Induced Lesion. *Mar. Drugs* **2020**, *18*, 468. [CrossRef]
27. Chi, C.-F.; Wang, B.; Deng, Y.-Y.; Wang, Y.-M.; Deng, S.-G.; Ma, J.-Y. Isolation and characterization of three antioxidant pentapeptides from protein hydrolysate of monkfish (*Lophius litulon*) muscle. *Food Res. Int.* **2014**, *55*, 222–228. [CrossRef]
28. Greyling, N.; Bordoloi, A.; Goosen, N.J. Optimising enzymatic conditions of monkfish (*Lophius vomerinus*) heads hydrolysis towards potential waste biomass valorisation. *Biomass Convers. Biorefinery* **2020**, *11*, 2711–2722. [CrossRef]
29. Nakamaru-Ogiso, E.; Han, H.; Matsuno-Yagi, A.; Keinan, E.; Sinha, S.C.; Yagi, T.; Ohnishi, T. The ND2 subunit is labeled by a photoaffinity analogue of asimicin, a potent complex I inhibitor. *FEBS Lett* **2010**, *584*, 883–888. [CrossRef]
30. Sadia, H.; Akter, Q.S.; Afroz, R.; Siddika, T. Effect of Punica Granatum (Pomegranate) on serum ALT and AST in Carbon tetrachloride induced liver damage in Wistar Albino Rats. *J. Bangladesh. Soc. Physiol.* **2016**, *11*, 23. [CrossRef]
31. Braud, L.; Battault, S.; Meyer, G.; Nascimento, A.; Gaillard, S.; de Sousa, G.; Rahmani, R.; Riva, C.; Armand, M.; Maixent, J.M.; et al. Antioxidant properties of tea blunt ROS-dependent lipogenesis: Beneficial effect on hepatic steatosis in a high fat-high sucrose diet NAFLD obese rat model. *J. Nutr. Biochem.* **2017**, *40*, 95–104. [CrossRef] [PubMed]
32. Nagata, N.; Xu, L.; Kohno, S.; Ushida, Y.; Aoki, Y.; Umeda, R.; Fuke, N.; Zhuge, F.; Ni, Y.; Nagashimada, M.; et al. Glucoraphanin Ameliorates Obesity and Insulin Resistance Through Adipose Tissue Browning and Reduction of Metabolic Endotoxemia in Mice. *Diabetes* **2017**, *66*, 1222–1236. [CrossRef] [PubMed]
33. Shin, S.; Wakabayashi, J.; Yates, M.S.; Wakabayashi, N.; Dolan, P.M.; Aja, S.; Liby, K.T.; Sporn, M.B.; Yamamoto, M.; Kensler, T.W. Role of Nrf2 in prevention of high-fat diet-induced obesity by synthetic triterpenoid CDDO-imidazolide. *Eur. J. Pharm.* **2009**, *620*, 138–144. [CrossRef] [PubMed]
34. Yang, Y.C.; Lii, C.K.; Lin, A.H.; Yeh, Y.W.; Yao, H.T.; Li, C.C.; Liu, K.L.; Chen, H.W. Induction of glutathione synthesis and heme oxygenase 1 by the flavonoids butein and phloretin is mediated through the ERK/Nrf2 pathway and protects against oxidative stress. *Free Radic. Biol. Med.* **2011**, *51*, 2073–2081. [CrossRef]
35. Day, C.P.; James, O.F. Steatohepatitis: A tale of two "hits"? *Gastroenterology* **1998**, *114*, 842–845. [CrossRef]
36. Arumugam, V.; Venkatesan, M.; Ramachandran, S.; Sundaresan, U. Bioactive Peptides from Marine Ascidians and Future Drug Development—A Review. *Int. J. Pept. Res. Ther.* **2017**, *24*, 13–18. [CrossRef]
37. Mendis, E.; Rajapakse, N.; Byun, H.G.; Kim, S.K. Investigation of jumbo squid (*Dosidicus gigas*) skin gelatin peptides for their in vitro antioxidant effects. *Life Sci.* **2005**, *77*, 2166–2178. [CrossRef]
38. Leamy, A.K.; Egnatchik, R.A.; Young, J.D. Molecular mechanisms and the role of saturated fatty acids in the progression of non-alcoholic fatty liver disease. *Prog. Lipid Res.* **2013**, *52*, 165–174. [CrossRef]
39. Malhi, H.; Gores, G.J. Molecular mechanisms of lipotoxicity in nonalcoholic fatty liver disease. *Semin. Liver Dis.* **2008**, *28*, 360–369. [CrossRef]
40. Gao, J.; Song, J.; Du, M.; Mao, X. Bovine α-lactalbumin hydrolysates (α-LAH) attenuate high-fat diet induced nonalcoholic fatty liver disease by modulating hepatic lipid metabolism in C57BL/6J mice. *J. Funct. Foods* **2019**, *54*, 254–262. [CrossRef]
41. Mota, M.; Banini, B.A.; Cazanave, S.C.; Sanyal, A.J. Molecular mechanisms of lipotoxicity and glucotoxicity in nonalcoholic fatty liver disease. *Metabolism* **2016**, *65*, 1049–1061. [CrossRef] [PubMed]
42. Wu, Z.; Zhang, Y.; Gong, X.; Cheng, G.; Pu, S.; Cai, S. The preventive effect of phenolic-rich extracts from Chinese sumac fruits against nonalcoholic fatty liver disease in rats induced by a high-fat diet. *Food Funct.* **2020**, *11*, 799–812. [CrossRef] [PubMed]
43. Hendy, O.M.; Elsabaawy, M.M.; Aref, M.M.; Khalaf, F.M.; Oda, A.M.A.; El Shazly, H.M. Evaluation of circulating zonulin as a potential marker in the pathogenesis of nonalcoholic fatty liver disease. *Apmis* **2017**, *125*, 607–613. [CrossRef] [PubMed]
44. Lin, X.; Zhang, Z.; Chen, J.M.; Xu, Y.Y.; Ye, H.R.; Cui, J.; Fang, Y.; Jin, Y.; Zhu, D.R.; Yuan, L. Role of APN and TNF-α in type 2 diabetes mellitus complicated by nonalcoholic fatty liver disease. *Genet. Mol. Res.* **2015**, *14*, 2940–2946. [CrossRef] [PubMed]
45. Agrawal, S.; Gollapudi, S.; Su, H.; Gupta, S. Leptin activates human B cells to secrete TNF-α, IL-6, and IL-10 via JAK2/STAT3 and p38MAPK/ERK1/2 signaling pathway. *J. Clin. Immunol.* **2011**, *31*, 472–478. [CrossRef] [PubMed]
46. Hu, X.; Liu, L.; Song, Z.; Sheikhahmadi, A.; Wang, Y.; Buyse, J. Effects of feed deprivation on the AMPK signaling pathway in skeletal muscle of broiler chickens. *Comp. Biochem. Physiol. B Biochem. Mol. Biol.* **2016**, *191*, 146–154. [CrossRef]
47. Brown, Z.J.; Fu, Q.; Ma, C.; Kruhlak, M.; Zhang, H.; Luo, J.; Heinrich, B.; Yu, S.J.; Zhang, Q.; Wilson, A.; et al. Carnitine palmitoyltransferase gene upregulation by linoleic acid induces CD4(+) T cell apoptosis promoting HCC development. *Cell Death Dis.* **2018**, *9*, 620. [CrossRef]
48. Ortiz, M.; Soto-Alarcón, S.A.; Orellana, P.; Espinosa, A.; Campos, C.; López-Arana, S.; Rincón, M.A.; Illesca, P.; Valenzuela, R.; Videla, L.A. Suppression of high-fat diet-induced obesity-associated liver mitochondrial dysfunction by docosahexaenoic acid and hydroxytyrosol co-administration. *Dig. Liver Dis.* **2020**, *52*, 895–904. [CrossRef]
49. Choi, B.K.; Kim, T.W.; Lee, D.R.; Jung, W.H.; Lim, J.H.; Jung, J.Y.; Yang, S.H.; Suh, J.W. A polymethoxy flavonoids-rich Citrus aurantium extract ameliorates ethanol-induced liver injury through modulation of AMPK and Nrf2-related signals in a binge drinking mouse model. *Phytother. Res.* **2015**, *29*, 1577–1584. [CrossRef]
50. Chen, Q.; Wang, T.; Li, J.; Wang, S.; Qiu, F.; Yu, H.; Zhang, Y.; Wang, T. Effects of Natural Products on Fructose-Induced Nonalcoholic Fatty Liver Disease (NAFLD). *Nutrients* **2017**, *9*, 96. [CrossRef]

51. Shen, B.; Zhao, C.; Wang, Y.; Peng, Y.; Cheng, J.; Li, Z.; Wu, L.; Jin, M.; Feng, H. Aucubin inhibited lipid accumulation and oxidative stress via Nrf2/HO-1 and AMPK signalling pathways. *J. Cell Mol. Med.* **2019**, *23*, 4063–4075. [CrossRef] [PubMed]
52. Huang, F.; Wang, J.; Yu, F.; Tang, Y.; Ding, G.; Yang, Z.; Sun, Y. Protective Effect of *Meretrix meretrix* Oligopeptides on High-Fat-Diet-Induced Non-Alcoholic Fatty Liver Disease in Mice. *Mar. Drugs* **2018**, *16*, 39. [CrossRef] [PubMed]
53. Tang, Y.; Yu, F.; Zhang, G.; Yang, Z.; Huang, F.; Ding, G. A Purified Serine Protease from *Nereis virens* and Its Impaction of Apoptosis on Human Lung Cancer Cells. *Molecules* **2017**, *22*, 1123. [CrossRef] [PubMed]

marine drugs

MDPI

Article

Extraction and Identification of Three New *Urechis unicinctus* Visceral Peptides and Their Antioxidant Activity

Jingjing Li [1,†], Jiajun Lu [1,†], Charles Asakiya [1], Kunlun Huang [1,2], Xiuzhi Zhou [3], Qingliang Liu [3] and Xiaoyun He [1,2,*]

1 Key Laboratory of Precision Nutrition and Food Quality, Ministry of Education, College of Food Science and Nutritional Engineering, China Agricultural University, Beijing 100083, China; 17861120538@163.com (J.L.); 17768116970@163.com (J.L.); asakiya@cau.edu.cn (C.A.); huangkl@cau.edu.cn (K.H.)
2 Key Laboratory of Safety Assessment of Genetically Modified Organism (Food Safety), The Ministry of Agriculture and Rural Affairs of the P.R. China, Beijing 100083, China
3 Shandong Baier Testing Corp., Ltd., Weifang 261061, China; 18764613510@163.com (X.Z.); 13666361630@163.com (Q.L.)
* Correspondence: hexiaoyun@cau.edu.cn
† These authors contributed equally to this work.

Citation: Li, J.; Lu, J.; Asakiya, C.; Huang, K.; Zhou, X.; Liu, Q.; He, X. Extraction and Identification of Three New *Urechis unicinctus* Visceral Peptides and Their Antioxidant Activity. *Mar. Drugs* **2022**, *20*, 293. https://doi.org/10.3390/md20050293

Academic Editors: Bin Wang and Chang-Feng Chi

Received: 22 March 2022
Accepted: 13 April 2022
Published: 27 April 2022

Abstract: The viscera of *Urechis unicinctus* with polypeptides, fatty acids, and amino acids are usually discarded during processing to food. In order to improve the utilization value of the viscera of *Urechis unicinctus* and avoid resource waste, antioxidant polypeptides were isolated from the viscera of *Urechis unicinctus*. First, a protein hydrolysate of *Urechis unicinctus* (UUPH) was prepared by ultrasonic-assisted enzymatic hydrolysis, and the degree of hydrolysis was as high as 79.32%. Subsequently, three new antioxidant peptides (P1, P2, and P3) were purified from UUPH using ultrafiltration and chromatography, and their amino acid sequences were identified as VTSALVGPR, IGLGDEGLRR, TKIRNEISDLNER, respectively. Then, the antioxidant activity of the polypeptide was predicted by the structure–activity relationship and finally verified by experiments on eukaryotic cells. The P1 peptide exhibited the strongest antioxidant activity among these three antioxidant peptides. Furthermore, P1, P2, and P3 have no toxic effect on RAW264.7 cells at the concentration of 0.01~2 mg/mL and can protect RAW264.7 cells from H_2O_2-induced oxidative damage in a concentration-dependent manner. These results suggested that these three new antioxidant peptides were isolated from the viscera of *Urechis unicinctus*, especially the P1 peptide, which might serve as potential antioxidants applied in health-derived food or beverages. This study further developed a new use of the by-product of *Urechis unicinctus*, which improved the comprehensive utilization of marine biological resources.

Keywords: internal organs of *Urechis unicinctus*; ultrasound-assisted enzymatic hydrolysis; polypeptide; antioxidant activity

1. Introduction

Urechis unicinctus, also known as "sea intestine", belongs to echiurioidea, echiurida, xenopneusta, and urechidae [1,2]. Studies have shown that *Urechis unicinctus* is rich in multiple substances such as polypeptides, fatty acids, amino acids [3], and crude protein accounts for about 22.84% of the total. The protein can be hydrolyzed into bioactive polypeptides, which have antihypertensive effects, lowering blood sugar and antimicrobial and antioxidant activity [4–6]. At present, the extraction of *Urechis unicinctus* polypeptide is mainly concentrated in the body's wall muscle [7,8], and its internal organs are directly thrown away as waste, which not only causes environmental pollution but also leads to a waste of resources. Therefore, polypeptides were extracted from the viscera of *Urechis unicinctus* in this study.

Antioxidants alleviate the damage caused by oxidative stress by preventing the formation of free radicals, scavenging free radicals, and reactive oxygen species (ROS), activating the antioxidant defense system, and performing functional repair of cells with ROS-induced damage [9–12]. Many studies have shown that oxidative damage caused by free radicals or oxidative stress in the body is closely related to aging, Alzheimer's disease, Parkinson's disease, and cardiovascular disease [11]. Therefore, looking for potential natural antioxidants to replace synthetic products has become a research hotspot, especially some fish-processing by-products. Hydrolyzed protein has become a hot topic in pharmacy and health food [13]. Studies have shown that chickpea proteolytic peptides have chelating iron activity [14], and the use of vegetable protein hydrolysates as food additives is already allowed in the United States. The viscera of *Urechis unicinctus* are inedible and rich in protein, so it is a good raw material for the industrial production of active peptides.

Consequently, this study isolated and identified three novel antioxidant peptides from UUPH using ultrasonic-assisted enzymatic hydrolysis. In addition, the LC-MS/MS method was used to identify amino acid sequences of peptides. Then, molecular docking was used to verify the antioxidant mechanism of peptides. Finally, the cytoprotective effect of peptides on H_2O_2-damaged RAW264.7 cells was determined.

2. Results and Discussion

2.1. Degree of Hydrolysis (DH)

In this study, ultrasound-assisted enzymatic technology was used for the enzymolysis of *Urechis unicinctus* protein. The final DH of UUPH measured was 79.32%. On the other hand, Zhang et al. [15] did not use ultrasound-assisted enzymolysis technology to hydrolyze *Urechis unicinctus* protein, and its DH was only 17.8%. The results show that the ultrasound-assisted enzymatic hydrolysis process can significantly improve the enzymatic hydrolysis reaction speed of *Urechis unicinctus* protein, which is consistent with the effect of ultrasound reported in the literature. In addition, ultrasound plays a synergistic role by reducing steric hindrance and making the substrate (specific peptide sequences) more accessible [16].

2.2. Ultrafiltration and Determination of Antioxidant Activity before and after Simulated Gastrointestinal Digestion

Ultrafiltration is often used as the first step of isolation and purification to realize the crude separation of protein hydrolysates according to the molecular weight obtained from the desired antioxidative components [17]. The UUPH-1 was divided into three parts by the ultrafiltration tube: UUPH-2 (>30 kDa), UUPH-3 (10–30 kDa), UUPH-4 (<10 kDa).

Activities of the compounds were evaluated using their DPPH·scavenging activity, hydroxyl radicals (·OH) scavenging activity, and superoxide anion free radical ($\cdot O_2^-$) scavenging activity. As shown in Figure 1, at the concentration of 0.5 mg/mL, the antioxidant activity was UUPH-4 > UUPH-3 > UUPH-1 > UUPH-2 before digestion. The antioxidant activity of UUPH-1 was slightly higher than that of UUPH-2, which may be due to it containing a small amount of UUPH-1 and UUPH-4. The results showed that the antioxidant activity of compounds with smaller molecular weight (MW) is generally better than that of compounds with larger average MWs. The results were consistent with those of other studies. For example, Xing et al. [18] isolated the antioxidant peptide from ham and measured the antioxidant activity of each component. The results showed that the component with MW < 3 kDa had the highest antioxidant activity; Canabady Rochelle et al. [19] and Wang et al. [20] have shown that low molecular weight peptides can terminate free radical chain reactions and chelate transition metal ions better than high molecular weight peptides. After digestion, the antioxidant activity of each component changed, but the antioxidant activity of UUPH-4 was still the highest. Therefore, UUPH-4 components were collected for further study.

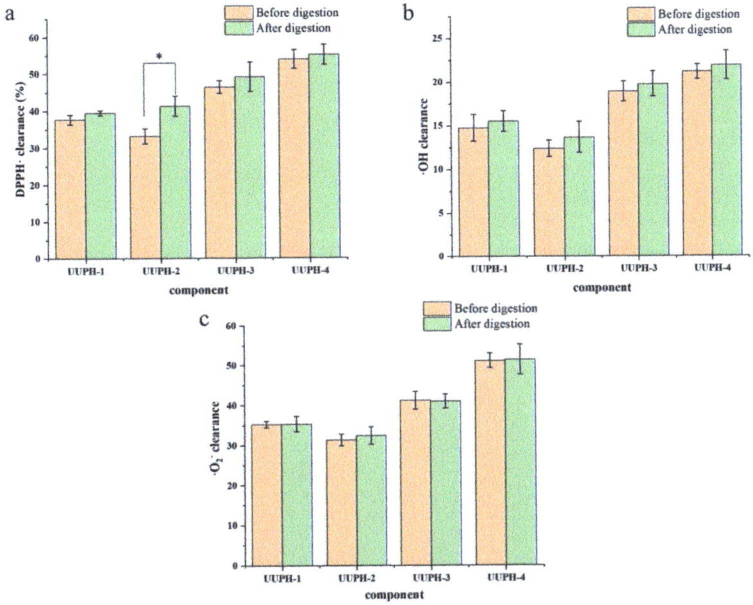

Figure 1. Determination of the antioxidant activity of each component. (**a**) DPPH clearance. (**b**) OH clearance. (**c**) $\cdot O_2$ clearance. Note: * indicates p value < 0.05.

2.3. Gel-Filtration Chromatography

Sephadex G-25 gel-filtration chromatography is an effective method for separating compounds according to the MW, widely used to isolate peptides in protein hydrolysates [21]. As shown in Figure 2, the UUPH-4 was separated on Sephadex G-25 to yield two fractions. The DPPH scavenging rate of UUPH-4-2 was 29.8%. On the other hand, the DPPH scavenging rates of UUPH-4-1 reached 58.5%, significantly higher than UUPH-4-2 (the protein concentration was 0.5 mg/mL). This result is consistent with previous reports that smaller MW of peptides have better antioxidant activities [22]. This result further proves that MW is a key factor affecting the antioxidant capacity of peptides [23].

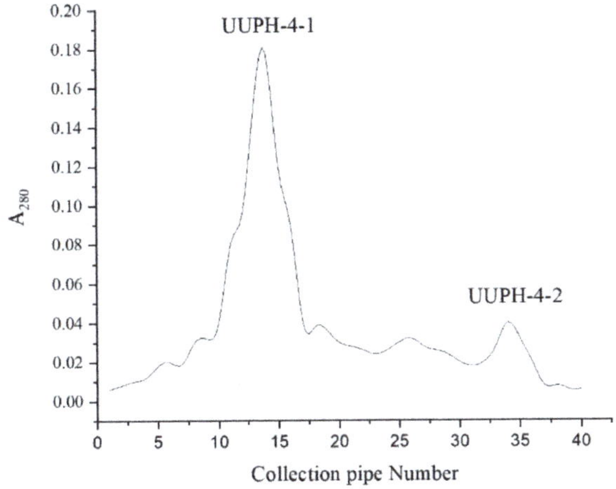

Figure 2. Sephadex G-25 gel column chromatography results.

2.4. Identification of Peptide Sequences

As shown in Figure 3, UUPH-4-1 was isolated by LC-MS/MS to afford three main peptides, named P1, P2, and P3. The sequence of each of the peptides was determined using the de nava algorithm in mascot software (version 2.2, Matrix Science, Boston, MA, USA). As shown in Table 1, P1, P2, and P3 sequences were identified as VTSALVGPR, IGLGDEGLRR, and TKIRNEISDLNER, respectively. Their MWs were 898.5, 1084.6, and 1586.8 Da. P1, P2, and P3 peptides contain amino acids related to antioxidant activity such as Pro, Gly, Ala, Val, or Leu [24].

P1

P2

P3

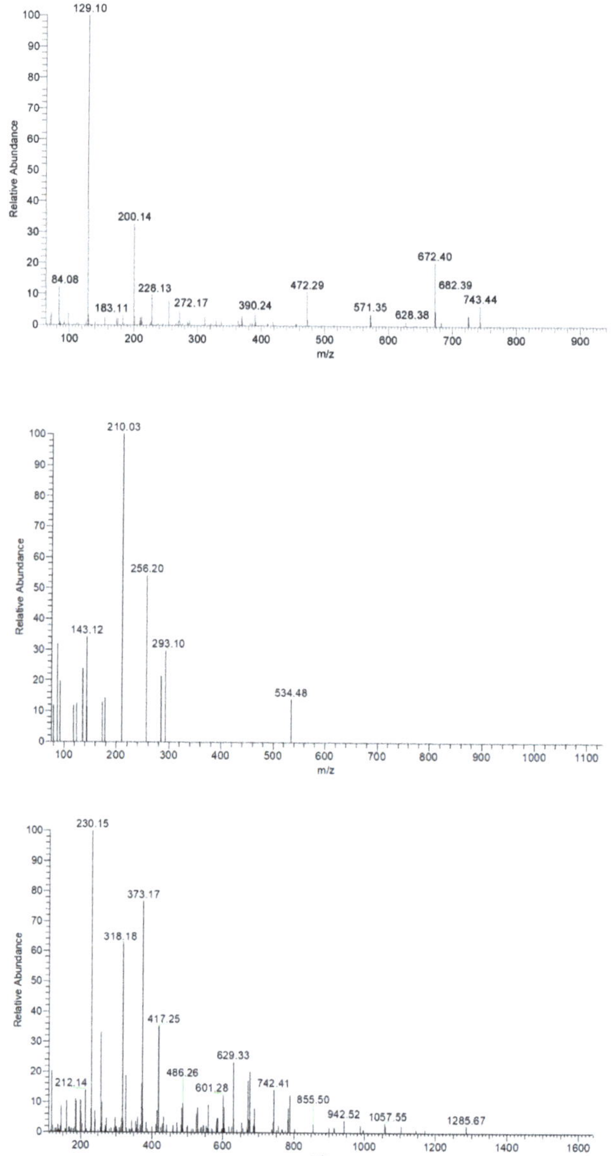

Figure 3. LC-MS/MS spectrogram analysis of peptides (P1, P2, and P3).

Table 1. Retention time (RT), amino acid sequence, and molecular weight (MW) of peptides.

No.	RT (min)	Amino Acid Sequence	MW (Da)
P1	31.52	VTSALVGPR	898.5
P2	43.87	IGLGDEGLRR	1084.6
P3	56.72	TKIRNEISDLNER	1586.8

2.5. The Structure–Activity Relationship

At present, there are two main research methods on the structure–activity relationship of antioxidant peptides; one is induction and the other is bioinformatics; that is, the molecular model of antioxidant peptides is constructed by a computer, and the interaction between antioxidant peptides and receptors is explored by molecular docking.

2.5.1. Induction

Firstly, the antioxidant activity of three peptides was predicted by induction. Many studies have proved that the antioxidant properties of peptides are related to their MW, composition, secondary structure, and hydrophobicity [25,26].

Studies found that the antioxidant activity of antioxidant peptides was negatively correlated with the MW of peptides, and the MW of most antioxidant peptides was less than 3 kDa [27]. As shown in Table 1, the MWs of P1, P2, and P3 were below 3 kDa, and the MW of P1 was the lowest. Therefore, it can be predicted from the MW that the antioxidant activity of P1 was the highest and P3 was the lowest.

In terms of amino acid composition, studies suggested that antioxidant peptides generally contain the following five amino acids: Pro, Gly, Ala, Val, and Leu [24]. The higher the total proportion of these five amino acids, the higher the antioxidant activity. It can be inferred from Table 2 that P1 had the highest antioxidant activity and P3 had the lowest.

Table 2. Proportion of amino acid composition of P1, P2, and P3.

Amino Acids	P1	P2	P3
A(Ala)	8.84	0	0
G(Gly)	7.2	18.05	0
L(Leu)	12.57	21.03	7.27
P(Pro)	11.04	0	0
V(Val)	22.46	0	0

Hydrophobic amino acid residues facilitate the interaction between antioxidant peptides and fat-soluble free radicals; thereby improving the ability to inhibit lipid peroxidation [25]. For example, in the study of oyster protein hydrolysates, Wang et al. found that the hydrophobic peptides can form complexes with zinc ions [28]. At the same time, hydrophobic amino acid residues located at the C-terminal or N-terminal contributed to the activities of antioxidant peptides. As shown in Figure 4, P1 had the greatest hydrophobicity, and the hydrophobic amino acid residues were mainly located at the N-end. P3 had the least hydrophobicity and had no hydrophobic amino acid residue. Therefore, in terms of hydrophobicity, P1 had the highest antioxidant activity and P3 had the lowest antioxidant activity.

Previous research suggested that the secondary structure of antioxidant peptides had more β-folding and irregular coils and less α-helix, which may be due to the fact that β-folding and irregular coils can expose more active sites of the peptides. At the same time, β-folding can also increase the structural stability of antioxidant peptides, so peptides are not easily affected by the environment [24]. As shown in Figure 5, P1 had the largest proportion of β-folding and irregular crimping structure and the least α-helix, followed by P3, and finally P2. Therefore, from the secondary structure, the antioxidant activity of P1 was the highest and P2 was the lowest.

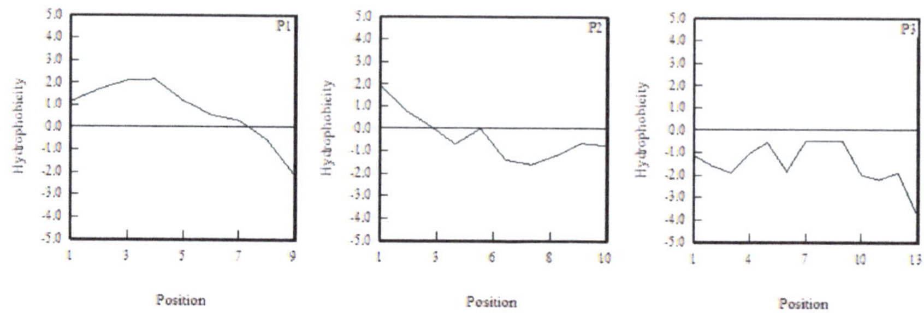

Figure 4. Hydrophobicity analysis of P1, P2, and P3.

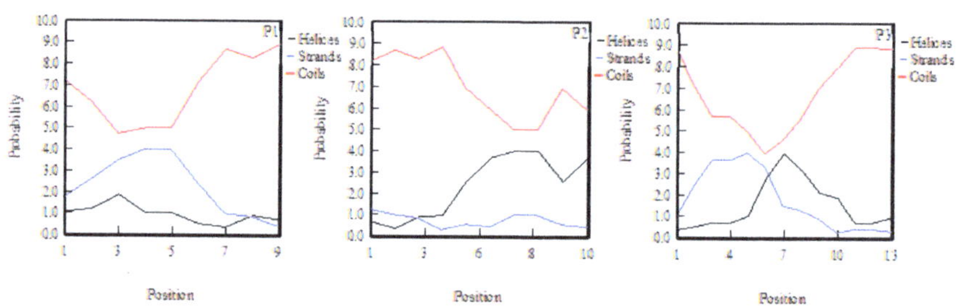

Figure 5. Results of secondary structure analysis of P1, P2, and P3.

Finally, in terms of MW, amino acid composition, hydrophobicity, and secondary structure, the order of antioxidant activity of P1, P2, and P3 was P1 > P2 > P3.

2.5.2. Molecular Docking

The Keap1-Nrf2 signal pathway is a classical signaling pathway of antioxidant damage in the human body [29]. The starting point of signaling pathway activation is the dissociation of Keap1 and Nrf2. The most important dissociation mode is competitive inhibition; that is, foreign molecules act on the binding region of keap1-Nrf2 to enhance the dissociation of Nrf2 and, in turn, promote the antioxidant damage of body cells.

The docking study was carried out by the kelch region bound by keap1-Nrf2 as the target. The results showed that only the P1 peptide interacted with the kelch region of Keap1 protein, the minimum binding free energy was −4.01 kcal/mol, and the main interaction between P1 and the kelch region was hydrogen bonding. The action sites shown in Figure 6 are Thr2 of P1 and Gly423 of the kelch region; Ala4 of P1 and Val420 of the kelch region; and Arg9 of P1 and Asn469 of the kelch region, respectively. The results showed that among the three peptides, the P1 peptide might play an antioxidant role via activation of the keap1-Nrf2 pathway, and the other two peptides may play an antioxidant role through other mechanisms.

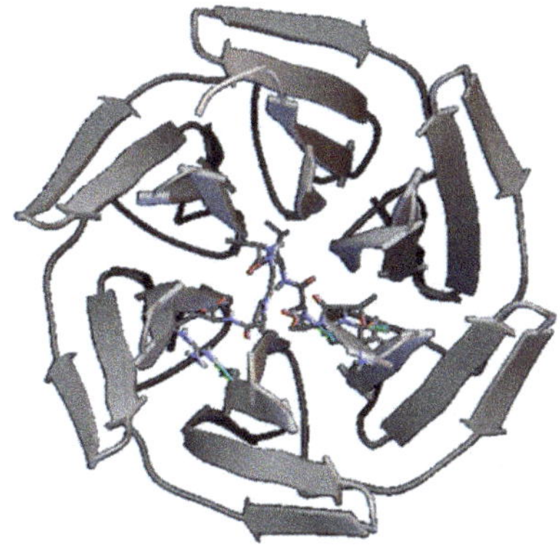

Figure 6. Three-dimensional structure of P1 combined with the kelch region.

2.6. Cytoprotective Activity of Peptide on H_2O_2-Damaged RAW264.7 Cells

2.6.1. Cytotoxicity

Cytotoxic effects of the three isolated peptides (P1, P2, and P3) at the concentration of 0.01–2 mg/mL were determined in RAW264.7 cells by CCK-8 assay. As shown in Figure 7, three peptides exhibited no significant effect on the viability of RAW264.7 cells compared to the blank control group at the test concentration. The result indicated that the three peptides could serve as potential antioxidants applied to food.

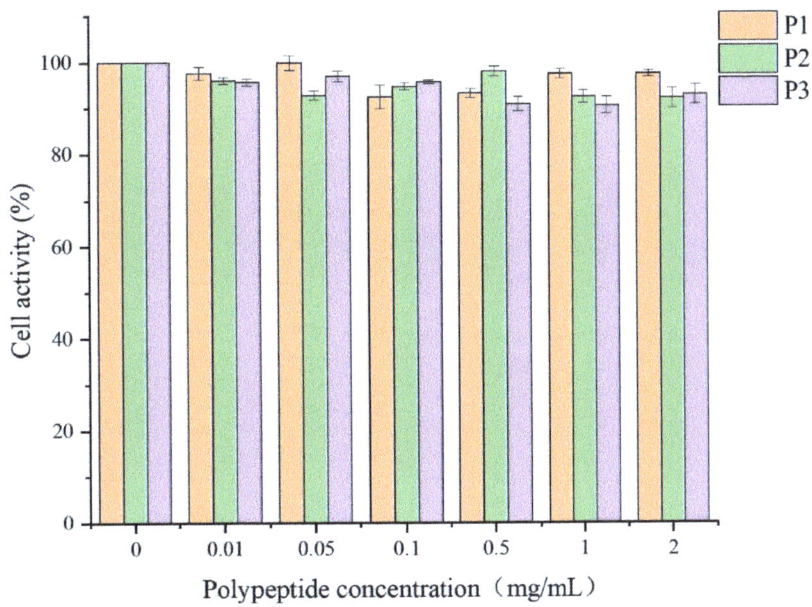

Figure 7. Effect of antioxidant peptides on the activity of RAW264.7 cells.

2.6.2. Protection of Peptide on H_2O_2-Induced Oxidative Damage RAW264.7 Cells

The RAW264.7 cells were treated for 24 h with the peptides and ascorbic acid; then, incubated with hydrogen peroxide for another 24 h. Figure 8 shows the influences of three peptides and ascorbic acid on H_2O_2-induced oxidative damage RAW264.7 cells. Three isolated peptides treated groups were gradually increased in a concentration-dependent manner. The P1 treated group increased the RAW264.7 cell viability from 54.52% to 55.23%,

66.18%, and 83.62% at the concentrations of 0.1, 0.5, and 1 mg/mL, respectively. Moreover, cells treated with 2 mg/mL of P1, P2, P3, and ascorbic acid restored cell viability up to 174.6%, 172.5%, 134.5%, and 180.2% (the 100% viability value refers to untreated control cells), which strongly protect H_2O_2-induced oxidative damage of RAW264.7 cells and promote cell proliferation, especially at the high concentrations. This is consistent with the report of Li et al. [30]. Compared with Figure 7, cells treated with 2 mg/mL peptide for 12 h did not promote cell proliferation, which may be due to the insensitive absorption of peptides. In general, the antioxidant activity of P1 was the best, which was close to ascorbic acid, followed by P2.

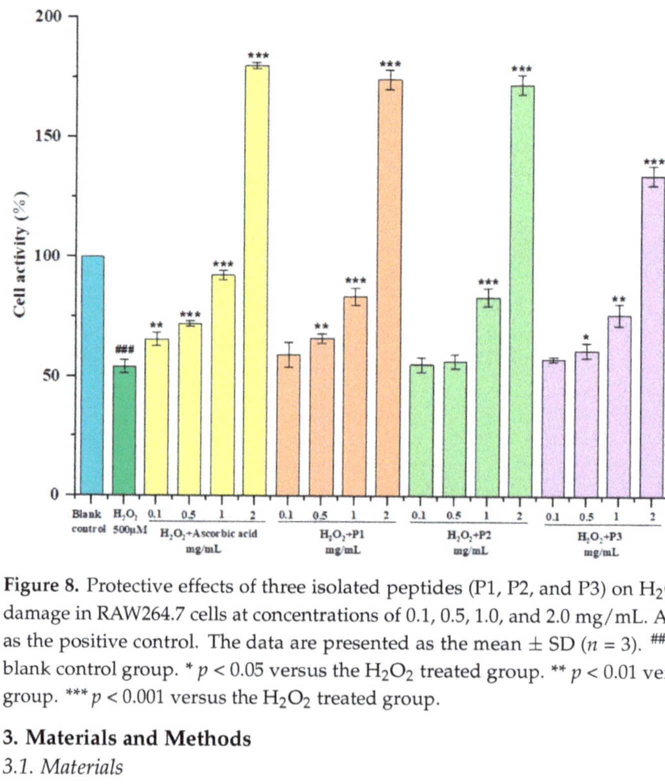

Figure 8. Protective effects of three isolated peptides (P1, P2, and P3) on H_2O_2-induced oxidative damage in RAW264.7 cells at concentrations of 0.1, 0.5, 1.0, and 2.0 mg/mL. Ascorbic acid was used as the positive control. The data are presented as the mean ± SD (n = 3). ### $p < 0.001$ versus the blank control group. * $p < 0.05$ versus the H_2O_2 treated group. ** $p < 0.01$ versus the H_2O_2 treated group. *** $p < 0.001$ versus the H_2O_2 treated group.

3. Materials and Methods

3.1. Materials

Urechis unicinctus was provided by the Yantai breeding base. Papain, trypsin, alcalase, pepsin, and compound protease were purchased from Anning Dongheng Huadao Biotechnology Co. Ltd. (Nanning, China). Superoxide anion free radical assay kit was purchased from the Beijing Solabao Technology Co. Ltd. (Beijing, China). Sephadex G-25 was purchased from Shanghai Yuanye Biotechnology Co., Ltd. (Shanghai China). DPPH was purchased from Sigma Corporation (St. Louis, MO, USA). RAW264.7 cells were purchased from Shanghai Biyuntian Biotechnology Co. Ltd. (Shanghai, China).

3.2. Preparation of Protein Hydrolysate from Urechis unicinctus Viscera (UUPH)

After degreasing with ethyl acetate, the viscera of *Urechis unicinctus* were dried and crushed. The visceral degreasing powder was prepared into a solution by adding water according to the material–liquid ratio of 27:1 (mL/g), adjusting pH = 7. UUPH samples were prepared by enzymatic hydrolysis using papain, trypsin, and alkaline protease at ultrasonic power of 675 W for 33 min; then hydrolyzed in a water bath at 50.0 °C for 2.0 h (the addition of papain was 0.6%, trypsin was 1.44%, and alkaline protease was 0.96%). After the reaction, the mixture was heated in 95 °C water for 15 min to inactivate the enzyme. Next, the hydrolysate was centrifuged at 5000× *g* for 10 min, and the supernatant was added in 2% granular activated carbon to decolorize at 60 °C for 60 min. The filtrate was collected by vacuum suction filtration, and subsequently, the filtrate was freeze-dried to obtain powdery material, which was stored at 20 °C for further use. The ultrasonic-assisted enzymatic hydrolysis conditions and enzymatic hydrolysis parameters in this experiment were optimized.

3.3. Degree of Hydrolysis (DH)

The DH of UUPH was calculated based on formaldehyde titration in GB 5009.235-2016 [31] using the following formula:

$$\text{Ammonia nitrogen content (g/100 mL)} = C \times (V_1 - V_2) \times 0.014 \times 100$$

where C denotes the concentration of NaOH solution (mol/L), V_1 stands for NaOH volume (mL), and V_2 is the volume of NaOH (mL) in the blank.

The degree of hydrolysis was calculated via the following equation:

$$\text{DH (\%)} = m/M \times 100$$

where m is the mass of ammonia nitrogen in UUPH and M stands for the total nitrogen mass in the sample.

3.4. Isolation and Purification of UUPH

3.4.1. Ultrafiltration Separation

The UUPH fraction was intercepted through an ultrafiltration tube using molecular weight cut-offs of 10 and 30 kDa. UUPH was fractionated into four fractions, including UUPH-1, UUPH-2 (>30 kDa), UUPH-3 (10–30 kDa), and UUPH-4 (<10 kDa).

3.4.2. Simulation of Gastrointestinal Digestion In Vivo

Freeze-dried powders of 4 components were prepared in 0.5 mg/mL protein solution. Pepsin was added at 2%, the pH value was adjusted to 2 with 1 mol/L HCl solution, and the system temperature was kept at 37 °C for enzymatic hydrolysis for 2 h. Then, the pH value was adjusted to 7 with the NaOH solution (1 mol/L), and the trypsin was added at 4%. The system's temperature was kept at 37 °C for 4 h, and then the antioxidant activity of each component after simulated digestion was determined. See step 3.7 for the antioxidant activity determination. The components with the highest antioxidant activity were selected for subsequent separation and purification.

3.4.3. Gel Filtration Chromatography (GFC)

The UUPH-4 fraction was further separated into two fractions (UUPH-4-1 and UUPH-4-2) using a Sephadex G-25 column. The elution conditions were as follows: ultrapure water and the flow rate was 0.5 mL/min. The elution flow rate was controlled at 0.5 mL/min. This eluted solution was collected every 5 min and evaluated at 280 nm. Taking the DPPH·scavenging activity as an indicator, the component with the strongest hydroxyl radical scavenging rate was selected for the next separation.

3.5. Peptide Identification by LC-MS/MS

Desalted UUPH aqueous solutions were filtered using a 0.22 μm membrane and the extract (10 μL) was injected into the chromatographic column (Acclaim PePmap 100 C18 traps) through an auto-sampler. The mobile phase was water with 0.1% formic acid (solvent A) and acetonitrile with 0.1% acetic acid (solvent B); the flow rate was 0.4 μL/min. The gradient elution of 0–6 min/5–8% B, 6–40 min/8–30% B, 40–45 min/30–60% B, 45–48 min/60–80% B, 48–56 min/80% B, 56–58 min/80–5% B, 58–65 min/5% B was applied. The amino acid sequence of peptides was determined using LC-MS/MS. The positive ion mode used for analysis with an ion source voltage was 1800 V and the capillary temperature was 360 °C.

Primary mass spectrometry parameters: the scanning range was 350–20,000 DA and the scanning resolution was 70,000; secondary mass spectrometry parameters: the scanning range depends on the mass charge ratio of primary parent ions and the scanning resolution was 17,500.

The mass spectra were retrieved by mascot software (version 2.2) and analyzed using the de nava algorithm.

3.6. Molecular Modeling

The three-dimensional structure of the peptide was downloaded from the PEP-FOLD3 (https://bioserv.rpbs.univ-paris-diderot.fr/services/PEP-FOLD3/, 10 December 2020) and used as a ligand. The PDB file of the kelch region of the Keap1 protein (PDB ID: 1u6d) was downloaded using PDB (http://www.rcsb.org/, 10 December 2020) and used as a receptor. All the water molecules were removed, and the construction structures of the peptide were optimized using AutoDockTools software. The AutoGrid and AutoDock were run, the relationship between the polypeptide and the Keap1-Nrf2 signal pathway was judged according to the binding free energy of the receptor and ligand. The smaller binding free energy indicated that the polypeptide was likely to activate the Keap1-Nrf2 signal pathway and play an antioxidant role.

3.7. Antioxidant Activity of the Peptides

3.7.1. DPPH· Scavenging Activity

The DPPH· scavenging activity was determined as described by Song et al. [32]. First, 0.1 mmol/L DPPH·solution was prepared with anhydrous ethanol. Then, 2 mL samples were mixed with 2 mL of fresh DPPH solution. The mixture was incubated for 30 min in a dark environment. The absorbance was measured at 517 nm. Subsequently, anhydrous ethanol and DPPH· solution were used as the blank and control, respectively. The DPPH scavenging rate was calculated via the following equation:

$$\text{DPPH scavenging rate } (\%) = \left(1 - \frac{A_1 - A_2}{A_0}\right) \times 100;$$

where A_1 is the sample absorbance, A_2 is the control absorbance, and A_0 is the blank absorbance.

3.7.2. Hydroxyl Radicals (·OH) Scavenging Activity

The·OH scavenging activity was determined as described by [33]. First, 9 mmol/L $FeSO_4$ solution was prepared with ultrapure water, and 9 mmol/L salicylic acid-ethanol solution was prepared with anhydrous ethanol. Then, 0.1 mL of 30% H_2O_2 was diluted with ultrapure water to 100 mL. Next, 1 mL of salicylic acid solution, 1 mL H_2O_2 solution, and 1 mL sample solution were mixed and incubated for 30 min in a dark environment. The absorbance was measured at 510 nm. Ultrapure water was used as the blank. The ·OH scavenging rate was calculated via the following equation:

$$\cdot\text{OH scavenging rate } (\%) = \left(1 - \frac{A_1 - A_2}{A_0}\right) \times 100$$

where A_1 is the sample absorbance, A_2 is the control absorbance, and A_0 is the blank absorbance.

3.7.3. Superoxide Anion Free Radical ($\cdot O_2^-$) Scavenging Activity

The$\cdot O_2^-$ scavenging assay was performed using a $\cdot O_2^-$ kit. In brief, the assay was performed according to the instructions accompanying the kit. The $\cdot O_2^-$ scavenging rate was calculated via the following equation:

$$\cdot O_2^{-} \text{ scavenging rate} = \left(1 - \frac{A_1 - A_2}{A_0}\right) \times 100$$

where A_1 is the sample absorbance, A_2 is the control absorbance, and A_0 is the blank absorbance.

3.8. Cell Cytotoxicity Assay

The isolated peptides were dissolved in the DMEM medium containing 10% fetal bovine serum with the concentrations of 0, 0.01, 0.05, 0.1, 0.5, 1, and 2 mg/mL, respectively. The RW264.7 cells were grown (1.0×10^4 cells/well) in a 96-well plate for 24 h. After that, RW264.7 cells were cultured at designed concentrations of peptide solution for 12 h. The cell viability was measured by the CCK-8 test. The WST-8 in the CCK8 kit can be reduced by dehydrogenases in mitochondria to produce orange yellow formazan, then can quantify the number of viable cells by colorimetry and, thus, the cell viability is detected.

3.9. The Cytoprotective Activity of Antioxidant Peptide on Oxidative Damaged RW264.7 Cells by H_2O_2

The *Urechis unicinctus* antioxidant peptide was synthesized by Beijing Zhongke Yaguang Biotechnology Co., Ltd. (Beijing, China) by solid-phase synthesis according to the sequence identification results of Section 2.4. The RW264.7 cells were grown (1.0×10^4 cells/well) in a 96-well plate for 24 h. Then, the supernatant was aspirated and 190 μL of peptide sample and ascorbic acid were added into the protection groups, respectively, for incubation for 24 h, 10 μL H_2O_2 (500 μmol/L) was added into the damage and protection groups and sequentially incubated for 24 h. The cell viability was measured by the CCK-8 test.

3.10. Statistical Analysis

The data are reported as the mean ± standard deviation (SD). Origin 2019 was used to draw the graphs. Sequence analysis was performed using DNAMAN software. Autodock4 software was used to simulate the interaction between antioxidant peptides and the kelch region of the Keap1 protein in the molecular docking experiment.

4. Conclusions

In this study, three antioxidant peptides (P1–P3) were isolated and purified from *Urechis unicinctus* visceral protein hydrolysate using ultrasound-assisted enzymatic hydrolysis. Their sequences were VTSALVGPR, IGLGDEGLRR, and TKIRNEISDLNER, respectively. Induction, molecular docking, and protection on H_2O_2-induced oxidative damage RAW264.7 cells were used to evaluate the antioxidant activity of three peptides. Among them, P1 peptide exhibited the strongest antioxidant activity. These results suggested that the three peptides could be applied as potential antioxidants in health-derived food or beverages. This study developed new uses for *Urechis unicinctus* by-products and improved the comprehensive utilization of marine biological resources. In the future, we will explore how to optimize the experimental conditions to improve the yield of these active peptides. In addition, animal feeding experiments on the three isolated peptides (P1, P2, and P3) will be conducted to evaluate their antioxidant effect and antioxidant mechanism in vivo in our lab.

Author Contributions: Writing—original draft, J.L. (Jingjing Li) and J.L. (Jiajun Lu); Writing—review & editing, C.A. and X.H.; Project administration and Supervision, K.H., X.H., X.Z. and Q.L. All authors provided critical feedback and helped shape the research, analysis, and manuscript. All authors have read and agreed to the published version of the manuscript.

Funding: This work was funded by Talent Development Program of China Agricultural University (2115) and Key Research and Development Project of Hebei Province (21372801D).

Institutional Review Board Statement: Not applicable.

Informed Consent Statement: Not applicable.

Data Availability Statement: The study did not report any data.

Conflicts of Interest: The authors declare no conflict of interest.

References

1. Ma, X.; Liu, X.; Zhou, D.; Bai, Y.; Gao, B.; Zhang, Z.; Qin, Z. The NF-κB pathway participates in the response to sulfide stress in *Urechis unicinctus*. *Fish Shellfish. Immunol.* **2016**, *58*, 229–238. [CrossRef] [PubMed]
2. Li, N.; Tang, Y.Z.; Song, S.L.; Wang, B.G. Studies on technique for artificial breeding of *Urechis unicinctus*. *Shandong Fish.* **1997**, *1*, 5–8.
3. Chen, W.; Zhang, S.; Sun, Y.; Tian, B.; Song, L.; Xu, Y.; Liu, T. Effects of substrate on the physiological characteristics and intestinal microbiota of Echiura worm (*Urechis unicinctus*) juveniles. *Aquaculture* **2021**, *530*, 735710. [CrossRef]
4. Ryu, B.M.; Kim, M.J.; Himaya, S.W.A.; Kang, K.H.; Kim, S.K. Statistical optimization of high temperature/pressure and ultra-wave assisted lysis of *Urechis unicinctus* for the isolation of active peptide which enhance the erectile function in vitro. *Process Biochem.* **2014**, *49*, 148–153. [CrossRef]
5. Kang, H.K.; Lee, H.H.; Seo, C.H.; Park, Y. Antimicrobial and Immunomodulatory Properties and Applications of Marine-Derived Proteins and Peptides. *Mar. Drugs* **2019**, *17*, 350. [CrossRef]
6. Harnedy, P.A.; FitzGerald, R.J. Bioactive peptides from marine processing waste and shellfish: A review. *J. Funct. Foods* **2012**, *4*, 6–24. [CrossRef]
7. Kim, K.S.; Bae, W.J.; Kim, S.J.; Kang, K.H.; Kim, S.K.; Cho, H.J.; Hong, S.H.; Lee, J.Y.; Kim, S.W. Improvement of erectile dysfunction by the active pepide from *Urechis unicinctus* by high temperature/pressure and ultra—Wave assisted lysis in Streptozotocin Induced Diabetic Rats. *Int. Braz. J. Urol.* **2016**, *42*, 825–837. [CrossRef]
8. Li, X.; Ma, Y.; Zuo, Y.; Liu, Z.; Wang, Q.; Ren, D.; He, Y.; Cong, H.; Wu, L.; Zhou, H. The efficient enrichment of marine peptides from the protein hydrolysate of the marine worm *Urechis unicinctus* by using mesoporous materials MCM-41, SBA-15 and CMK-3. *Anal. Methods* **2021**, *13*, 2405–2414. [CrossRef]
9. Chen, M.L.; Ning, P.; Jiao, Y.; Xu, Z.; Cheng, Y.H. Extraction of antioxidant peptides from rice dreg protein hydrolysate via an angling method. *Food Chem.* **2021**, *337*, 128069. [CrossRef]
10. Yang, Q.; Cai, X.; Yan, A.; Tian, Y.; Du, M.; Wang, S. A specific antioxidant peptide: Its properties in controlling oxidation and possible action mechanism. *Food Chem.* **2020**, *327*, 126984. [CrossRef]
11. Haider, K.; Haider, M.R.; Neha, K.; Yar, M.S. Free radical scavengers: An overview on heterocyclic advances and medicinal prospects. *Eur. J. Med. Chem.* **2020**, *204*, 112607. [CrossRef] [PubMed]
12. Dao, V.T.; Casas, A.I.; Maghzal, G.J.; Seredenina, T.; Kaludercic, N.; Robledinos-Anton, N.; Di Lisa, F.; Stocker, R.; Ghezzi, P.; Jaquet, V.; et al. Pharmacology and Clinical Drug Candidates in Redox Medicine. *Antioxid. Redox. Signal.* **2015**, *23*, 1113–1129. [CrossRef] [PubMed]
13. Mukhia, S.; Kumar, A.; Kumar, R. Generation of antioxidant peptides from soy protein isolate through psychrotrophic *Chryseobacterium* sp. derived alkaline broad temperature active protease. *LWT* **2021**, *143*, 111152. [CrossRef]
14. Torres-Fuentes, C.; Alaiz, M.; Vioque, J. Iron-chelating activity of chickpea protein hydrolysate peptides. *Food Chem.* **2012**, *134*, 1585–1588. [CrossRef]
15. Zhang, X.X.; Liu, F.; Liu, C.E.; Ji, Y.; Duan, D.; Yan, N. Optimization of enzymatic hydrolysis of visceral polypeptides of echinus unicyclicus by Response Surface Methodology. *Food Res. Dev.* **2018**, *39*, 52–57.
16. Jorge, S.; Pereira, K.; López-Fernández, H.; LaFramboise, W.; Dhir, R.; Fernández-Lodeiro, J.; Lodeiro, C.; Santos, H.M.; Capelo-Martínez, J.L. Ultrasonic-assisted extraction and digestion of proteins from solid biopsies followed by peptide sequential extraction hyphenated to MALDI-based profiling holds the promise of distinguishing renal oncocytoma from chromophobe renal cell carcinoma. *Talanta* **2020**, *206*, 120180. [CrossRef]
17. Wang, B.; Wang, Y.M.; Chi, C.F.; Luo, H.Y.; Deng, S.G.; Ma, J.Y. Isolation and characterization of collagen and antioxidant collagen peptides from scales of croceine croaker (*Pseudosciaena crocea*). *Mar. Drugs* **2013**, *11*, 4641–4661. [CrossRef]
18. Xing, L.; Liu, R.; Gao, X.; Zheng, J.; Wang, C.; Zhou, G.; Zhang, W. The proteomics homology of antioxidant peptides extracted from dry-cured Xuanwei and Jinhua ham. *Food Chem.* **2018**, *266*, 420–426. [CrossRef]
19. Canabady-Rochelle, L.L.; Harscoat-Schiavo, C.; Kessler, V.; Aymes, A.; Fournier, F.; Girardet, J.M. Determination of reducing power and metal chelating ability of antioxidant peptides: Revisited methods. *Food Chem.* **2015**, *183*, 129–135. [CrossRef]
20. Wang, X.; Chen, H.; Fu, X.; Li, S.; Wei, J. A novel antioxidant and ACE inhibitory peptide from rice bran protein: Biochemical characterization and molecular docking study. *LWT* **2017**, *75*, 93–99. [CrossRef]
21. Moayedi, A.; Mora, L.; Aristoy, M.C.; Safari, M.; Hashemi, M.; Toldrá, F. Peptidomic analysis of antioxidant and ACE-inhibitory peptides obtained from tomato waste proteins fermented using Bacillus subtilis. *Food Chem.* **2018**, *250*, 180–187. [CrossRef] [PubMed]
22. Jin, H.X.; Xu, H.P.; Li, Y.; Zhang, Q.W.; Xie, H. Preparation and Evaluation of Peptides with Potential Antioxidant Activity by Microwave Assisted Enzymatic Hydrolysis of Collagen from Sea Cucumber Acaudina Molpadioides Obtained from Zhejiang Province in China. *Mar. Drugs* **2019**, *17*, 169. [CrossRef] [PubMed]

23. Hu, F.; Ci, A.T.; Wang, H.; Zhang, Y.Y.; Zhang, J.G.; Thakur, K.; Wei, Z.J. Identification and hydrolysis kinetic of a novel antioxidant peptide from pecan meal using Alcalase. *Food Chem.* **2018**, *261*, 301–310. [CrossRef] [PubMed]
24. Wen, C.; Zhang, J.; Zhang, H.; Duan, Y.; Ma, H. Plant protein-derived antioxidant peptides: Isolation, identification, mechanism of action and application in food systems: A review. *Trends Food Sci. Technol.* **2020**, *105*, 308–322. [CrossRef]
25. Lu, X.; Zhang, L.; Sun, Q.; Song, G.; Huang, J. Extraction, identification and structure-activity relationship of antioxidant peptides from sesame (*Sesamum indicum* L.) protein hydrolysate. *Food Res. Int.* **2019**, *116*, 707–716. [CrossRef] [PubMed]
26. Ma, Y.; Wu, Y.; Li, L. Relationship between primary structure or spatial conformation and functional activity of antioxidant peptides from Pinctada fucata. *Food Chem.* **2018**, *264*, 108–117. [CrossRef] [PubMed]
27. Wu, D.; Li, M.; Ding, J.; Zheng, J.; Zhu, B.W.; Lin, S. Structure-activity relationship and pathway of antioxidant shrimp peptides in a PC12 cell model. *J. Funct. Foods* **2020**, *70*, 103978. [CrossRef]
28. Wang, Z.; Cheng, S.; Wu, D.; Xu, S.; Chen, H.; Du, M. Hydrophobic peptides from oyster protein hydrolysates show better zinc-chelating ability. *Food Biosci.* **2021**, *41*, 100985. [CrossRef]
29. Tonolo, F.; Folda, A.; Cesaro, L.; Scalcon, V.; Marin, O.; Ferro, S.; Bindoli, A.; Rigobello, M.P. Milk-derived bioactive peptides exhibit antioxidant activity through the Keap1-Nrf2 signaling pathway. *J. Funct. Foods* **2020**, *64*, 103696. [CrossRef]
30. Li, Y.; Li, J.; Lin, S.J.; Yang, Z.S.; Jin, H.X. Preparation of Antioxidant Peptide by Microwave- Assisted Hydrolysis of Collagen and Its Protective Effect Against H_2O_2-Induced Damage of RAW264.7 Cells. *Mar. Drugs* **2019**, *17*, 642. [CrossRef]
31. *GB5009.235-2016*; State Health and Family Planning Commission of the People's Republic of China. National Standard of the People's Republic of China–Determination of Amino Acid Nitrogen in Food. Standards Press: Beijing, China, 2016.
32. Song, Y.; Fu, Y.; Huang, S.; Liao, L.; Wu, Q.; Wang, Y.; Ge, F.; Fang, B. Identification and antioxidant activity of bovine bone collagen-derived novel peptides prepared by recombinant collagenase from *Bacillus cereus*. *Food Chem.* **2021**, *349*, 129143. [CrossRef] [PubMed]
33. Zhang, J.; Li, M.; Zhang, G.; Tian, Y.; Kong, F.; Xiong, S.; Zhao, S.; Jia, D.; Manyande, A.; Du, H. Identification of novel antioxidant peptides from snakehead (*Channa argus*) soup generated during gastrointestinal digestion and insights into the anti-oxidation mechanisms. *Food Chem.* **2021**, *337*, 127921. [CrossRef] [PubMed]

MDPI
St. Alban-Anlage 66
4052 Basel
Switzerland
Tel. +41 61 683 77 34
Fax +41 61 302 89 18
www.mdpi.com

Marine Drugs Editorial Office
E-mail: marinedrugs@mdpi.com
www.mdpi.com/journal/marinedrugs

www.ingramcontent.com/pod-product-compliance
Lightning Source LLC
Chambersburg PA
CBHW061558210926
51850CB00009B/2141
9783036582603